MICROBIAL PHYSIOLOGY

VOLUME FOUR OF

BASIC MICROBIOLOGY

VOLUME FOUR BASIC MICROBIOLOGY

Microbial Physiology

IAN W. DAWES BSc, DPhil

School of Biochemistry and Molecular Genetics
University of New South Wales

IAN W. SUTHERLAND BSc, PhD, DSc

Division of Biology
Institute of Cell and Molecular Biology
University of Edinburgh

SECOND EDITION

OXFORD

BLACKWELL SCIENTIFIC PUBLICATIONS

LONDON EDINBURGH BOSTON
MELBOURNE PARIS BERLIN VIENNA

©1976, 1992 by
Blackwell Scientific Publications
Editorial Offices:
Osney Mead, Oxford OX2 0EL
25 John Street, London WC1N 2BL
23 Ainslie Place, Edinburgh EH3 6AJ
3 Cambridge Center, Cambridge
  Massachusetts 02142, USA
54 University Street, Carlton
  Victoria 3053, Australia

Other Editorial Offices:
Arnette SA
2, rue Casimir-Delavigne
75006 Paris
France

Blackwell Wissenschaft
Meinekestrasse 4
D-1000 Berlin 15
Germany

Blackwell MZV
Feldgasse 13
A-1238 Wien
Austria

First published 1976
German edition 1978
Spanish edition 1978
Reprinted 1980
Second edition 1992

Set by Excel Typesetters Limited,
Hong Kong
Printed and bound in Great Britain
by Hartnolls Ltd, Bodmin, Cornwall

DISTRIBUTORS

Marston Book Services Ltd
PO Box 87
Oxford OX2 0DT
(Orders: Tel: 0865 791155
        Fax: 0865 791927
        Telex: 837515)

USA
Blackwell Scientific Publications,
Inc.
3 Cambridge Center
Cambridge, MA 02142
(Orders: Tel: 800 759-6102)

Canada
Oxford University Press
70 Wynford Drive
Don Mills
Ontario M3C 1J9
(Orders: Tel: 416 441-2941)

Australia
Blackwell Scientific Publications
(Australia) Pty Ltd
54 University Street
Carlton, Victoria 3053
(Orders: Tel: 03 347-0300)

British Library
Cataloguing in Publication Data
  Microbial physiology. 2nd. ed.
  1. Microorganisms. Physiology
  I. Title   II. Sutherland, Ian W.
  III. British Society of Plant
  Pathology   IV. Series
  576.11

  ISBN 0-632-02463-1

Library of Congress
Cataloging-in-Publication Data
  Dawes, Ian W.
    Microbial physiology/Ian W.
  Dawes, Ian W. Sutherland.—
  2nd ed.
        p.   cm.—(Basic
  microbiology; v. 4)
  Includes bibliographical
  references and index.
  ISBN 0-632-02463-1
  1. Microorganisms—
  Physiology.   I. Sutherland, Ian W.
  II. Title.   III. Series.
  QR84.D29 1991
  576'.11—dc20

Contents

Preface to the second edition

The obvious preface for a second edition would seem to be 'Plus ca change, plus ça la meme chose', however, this is not strictly true. Microbiology has advanced considerably since the first edition, as can be seen in the following pages, and the authors have aged in the meantime. Also, a careful scrutiny of their addresses will reveal that the senior author has departed Edinburgh for the delights of his native Oz. Thus any delays in producing this new edition must be blamed on the intervening distance between Scotland and Australia. A further advantage of the time elapsed since the first edition is that families have grown up in the meantime. Thus, the assistance of Karen Sutherland in reading the manuscript and in typing considerable parts of it, is gratefully acknowledged.

Ian W. Dawes
Ian W. Sutherland
Kensington & Edinburgh

Preface to the first edition

Most prefaces begin with 'This book is . . .' followed by an apology for its existence, a statement of the aims of the authors, an acceptance of responsibility for all errors and omissions, and a grateful acknowledgement of the patience of the authors' spouses.

The title of this book is obvious, and we have no intention of putting off potential customers by apologizing for any shortcomings. Errors are inevitably the result of the other author. The size was set by our genial publisher who must therefore accept all kudos for the delightful brevity of the book, its lack of boring detail, and of course any omissions. Our wives are no more, nor less, patient than they were when we began and we remain happily married to them.

A final word of warning to our readers. This book is intended (it had to come in somewhere) as an introduction to microbial physiology to cover a broad spectrum of course requirements. It provides a foundation upon which to build by judicious reading of other sources. We trust our readers find the book useful and we would be delighted to receive any comments in case we have the opportunity to prepare another edition.

Ian W. Dawes
Ian W. Sutherland
Edinburgh 1976

Introduction

Physiology, according to the *Concise Oxford Dictionary*, is the science of normal functions and phenomena of living things, in other words the science of the processes of life. Even when restricted to microorganisms, our present knowledge is very extensive and it resembles microorganisms in a nutrient culture, in that it is expanding exponentially. There are many reasons for this interest. Microorganisms have become basic tools in the understanding of life processes, largely because they can be grown and manipulated with relative ease. The choice of experimental organism has frequently been *Escherichia coli*, since biochemical and genetic techniques have been developed to a level of sophistication unmatched in most other organisms. There are, however, a number of major differences between prokaryotic and eukaryotic organisms, and a number of eukaryotic microorganisms (notably the slime mould *Dictyostelium*; the yeast *Saccharomyces cerevisiae*; fungi such as *Neurospora* and *Aspergillus*; algae *Chlamydomonas* and *Chlorella*; and the protozoan *Tetrahymena*) are representative and amenable to detailed study.

Escherichia coli is not a typical prokaryotic cell. Different groups of bacteria have adapted to grow in different environments to the extent that they can be isolated from almost any ecological niche. This diversity is reflected in the range of activities to be found in different groups, and in their response to particular environmental conditions. Bacteriologists, ecologists, many industrial microbiologists, taxonomists and developmental biologists are therefore more likely to be interested in the differences between various microorganisms, as well as their similarity to *E. coli* or their conformity to the notion of a 'generalized microbial cell'.

In this book there is an attempt to strike a balance between the approaches of studying a few organisms in depth, and discussing the different activities to be found among diverse groups of microorganisms. Where possible, eukaryotes are introduced into the discussion to emphasize the differences between them and prokaryotes. It is assumed that the reader has a basic knowledge of biochemistry. Consequently less space has been allotted to common biological processes, and more to those aspects in which microorganisms differ from plant and animal cells.

Since the first edition of this volume was produced, there have been many very significant advances in microbial physiology. A wide range of new isolates has been discovered, including some from extreme environments such as 'black smokers' (thermal vents from deep ocean troughs) and also prokaryotic cells with unusual mechanisms of division (Fig. i). Microbial genetics, in particular, has almost developed into a separate discipline in its

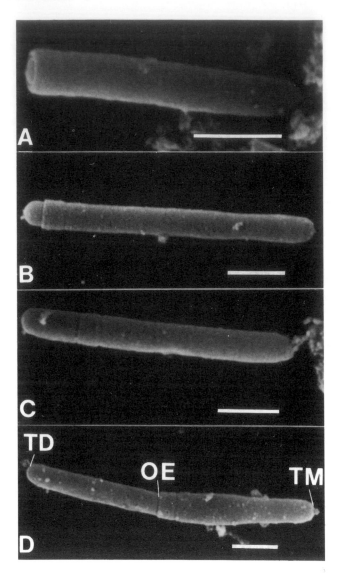

Fig. i Scanning electron micrographs of a Gram-negative sulphate-reducing bacterium showing a unique collar structure in various locations. TD = terminus of daughter cell; OE = open end of collar; TM = terminus of mother cell. Bar = 1 μm. (By courtesy of Professor Tiedje.)

own right. It has, however, produced much information about the processes involved in the physiology of microorganisms and enabled us to understand the mechanisms of control and regulation considerably better than we did 15 years ago. Thus any volume on microbial physiology must contain an appreciable quantity of background information on microbial genetics. At the same time, the methods of enzyme purification and analysis also produce a clearer picture of many processes, but we should not forget that other information has come from careful studies of hitherto unrecognized systems. Nitrogen fixation provides an excellent example of all these advances—genetics, physiology and biochemistry—but it is only one area in which our overall knowledge has increased.

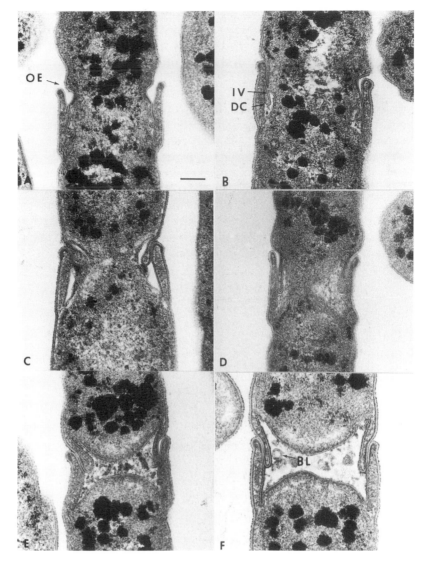

Fig. ii Transmission electron micrographs showing the collar region of dividing cell OE = open end of collar; IV = invagination; DC = daughter cell collar; BL = blebs. Bar = 0.1 μm. (By courtesy of the American Society of Microbiology.)

We should also not forget that many new microbial species have been identified in the last few years. This is particularly true of novel members of the Archaebacteria living in extreme environmental conditions, but also applies to many other types including the unusual collared bacterium reported recently by Tiedje (Fig. ii).

Along with the academic developments in microbiology, one has seen the intense interest of the biotechnologist in utilizing knowledge gained from basic microbiology to develop or to improve industrial products. Many of the skills needed for such developments are those already available to the microbial physiologist. This has increased interest in, and demand for, courses at all levels of microbiology. Hopefully, this volume will prove useful to some of the students taking these courses.

The reader will realize that any book of this size can only act as an introduction to the subject and provide a basis for further reading. For those wanting to obtain a broader coverage of the topics outlined here, or to delve into other developing areas of microbiology, a list of references to useful review articles is provided at the end of the book. In addition to these, the following review journals are important sources of information and act as indicators of current trends in the study of microbiology: *Annual Reviews of Microbiology, Annual Reviews of Biochemistry, Advances in Microbial Physiology, Symposia of the Society for General Microbiology, Microbiological Reviews, FEMS Reviews in Microbiology* and *Critical Reviews in Microbiology*. In addition several of the leading journals in the field, including *Journal of Bacteriology, Journal of General Microbiology* and *Molecular Microbiology*, regularly publish minireviews which expand and update some of the information provided here.

Abbreviations

ACL	antigen carrier lipid
ACLP	antigen carrier lipid phosphate
ACP	acyl carrier protein
ADP	adenosine diphosphate
ala	alanine
AMP	adenosine monophosphate
APS	adenosine phosphosulphate
ATP	adenosine triphosphate
CAC	citric acid cycle (Krebs cycle)
cAMP	cyclic adenosine monophosphate
CMP	cytosine monophosphate
CoA	coenzyme A
CTP	cytosine triphosphate
	cytidine triphosphate
DAP	diaminopimelic acid
DNA	deoxyribonucleic acid
DPA	dipicolinic acid
fd	ferredoxin
FMN	flavin mononucleotide
Fuc	L-fucose
Gal	D-galactose
GDH	glutamate dehydrogenase
GDP-man	guanosine diphosphate mannose
Glc	D-glucose
GlcA	D-glucuronic acid
GlcNAc	N-acetyl-D-glucosamine
glu	glutamic acid
GMP	guanosine monophosphate
GOGAT	glutamine oxoglutarate aminotransferase
GS	glutamine synthetase
GTP	guanosine triphosphate
Hep	heptose
IMP	inosine monophosphate
IPTG	isopropyl-thiogalactoside
KDO	2-keto-3-deoxyoctonic acid (3-keto-D-manno-octulosonic acid)
lys	lysine

Man	D-mannose
ManA	D-mannuronic acid
MCP	methyl-accepting protein
mRNA	messenger RNA
MurNAc	*N*-acetyl-D-muramic acid
NAD	nicotinamide adenine dinucleotide
NADP	nicotinamide adenine dinucleotide phosphate
PAB	*para*-aminobenzoic acid
PAPS	phosphoryladenylyl sulphate
PEP	phosphoenolpyruvate
PHB	poly-β-hydroxybutyrate
P_i	orthophosphate
PP_i	pyrophosphate
PRPP	phosphoribosyl pyrophosphate
PTS	phosphotransferase
rDNA	recombinant deoxyribonucleic acid
Rha	L-rhamnose
RNA	ribonucleic acid
rRNA	ribosomal RNA
RuMP	ribulose monophosphate
Ser	serine
Thr	threonine
TPP	thiamine pyrophosphate
tRNA	transfer RNA
TTP	thymidine triphosphate
UDP	uridine diphosphate
UDP-Glc	uridine diphosphate glucose
UMP	uridine monophosphate
UTP	uridine triphosphate
UV	ultraviolet light

1 Chemical cytology of the microbial cell

Microbial cells, whether prokaryotic or eukaryotic, are usually so small that important structures cannot be resolved by light microscopy. Consequently, much of our present knowledge of microbial cell structure derives from electron microscopy. Specimens for electron microscopy often require extensive pretreatment before they can be satisfactorily visualized, and care must be taken in interpreting the electron micrographs. During the preparation of thin sections, the techniques involved cause inactivation of cell constituents and are liable to introduce artifacts. There are thus problems in attempting to use cytochemical staining to locate some labile cell components, such as enzymes, within particular structures.

Techniques have been developed for disrupting cells so that some organelles or other particles can be isolated in a state which retains at least some of the *in vitro* structure and activity. Particular structures can usually be isolated from cell lysates by zonal centrifugation through sucrose density gradients. Again, care has to be taken in interpreting the results, since disruption of the cells often involves harsh physical procedures needed to overcome the strength of the cell wall which surrounds most microorganisms. Methods used to break cells include grinding with glass beads or sand, exposure to ultrasonic irradiation, or exposure to sudden changes in pressure. Alternatively, the cells may be subjected to osmotic lysis after removal of part or all of the rigid wall with lytic enzymes—lysozyme, lysostaphin or glusulase for *Micrococcus lysodeikticus*, *Staphylococcus aureus* or yeast, respectively. Thereafter, isopycnic sucrose gradient centrifugation can be used to resolve different membrane fractions.

Before discussing general cytological features found in microorganisms, one should remember that there are many fundamental differences between prokaryotes and eukaryotes. The eukaryotic cell differs from the prokaryote in the mode of chromosome replication and of cell division. In eukaryotes, chromosome duplication occurs at an early stage of mitosis and the duplicate copies are passed into the daughter cells. In the prokaryote, duplication of the chromosome occurs at the same time as the cell envelope is extended and the copies of the chromosome are separated. Eventually a septum forms and completely separates the two daughter cells.

The nature of the polymers found in the walls of eukaryotic microorganisms is also very different from those found in the prokaryotic cell envelope. Some of the surface polymers are unique to specific microbial groups, while others such as chitin are found both in fungal walls and as major components of the shells of marine

Table 1.1 Brief comparison of prokaryotic and eukaryotic cells.

Characteristic	Prokaryotic cell	Eukaryotic cell
Size	Usually around $1-5\,\mu m$	Usually greater than $5\,\mu m$
Movement	Flagellar or gliding motion, simple fibrillar arrangement of each flagellum	Flagellar or amoeboid motility, complex fibrillar arrangement of flagellum
Wall structure	Usually contains several polymers, almost always peptidoglycan	Contains a variety of organic or rarely inorganic polymers, never peptidoglycan
Vacuoles	Rarely present, if so gas vacuoles	Often present, range of different types and functions
Arrangement of nuclear DNA	No delineating nuclear membrane, single circular chromosome attached to cell membrane or mesosome	Within membrane-bound nucleus as several linear chromosomes; DNA complexed to basic proteins, histones
Replication of DNA and segregation	Bidirectional from single replication origin; amitotic segregation	Bidirectional replication from multiple origins; limited to part of cell cycle and segregation by mitosis or meiosis
Protein synthesis	Translation simultaneous with transcription; only one RNA polymerase known, with modifying proteins; ribosomes are 70S and inhibited by a group of antibiotics specific for prokaryotes	Translation of nuclear genes occurs in cytoplasm; three RNA polymerases; cytoplasmic ribosomes are 80S and inhibited by cycloheximide; mitochondrial and chloroplast ribosomes resemble those of prokaryotes
Energy production	Respiration, fermentation or photosynthesis; wide range of substrates; respiratory chain associated with plasma membrane; photosynthesis on invaginations	Some fermentative, but usually either respiratory or by photosynthesis; respiration in mitochondria, photophosphorylation in chloroplasts
Reproduction	Asexual, by binary fission; conjugation is rare, leads only to partial diploids and is not associated with reproduction	Sexual or asexual; many ways, including budding, binary fission, hyphal extension and sporulation; conjugation part of reproduction and leads to diploids

crustaceans, but not in prokaryotes. However, both eukaryotic and prokaryotic microbial cells generally derive their shape and wall structures from different types of carbohydrate-containing macro-molecules. The eukaryotic cells contain various intracellular components bounded by membranes. Prokaryotes lack organelles surrounded by subunit membranes and are simpler in the structure and composition of the cytosol.

The major differences between the two groups of cells are sum-marized in Table 1.1, while Fig. 1.1 illustrates structures which can be found in prokaryotic and eukaryotic microorganisms. There

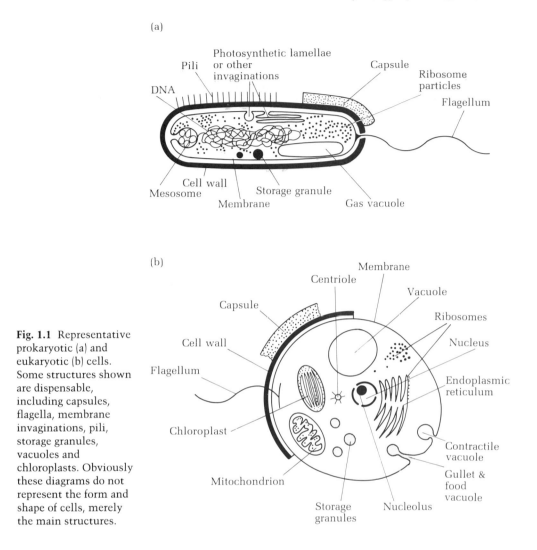

Fig. 1.1 Representative prokaryotic (a) and eukaryotic (b) cells. Some structures shown are dispensable, including capsules, flagella, membrane invaginations, pili, storage granules, vacuoles and chloroplasts. Obviously these diagrams do not represent the form and shape of cells, merely the main structures.

is a very wide range of cytological features found in microbes and those outlined in Fig. 1.1 and in the subsequent discussion need not occur in all species. There may also be extensive differences between cells of the same species grown under different physiological conditions. Thus, where quantitative results are important, they must include a definition of the culture conditions used.

CELL SURFACE AND ITS APPENDAGES

Flagella and cilia

Cell motility is found in both eukaryotic and prokaryotic micro-organisms and is usually dependent on specialized organelles protruding from the cell surface. In bacteria, these are flagella; in

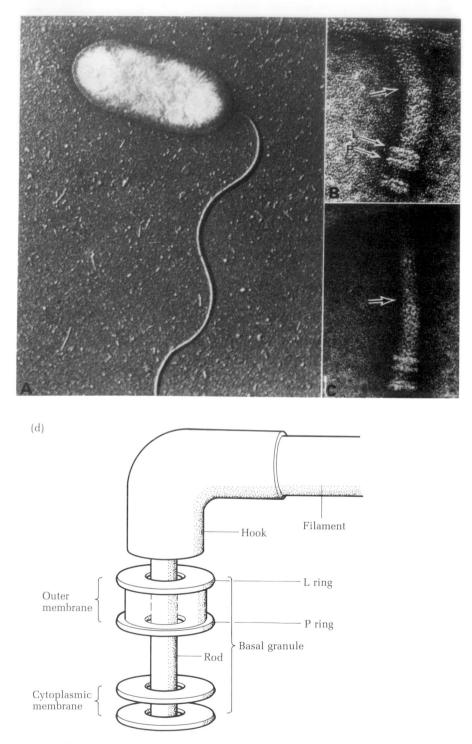

Fig. 1.2 The bacterial flagellum: (a) cell with a single polar flagellum, electron micrograph of a shadowed cell; (b) basal granule, negatively stained; (c) some subunit structure of the flagellum revealed by negative staining; (d) interpretation of the basal body structure. ((a) By courtesy of Professor Duguid; (b), (c) and (d) by courtesy of Dr Adler and the *Journal of Bacteriology*.)

eukaryotes, the terms flagella and cilia have both been used, although the structures are essentially similar.

Bacterial flagella

Flagella are helical structures several times the length of the bacterial cell (Fig. 1.2), and if sheared off by ultrasonic treatment or in a high-speed vortex mixer, motility is lost. It is, however, regained as new flagella are resynthesized. The pitch, wavelength and arrangement of the flagella on the cell surface are characteristic to each species. In cells of *Pseudomonas* species, there may be one or two polar flagella, while in other genera they may be peritrichous, found in large numbers over the whole surface of the cell. *Rhodobacter spheroides* is unusual in that it possesses a single *central* flagellum. In spirochaetes, a modified form of flagellum is present as an *axial filament*; two sets of fibrils are fixed at the poles of the cell and run the length of the cell, enclosed within the outer layer of the cell surface. This arrangement enables these spirally shaped microorganisms to move by a flexing motion.

Flagella are composed of subunits of a single protein, flagellin, which in the electron microscope are seen to be aggregated into rigid chains of molecules arranged helically. Flagellins from various species differ in their amino acid composition and serological properties. In some *Salmonella* species and in *Spirillum serpens*, an unusual amino acid—ε-*N*-methyllysine—is found in the flagellin, but mutants lacking the methyl amino acid still form functional flagella.

Flagellar assembly provides a simple and interesting model of the assembly of biological structures from their chemical components. Under acid conditions, *Bacillus pumilis* flagellar filaments can be dissociated into their subunit polypeptide of relative molecular mass 30 000–40 000. On slowly raising the pH, these subunits reaggregate to yield straight filaments as well as the wavy, flagellum-like structure. The straight form undergoes rearrangement to the more stable wavy form. The flagellar filaments are very rigid. Experiments using *p*-fluorophenylalanine, the incorporation of which leads to the formation of abnormal flagella, have shown that they grow by condensation of the tip distal to the cell membrane. This raises the intriguing question as to how the subunits are transported there—through the hollow core of the flagellum?

The filament of each flagellum is attached to the cell membrane at a structure known as the *basal granule* or disc. The precise structure varies between species, but a typical example is shown in Fig. 1.2. A filament is joined by a hook to a rod and set of rings located in the cell envelope. Typically, in a Gram-negative cell, a set of four rings (L, P, S and M) is associated with lipopolysaccharide, peptidoglycan and the inner face of the cytoplasmic

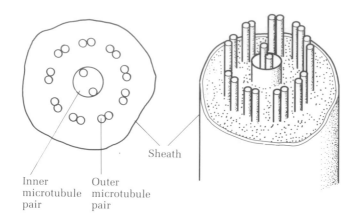

Sheath

Inner
microtubule
pair

Outer
microtubule
pair

Fig. 1.3 Cross-section
and diagrammatic
representations of a
eukaryotic flagellum.

membrane respectively. The M ring is an integral part of the inner
membrane, while the S or supramembrane ring is distal to it. The L
and P rings form the outer cylinder of the flagellum, forming
a large pore through which the rod passes. In *Caulobacter* and
in *Rhodobacter spheroides*, each of which possesses a single
flagellum, *five* rings are observed. The basal granule is probably
involved in the transduction of energy from the cytoplasm
or membrane to the flagellum. The complete assembly and
functioning of the bacterial flagellum is quite complicated; in
Escherichia coli and *Salmonella typhimurium*, some 40 genes
organized in a regulon of 13 operons are involved. They include
the gene for flagellin and those determining rotation of the
'motor', including whether or not it turns the flagellum, and if so,
whether it can go both clockwise and anticlockwise. Most of the
genes are clustered in three regions of the chromosome, one of
which codes for all except one of the known components of the
basal body. About nine of the genes are involved in the chemotactic
response, while 16 genes of as yet unknown function are needed
before structural flagellar components appear.

Eukaryotic flagella and cilia

Eukaryotic flagella and cilia are much larger and more complex
than the corresponding prokaryotic organs and are always attached
to cylindrical basal bodies within the cytoplasm. An extension
of the plasma membrane surrounds the flagella and encloses a
system of microtubules (each resembling a bacterial flagellum)
arranged as two central tubules surrounded by a further nine pairs
(Fig. 1.3). The only difference between flagella and cilia is their
length, up to 200 μm and up to 10 μm respectively; a far greater
number of cilia are found on the cell.

Mechanisms of motility

How do flagella move cells? In electron micrographs, bacterial
flagella appear as sinusoidal structures, but this is really a two-

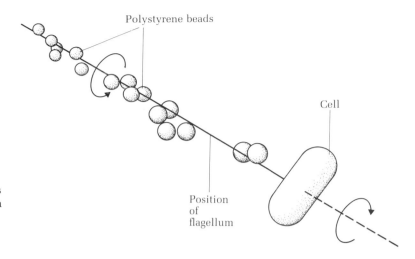

Polystyrene beads

Cell

Position
of
flagellum

Fig. 1.4 Rigid rotation
of the bacterial
flagellum shown by
fixing polystyrene beads
to the straight flagellum
of an *Escherichia coli*
mutant. (By courtesy of
Dr Berg and *Nature*.)

dimensional visualization of a three-dimensional shape. Eukaryotic
flagella, on the other hand, are straighter. Eukaryotes and prokaryotes also differ in the way in which they move cells. There are
several ways by which such helices can move cells. Eukaryotic
flagella contain complicated bending machinery, and an input of
energy derived from ATP causes a protein called dynein attached
to one set of microtubules to slide along another set, leading to
localized bending of the flagellum. Some flagella whip by transmission of this bending along their length; others move more like
an oar.

Bacterial flagella, on the other hand, rotate rigidly. When the
distal end of the straight filament is fixed to a glass slide with an
antifilament antibody, the cell rotates at several revolutions per
second. Similarly, after fixing polystyrene beads to mutant cells
with a straight filament, the beads rotate about the axis of the
filament in one direction, while the cells rotate in the other (Fig.
1.4). Bacterial swimming is modulated by switching the direction
of the flagellar motor.

The mechanisms of energy supply to each system probably differ;
in eukaryotes ATP may be involved, since detached eukaryotic
flagella beat if ATP is added. This ATP is hydrolysed by an ATPase,
thereby affording a source of energy. Bacterial flagella do not
possess ATPase activity, and although ATP does cause an interconversion between two arrangements of flagellin subunits isolated
from *Salmonella typhimurium* it is not hydrolysed. The bacterial
'motor' may well reside in the cell membrane with the basal body
acting as an energy transducer using a proton gradient to produce
the energy in the form used for the flagellar rotation. The source of
the proton motive force under respiratory conditions is the electron transport chain located either in the bacterial membrane or
closely associated with it. The coupling of energy released in the

respiratory chain does not require ATP as an intermediate; rather, as we shall see later, solute and ion transport, ATP biosynthesis and flagellar rotation are alternatives for linking into the respiratory chain.

Most bacteria move steadily, tumbling end over end, almost in straight lines, then alter direction abruptly. In some organisms, including *E. coli*, the choice of new direction seems random but overall movement can be influenced by chemicals acting as attractants and repellants for *chemotaxis* (p. 72). Photosynthetic species similarly show phototaxis, light being the attractant. A small number of Gram-negative bacteria show *magnetotaxis* under the influence of a magnetic field. These bacteria possess uniformly shaped crystals of magnetite—magnetosomes—which orientate the cells in a magnetic field. They then swim downwards into the microaerophilic environment which they require for growth.

Another form of movement, gliding motility, is of relatively common occurrence in Gram-negative eubacteria including *Cytophaga*, cyanobacteria and related species, and myxobacteria. The cells move slowly over solid surfaces (2 μm/min for *Myxococcus xanthus*) although no recognizable organs of motility can be seen. The only common property found in such bacteria, which might be involved in this movement, is the secretion of mucilage over the exterior of the cells and on to the surface of the medium. Time-lapse photographs reveal 'paths' towards which the cells move, eventually forming streams of many bacteria. In *M. xanthus*, two separate gene systems coding for different types of motility have been identified. One is required for movement of individual cells; the other is needed for the movement of cells in swarms. However, more than one mechanism of gliding motility may exist. In eukaryotes, amoeboid movement is found in slime moulds and in some protozoans. This is the result of *cytoplasmic streaming* in organisms without a rigid wall and also occurs on solid surfaces.

Pili and fimbriae

At the surface of many Gram-negative bacteria, numerous filamentous appendages called pili or fimbriae may be found; these are up to 3 μm long and have a diameter of 5–10 nm (Fig. 1.5). Other types of pilus are found on the male or donor cells of bacteria which undergo conjugation; some of these 'sex pili' are much larger than the common 'type I' pili or fimbriae. They may be 25–30 nm thick and intermediate in length between common fimbriae and flagella, although the nature, size and shape of sex pili are determined by the different conjugative plasmids which specify them. Only one or two sex pili are present on each cell.

Pili or fimbriae resemble flagella in being composed of proteins which can be disaggregated and show spontaneous self-assembly, but they can be readily distinguished from flagella by their smaller

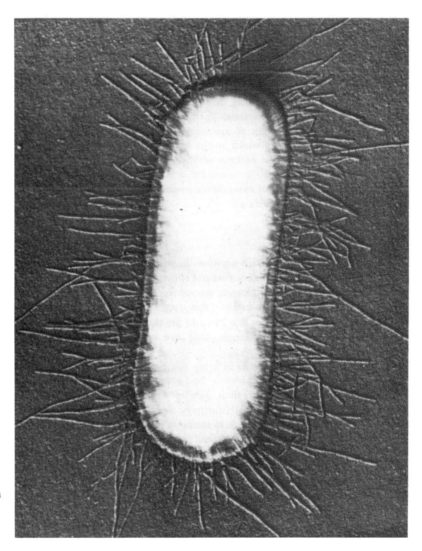

Fig. 1.5 Pili at the surface of *Escherichia coli*. Shadowed electron micrograph. (By courtesy of Professor Duguid.)

diameter and the absence of wave structure. All types of pili are hollow. During bacterial conjugation, the sex pili permit the formation of stable pairs of mating cells. The genetic material then passes from donor to recipient cell through a conjugation bridge formed by fusion of the cell envelopes. The sex pili are also the sites of adsorption of a group of highly specialized bacteriophages. Some adsorb at the tip and others along the length of the pilus.

Pili or fimbriae may play a part in adhesion of bacteria either to cells, especially the epithelial cells of a host organism, or to particulate material. This is obviously important for the utilization of solid substrates as well as in the more specialized process of bacterial conjugation and transfer of genetic material. The fimbriae provide a means of attachment of the bacteria in aqueous environments, including the gut. They may have a major role in colonization and subsequent infection. Their involvement in attachment to epithelial cells is part of the infective process of *Neisseria gonorrhoeae*. Some of the fimbriae are lectin-like molecules with an affinity for surface polymers containing D-mannosyl residues, a feature of which is their agglutination of erythrocytes and of yeast cells. Other types have different specificities. The newly discovered *E. coli* type P fimbriae have lectin specificity towards a D-galactosyl 1,4 α-D-galactose disaccharide; those in *Mycoplasma* are sialic acid-specific.

Capsules and slime

Many microorganisms have a discrete external layer of mucilaginous material called a capsule, which completely surrounds the cells and occludes the cell walls. The size of the capsule and the amount of capsular material produced is markedly dependent on the cultural conditions. It is often favoured by a high degree of aeration and a high ratio of utilizable carbon to a limiting nutrient such as nitrogen, phosphorus or sulphur in the growth medium. In some microorganisms only cell-free slime is formed. In most microbial species in which they are synthesized, capsules and slime are polysaccharides, termed *extracellular polysaccharides* or *exopolysaccharides*, to distinguish them from others found within the cell walls and the cell itself (Table 1.2).

Microbial extracellular polysaccharides may be homopolysaccharides formed from a single sugar, or heteropolysaccharides composed of two or more sugars. A large number of different monosaccharides have been identified in extracellular poly-

Table 1.2 Chemical composition of microbial capsules and slime.

Organism	Polymer	Capsule/slime	Monomers
Bacillus anthracis	Polypeptide	Capsule	D-glutamic acid
Leuconostoc mesenteroides	Dextran (homopolysaccharide)	Slime	D-glucose
Streptococcus pneumoniae type 3	Heteropolysaccharide	Capsule	D-glucose, D-glucuronic acid
Enterobacter aerogenes type 1	Heteropolysaccharide	Capsule/slime	D-glucose, D-glucuronic acid, L-fucose, pyruvate
Escherichia coli K12	Colanic acid (heteropolysaccharide)	Slime	D-glucose, D-glucuronic acid, D-galactose, L-fucose, acetate, pyruvate
Azotobacter vinelandii	Alginate (heteropolysaccharide)	Capsule/slime	D-mannuronic acid, acetate, L-guluronic acid
Escherichia coli K1	Sialic acid (homopolysaccharide)	Slime	*N*-acetyl-neuraminic acid
Sclerotium spp.	Scleroglucan (homopolysaccharide)	Slime	D-glucose

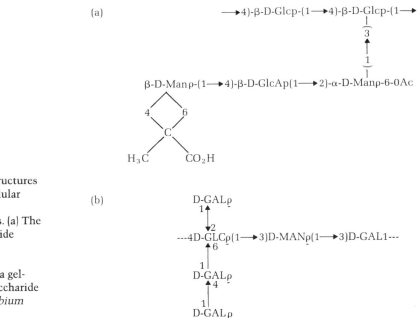

(a)

$\longrightarrow$4)-β-D-Glcp-(1$\longrightarrow$4)-β-D-Glcp-(1$\longrightarrow$

β-D-Manρ-(1$\longrightarrow$4)-β-D-GlcAp(1$\longrightarrow$2)-α-D-Manρ-6-0Ac

H₃C   CO₂H

(b)

D-GALρ

---4D-GLCρ(1$\longrightarrow$3)D-MANρ(1$\longrightarrow$3)D-GAL1---

D-GALρ

D-GALρ

Fig. 1.6 The structures of two extracellular bacterial polysaccharides. (a) The exopolysaccharide xanthan from *Xanthomonas campestris*; (b) a gel-forming polysaccharide found in *Rhizobium* species.

saccharides, including: neutral sugars—D-glucose, D-galactose and D-mannose (all hexoses); L-fucose and L-rhamnose (methylpentoses or 6-deoxyhexoses); amino sugars—N-acetyl-D-glucosamine and N-acetyl-D-galactosamine; and uronic acids—D-glucuronic acid, D-galacturonic acid and (rarely) D-mannuronic acid (Table 1.2). Pentoses such as D-ribose and D-xylose are seldom found in bacterial capsules and slime but are frequently components of the extracellular polysaccharides of yeasts and algae. In addition, numerous extracellular polysaccharides contain phosphate, ester-linked acetate and succinate and ketal-linked pyruvate. The hetero-polysaccharides, many of which are polyanionic, are normally composed of regular sequences of repeating units, varying in size from disaccharides to octasaccharides (Fig. 1.6). An increasing number of bacterial species have been shown to produce two or more distinct types of extracellular polysaccharide.

There may be many possible functions for microbial capsules, but non-capsulate mutants grow as well under laboratory conditions as do capsulate, wild-type strains. The capsule is highly hydrated, representing about 99% water; in natural environments, a capsule may protect an organism against desiccation, phage infection or phagocytosis. For pathogenic species such as *Streptococcus pneumoniae* or *Neisseria meningitidis*, capsule formation is associated with virulence, affording protection against attack by both antibodies and macrophages. Some of the capsular polysaccharides mimic eukaryotic polymers in their structure and are thus poor immunogens. Exopolysaccharides are also involved in the formation of microcolonies on solid surfaces exposed to

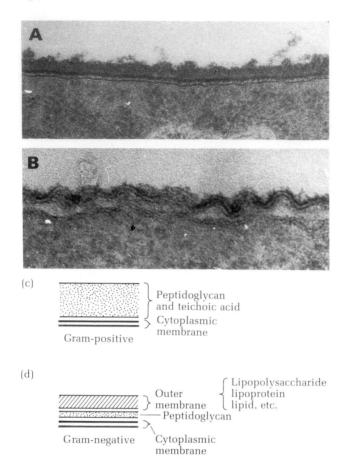

Fig. 1.7 Cell wall structures seen in thin-section electron microscopy. (a) Gram-positive *Bacillus subtilis* (× 60 000); (b) Gram-negative *Escherichia coli* (× 120 000); (c) and (d) diagrammatic representations of the Gram-positive and Gram-negative wall respectively. The location of various wall components is indicated. (By courtesy of Dr Highton.)

aqueous environments and may bind cations, sometimes with relatively high specificity.

The cell envelope

The shape of most microbial cells is due to the presence of rigid components of the cell envelope, which have the major function of protecting the fragile protoplast (cell membrane and its contents) from osmotic lysis. Microorganisms usually live in an environment which is hypotonic to the cell cytoplasm and, unless the protoplast is supported by the rigid layer, it expands and lyses. The rigidity is mainly conferred by a single polysaccharide or related component in combination with one or more proteins; other polysaccharides, proteins and lipoproteins are present and these are generally characteristic of particular groups of organisms or even strains of one species. The polymeric cell envelope components are organized into complicated multilayer structures; some bacterial examples are shown in Fig. 1.7.

On their surface, a number of bacterial cells have regular paracrystalline surface layers (*S layers*) composed of a single species of

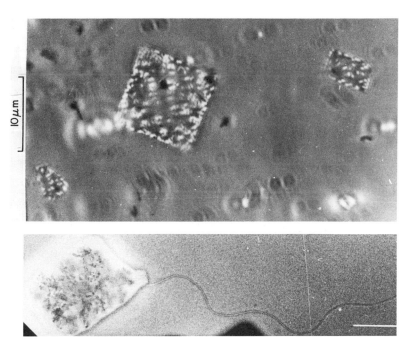

Fig. 1.8 Square bacterial cells with S layers. One non-flagellated bacterium is seen, the other possesses a single attached flagellum. (By courtesy of Professor Walsby and Dr Oesterheld.)

protein or glycoprotein. These molecules can be translocated through the cell envelope and can then self-assemble into a two-dimensional array. The proteins are composed predominantly of acidic amino acids and are deficient in sulphur-containing amino acids. The S layer is readily lost during laboratory culture but is found in a considerable number of freshly isolated Gram-positive and Gram-negative bacterial species and in some archaebacteria, including the unusual square bacterium discovered by Walsby (Fig. 1.8). The role of the S layers is uncertain. It has been suggested that they may protect against proteolysis and against bacteriophage infection.

The cell envelope has other functions; the highly charged polymers may provide an ion-exchange mechanism assisting in the uptake of ions and nutrients. It is also effectively a molecular sieve providing a barrier to entry of some molecules and retaining proteins found in the periplasm, the region between the outer membrane and the cytoplasmic (inner) membrane in Gram-negative bacterial cells. The pores of the sieve are in the form of components of the outer membrane, which have been termed porins; these vary in size in different Gram-negative bacteria. In *E. coli* molecules up to *c.* 600 Da enter, whereas in *Pseudomonas aeruginosa*, the exclusion limit is nearer 4000 Da. The respective pore sizes are thought to be 1.2 nm and 2 nm respectively. Thus small hydrophilic molecules can pass through the outer membrane by means of these non-specific, water-filled channels or porins. The porins found in any one bacterial species are dependent on the physiological conditions used for cell growth and are also markedly affected by osmotic pressure, by temperature and by nutrient limitations.

Prokaryotic cell wall

Most bacteria and cyanobacteria, apart from *Mycoplasma* spp. and other mollicutes, which lack defined cell walls, and halobacteria, which have an unusual wall structure, can be allocated to one of two groups, Gram-positive or Gram-negative, according to the structure and composition of the cell envelope. The difference was originally based on the ability of the organisms to retain crystal violet during Gram's staining procedure, but with electron microscopic and chemical analysis of the envelope structures, it became clear that the staining reflected an intrinsic difference in the chemistry and arrangement of the wall layers between the two groups.

Cytological differences between Gram-positive and Gram-negative bacteria are indicated in Fig. 1.9. Gram-positive walls are thicker and appear relatively amorphous, whereas Gram-negative 'envelopes' are much more complicated and show a multilayered structure. This is also seen in the chemical composition of the respective surface components (Table 1.3) and in their localization (Fig. 1.7). Several of the polymers found in bacterial cell envelopes are unique to prokaryotes. These are discussed below.

Polysaccharide components of the bacterial cell envelope

Peptidoglycan (syn. murein). Peptidoglycan is found in most prokaryotes (except *Mycoplasma* spp. and archaebacteria) and is not only unique in itself to the bacterial cell, but contains up to three components which are not found in eukaryotic polymers: D-amino acids, N-acetyl-D-muramic acid and diaminopimelic acid. Peptidoglycan is the polymer conferring rigidity on the bacterial cell, determining shape and resistance to osmotic lysis. When peptidoglycan is removed by lysozyme in hypotonic medium, the cells lyse. In hypertonic medium, rounded spheroplasts or protoplasts are formed, depending on whether part or all of the wall is removed. Peptidoglycan is essentially a linear polymer of alternating residues of N-acetyl-D-muramic acid and N-acetyl-D-glucosamine with the separate chains crosslinked to varying degrees by short peptide bridges. The polysaccharide backbone of the macromolecule, which is shown in Fig. 1.9, is ubiquitous to prokaryotes containing the polymer. Attached to the lactyl moiety of the muramic acid residues are peptide side-chains containing four amino acids in a characteristic sequence:

$$\text{L-alanyl–D-glutamyl–X–D-alanine}$$

X may be neutral (e.g. homoserine) but is more commonly a

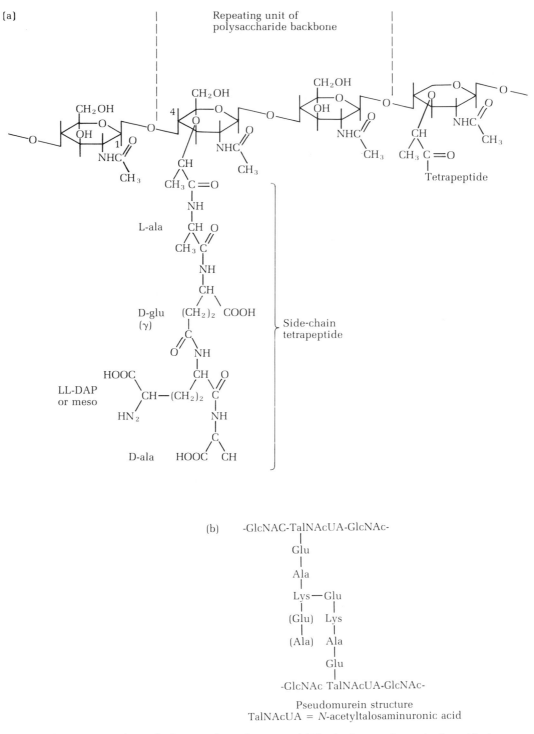

(b)   -GlcNAC-TalNAcUA-GlcNAc-
|
Glu
|
Ala
|
Lys—Glu
| |
(Glu)   Lys
| |
(Ala)   Ala
|
Glu
|
-GlcNAc TalNAcUA-GlcNAc-

Pseudomurein structure
TalNAcUA = *N*-acetyltalosaminuronic acid

Fig. 1.9 The structure of peptidoglycan and pseudomurein. (a) The basic repeating unit of peptidoglycan; (b) pseudomurein found in some archaebacteria.

Table 1.3 Composition of microbial cell walls.

	Peptidoglycan	Teichoic acid	Lipopolysaccharide	Lipid	Protein
BACTERIA					
Gram-positive	40–50%	+	–	2%	*c.* 10%
Gram-negative	5–15%	–	+	20%	*c.* 60%

	Wall components
FUNGI	
Acrasiales	Cellulose
Oomycetes	Cellulose, glucan
Zygomycetes	Chitosan, chitin
Ascomycetes (most)	Chitin, glucan
Basidiomycetes (most)	Chitin, glucan
Deuteriomycetes	Chitin, glucan
Saccharomycetaceae	Mannoprotein, glucan and (in bud scars) chitin
Sporbolomyceteae	Mannan, chitin

diamino acid such as L-ornithine, L-lysine, L-diaminobutyric acid, or is diaminopimelic acid as the *meso-* or LL-isomer.

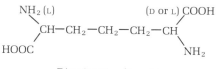

Diaminopimelic acid

In Gram-negative bacteria, the peptidoglycan is of one type only and is probably present as a thin layer 2–3 molecules thick. The chains are not extensively crosslinked (see Fig. 1.10). Only diaminopimelic acid is found as the third side-chain residue. In Gram-positive bacteria, the wall appears to be composed of multiple layers of peptidoglycan chains (about 20 in *Bacillus subtilis*) and, particularly in cocci, the side-chains are extensively crosslinked. Crosslinkage occurs between carboxyl groups of the terminal D-alanine residue and *either* a free amino acid of the tetrapeptide *or* the terminal amino acid in an additional peptide sequence. The bridge between the two chains can thus be: (i) a direct peptide bond (*E. coli*); (ii) by incorporation of a single additional amino acid (many Gram-positive bacteria); (iii) by a peptide of up to five amino acid residues, commonly of glycine but sometimes also containing serine or alanine (many Gram-positive species); or (iv) by an extra peptide with essentially the same composition as the tetrapeptide already attached to a muramic acid residue (*Micrococcus lysodeikticus*). The whole peptidoglycan structure in some bacteria may be envisaged as a giant net-like molecule of considerable strength.

In contrast to eubacteria, the archaebacteria lack peptidoglycan

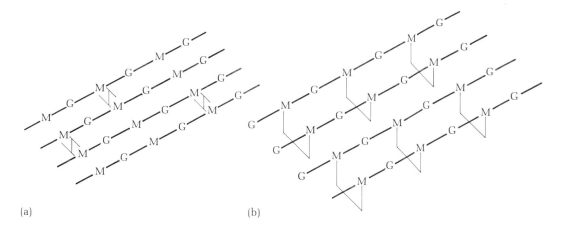

(a)   (b)

Fig. 1.10 The cross-linking in peptidoglycan of (a) Gram-negative *Escherichia coli*; (b) Gram-positive *Staphylococcus aureus*. G = *N*-acetylglucosamine; M = *N*-acetylmuramic acid.

and no common wall polymer is found. In the methanogens (methane-synthesizing bacteria) murein is replaced by a polymer, termed pseudomurein, which does have some features in common with peptidoglycan (Fig. 1.9). The envelopes of *Methanosarcina* spp. contain an acid polysaccharide resembling non-sulphated chondroitin. Some species of *Halococcus* are probably among the few prokaryotes to contain a sulphated polysaccharide as part of the structure of the cell envelope. Other archaebacteria possess proteinaceous structures.

Teichoic acids. These unusual anionic polymers of glycerol phosphate, ribitol phosphate or other sugar phosphates (Fig. 1.11) are found in Gram-positive bacteria covalently linked through a specific linkage unit of glycerol phosphate residues and *N*-acetylglucosamine phosphate to muramic acid residues of peptidoglycan. Glycerol-containing *lipoteichoic acids*, found associated with the cell membranes, contain glycerol phosphate residues covalently attached to glycolipid in the membrane. The precise function of teichoic acids is not clear, although they may provide an essential negatively charged environment in the cell envelope for binding ions such as Mg^{2+} or for regulating enzyme activity. Teichoic acids bind to autolytic enzymes present in the cell envelope, and may also be involved in the regulation of lytic modification of peptidoglycan necessary for normal cell division (see Chapter 2). When phosphate is a limiting component in the growth medium, wall teichoic acids (but not lipoteichoic acids) are replaced by other negatively charged polymers. These are the *teichuronic acids*, which lack phosphate groups and are composed of D-glucuronic acid and *N*-acetyl-D-glucosamine (Fig. 1.11), or by other structures.

Lipopolysaccharides. Lipopolysaccharides form one component of the outer membrane of Gram-negative bacteria. They are very variable in chemical structure from one group of organisms

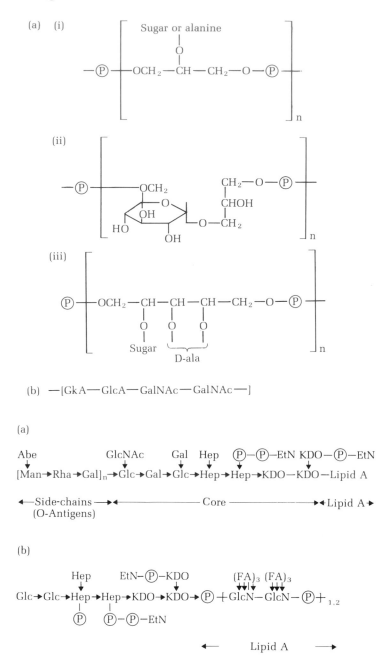

(a) (i)

(ii)

(iii)

(b) —[GkA—GlcA—GalNAc—GalNAc—]

Fig. 1.11 (a) Teichoic acid structures. (i) Glycerol teichoic acid; (ii) glycerol teichoic acid with glucose in backbone chain; (iii) ribitol teichoic acid. (b) A teichnronic acid structure.

(a)

Abe   GlcNAc   Gal   Hep P—P—EtN   KDO—P—EtN

[Man→Rha→Gal]$_n$→Glc→Gal→Glc→Hep→Hep→KDO—KDO—Lipid A

◄—Side-chains—►◄————— Core —————►◄Lipid A►
    (O-Antigens)

(b)

      Hep   EtN–P–KDO   (FA)$_3$ (FA)$_3$

Glc→Glc→Hep→Hep→KDO→KDO→P + GlcN–GlcN–P +$_{1,2}$
          | |
         P P–P–EtN

◄———— Lipid A ————►

Fig. 1.12 The structure of lipopolysaccharides of (a) *Salmonella typhimurium* and (b) *Escherichia coli.* Man = mannose; Glc = glucose; GlcNAc = *N*-acetylglucosamine; Rha = rhamnose; Gal = galactose; Hep = heptose; KDO = ketodeoxyoctonate; Abe = abequose; GlcN = glucosamine; EtN = ethanolamine; P = phosphate; FA = fatty acids (usually β-hydroxymyristic acid).

to another, but usually contain between five and nine different sugars, including some not found in other microbial polymers (e.g. 3,6-dideoxyhexoses) and a lipid (lipid A) which has the unusual structure shown in Fig. 1.12. Almost all enterobacterial lipopolysaccharides contain D-glucose, D-galactose and *N*-acetyl-D-glucosamine, as well as two sugars which are only rarely found in other polysaccharides—L-glycero-D-mannoheptose and 2-keto-3-deoxyoctonic acid (KDO)—i.e. a 7-carbon sugar and an 8-carbon sugar acid respectively. While KDO has been found in all lipopoly-saccharides examined, and also recently in the capsules of some pathogenic *E. coli* strains, heptoses are not always present. None have been found in the myxobacteria. The lipopolysaccharide molecules are formed from three components—lipid A, the core and the O-antigen. The function of the lipopolysaccharide is not known, but mutants lacking the O-antigens and much of the core are viable under laboratory conditions, although their phage sensitivity and serological specificity are altered. Loss of KDO or lipid A causes loss of viability. The complete structure is, however, necessary for pathogenicity, and different parts of it form recognition sites for bacteriophages and bacteriocins as well as antibodies. It can thus be visualized as being partly on the outer-most surface of the outer membrane of the Gram-negative bac-terium. The length of the side-chains varies considerably and may depend on the physiological conditions under which the bacteria were grown. Studies with a range of Gram-negative bacterial species indicate that some wild-type bacteria appear to contain some core molecules to which single repeat units or even no O-antigens are attached.

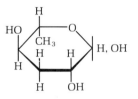
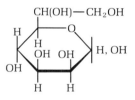

3,6-dideoxyhexose   L-glycero-D-mannoheptose

THE PROTOPLAST

Membranes

The cytoplasmic membrane of bacteria performs several functions which in eukaryotes are located in organelles. The two microbial groups will therefore be considered separately. Before doing so, however, the general concepts of membrane structure should be considered. These probably apply to most, if not all, membranes found in living systems.

General membrane structure

In thin sections examined by electron microscopy, the membrane has a 'unit membrane' structure; two densely staining layers sep-arated by a non-staining region (Figs 1.7 and 1.13). The classical concept of Davson and Danielli suggests that this unit structure is a bilayer of phospholipid molecules with polar groups facing out-wards into aqueous phases at the membrane surfaces, and the fatty acyl moieties forming a hydrophobic, semi-liquid phase to the

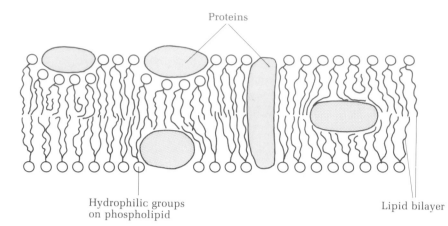

interior (it should be noted that membranes contain about 40% phospholipid). A variety of physical studies of mycoplasma membranes, in particular, tend to support this view of the membrane as a permeability barrier to ions and polar molecules.

Proteins also play an important part in membrane structure.

Fig. 1.13 Structure of membranes, a diagrammatic representation. The lipid molecules are probably in constant motion.

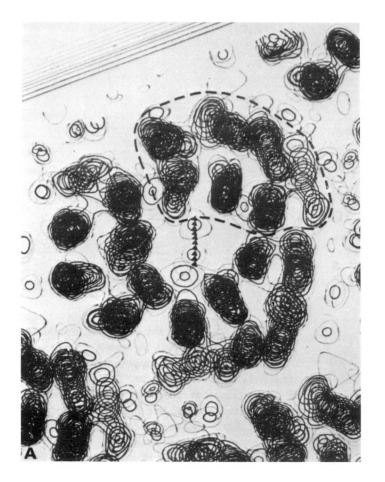

Fig. 1.14 (a) The purple membrane of *Halobacterium halobium*. Three-dimensional potential map of a region 5 nm thick spanning the membrane, showing protein molecules grouped around a threefold axis. One of these is indicated by the broken line; (b) the purple membrane of *Halobacterium halobium*—model of a single protein molecule in the membrane. The top and bottom are exposed to the solvent, the rest is in contact with lipid. (Courtesy of Dr Henderson, Dr Unwin, and *Nature*.)

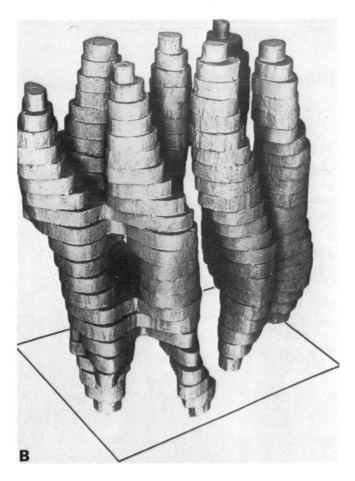

Fig. 1.14 Cont.

Much of the protein is apparently associated with the surfaces, but freeze-etch electron microscopy and amino acid sequence studies indicate that there may be particular regions of the membrane which have protein molecules embedded in, or across, the lipid bilayer.

The membrane is regarded as a fluid mosaic of small functional regions that are predominantly protein (*c.* 60% of the membrane by weight) embedded in a relatively homogeneous phospholipid bilayer matrix (Fig. 1.13). Hydrophobic bonds are thought to predominate and the phospholipid polar regions may largely be exposed. Many different proteins sediment with membranes during centrifugation. Some are enzymes bound to a greater or lesser extent to lipid. When proteins of intact cell membranes are chemically labelled by reaction with a molecule to which membranes are impermeable, some polypeptides are labelled, others are not, unless the membrane has been ruptured. This indicates that membranes have a distinct polarity with different proteins accessible to the aqueous environment on both sides. In the next chapter, we shall see that there is functional as well as structural polarity shown by the vectorial transport of compounds into and out of the microbial cell.

The above concept of membrane structure has been confirmed in an elegant, and technically very sophisticated electron microscopic study of the halophilic bacterium, *Halobacterium halobium*. This specialized membrane functions as a light-driven proton pump and is unusual in containing identical (rhodopsin) protein molecules of 26000 Da, comprising 75% of the total weight. These proteins have been visualized in a three-dimensional map of the membrane at 0.7 nm resolution, revealing the location of protein and lipid components, as shown in Fig. 1.14. The protein molecules are arranged in groups of three, each molecule extending across the membrane and contacting the aqueous solvent on both sides; the space between the protein molecules appears to be packed with phospholipid to form the classical bilayer configuration.

Prokaryotic membranes

The outer membrane of Gram-negative bacteria

The outermost layer of Gram-negative bacteria is the outer membrane. It protects the cell from toxic compounds in the extracellular environment and contains the proteins of the periplasm, preventing them from leaking out and becoming lost from the bacterium. The main constituents of the outer membrane are lipopolysaccharide (LPS), protein and phospholipid in an approximate ratio of 2:2:1. The phospholipid content is much lower than that of the cytoplasmic membrane. Most of the phospholipid (<85%) in the outer membrane of enterobacteria and many other species is phosphatidylethanolamine. The protein spectrum of the outer membrane is relatively simple; it contains multiple copies of a smaller number of so-called 'major polypeptides', some of which have characteristic molecular weights—between 35.8 and 37.2 kDa in *E. coli*. Additional outer membrane proteins are synthesized during growth in limiting concentrations of iron or phosphate or when induced by maltose (see p. 81). Further changes can be effected by altering the growth temperature or the osmolarity. As well as the major proteins, the outer membrane contains a number of minor proteins. While the major proteins are mainly involved in the passage of low-molecular weight solutes through the outer membrane into the periplasm, the minor proteins include receptors for phages, bacteriocins and some nutrients (Table 1.4).

The porins, which in *E. coli* include OmpC, OmpF, LamB and PhoE, exist as trimers which are fairly closely associated with the peptidoglycan layer. The total amount of porins in both *E. coli* and *S. typhimurium* is relatively constant, representing about 2% of the cell protein. Another major lipoprotein is the so-called Braun lipoprotein, which is the most abundant protein in the *E. coli*

Table 1.4 Some outer membrane proteins of Gram-negative bacteria.

Organism	Protein	Molecular mass (Da)	Conditions of production
Escherichia coli	TonA	78 000	Iron limitation
	K	40 000	—
	LamB	48 000	Maltose induction
	NmpC	39 500	—
	OmpF	37 200	Low osmolarity
	PhoE	36 800	Phosphate limitation
	OmpC	36 600	High osmolarity
	OmpA	35 200	
	Lipo-protein	7 200	
Salmonella typhimurium	OmpC	39 800	High osmolarity
	OmpF	39 300	Low osmolarity
	OmpD	38 000	—
	PhoE	34 000	Phosphate limitation
	(OmpA)	33 000	
	Lipo-protein	7 200	

outer membrane. It exists both covalently bound to the peptido-glycan ($\frac{1}{3}$) and as a free form ($\frac{2}{3}$). In the bound form, it links the inner face of the outer membrane to peptidoglycan. The outer membrane lacks ATPase or electron transfer-type reactions, indicating an inability to regulate a potential difference across the membrane. In this, it clearly differs from the cytoplasmic membrane.

The periplasm

The space between inner and outer membranes, occupied in part by peptidoglycan, is the periplasm or periplasmic space. Within the periplasm, a range of molecules is found, including enzymes, nutrient-binding proteins, membrane-derived oligosaccharides (MDO) and other osmoprotectants. The components of nutrient uptake systems ensure that specific metabolites can be taken into the cell, but detoxifying enzymes such as β-lactamases are also present, as are proteins which function in chemotaxis. Some are carbohydrate-binding proteins with dual functions: they also interact with proteins on the cytoplasmic membrane that are signal transducers for chemotaxis (p. 72).

Plasmolysis of Gram-negative cells by exposure to hypertonic sucrose solutions can be used to retract the cytoplasmic membrane from the peptidoglycan-outer membrane layer. Water passes from the cytoplasm to the periplasm increasing its volume. The expansion of the periplasmic space is confined to localized regions indicating the presence of a series of periplasmic compartments and a single open compartment. In wild-type bacterial cells, periplasmic bays are clustered at ¼ and ¾ cell lengths, possibly indicating that they are precursors of the periplasmic annuli which will participate in septation during the next growth cycle. Thus it is possible that division sites can be identified prior to the cell cycle in which they will function as the sites for septum formation.

The bacterial cytoplasmic membrane

Gram-positive cells possess a wall–membrane complex in which there is a single (cytoplasmic) membrane which has similar com-

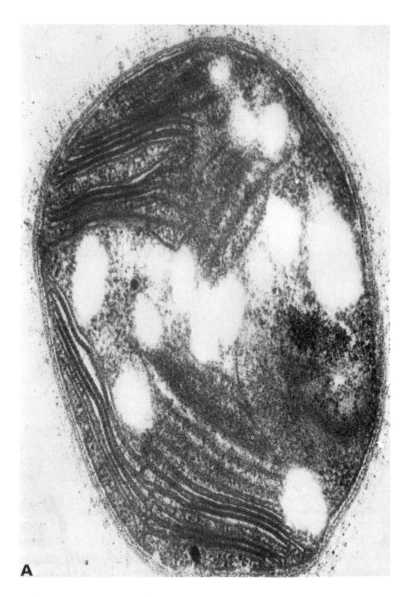

A

Fig. 1.15 Membrane invaginations in methane-utilizing bacteria. (a) Thin section; (b) freeze-etch electron micrograph. (Courtesy of Dr Watson and Professor Wilkinson.)

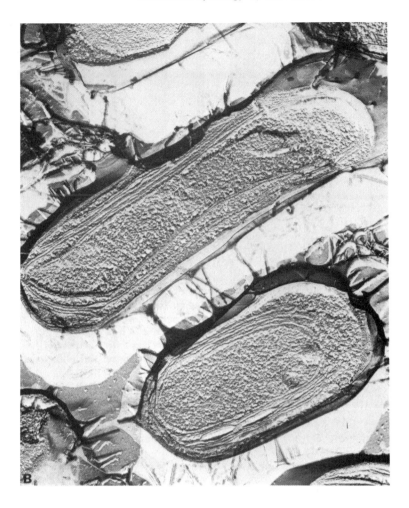

Fig. 1.15 Cont.

position and functions to the inner (cytoplasmic) membrane bounding the cytosol of the Gram-negative bacterium. The cytoplasmic membrane is much more complex than the outer membrane of Gram-negative bacteria. It contains three phospholipid species and about 100 major species of protein. The membrane lipid is structured into a lipid bilayer acting as a hydrophobic barrier and controlling the entry and exit of water-soluble solutes. Chemically the lipid component differs from that of eukaryotes in containing branched-chain and cyclopropane-containing fatty acids. Lecithin is rarely found in the phosphatides and sterols are normally absent.

In some Gram-positive bacteria it is easy to isolate membranes since the outer wall can be removed with lysozyme or other lytic enzymes to leave the osmotically fragile protoplast. Gram-negative bacteria are more resistant to lysozyme, although fragile spheroplasts can be obtained by treatment of plasmolysed cells with lysozyme in the presence of chelating agents. The membrane and wall together form a complex structure which can with difficulty be separated into component layers, including cytoplasmic and outer membrane fractions.

Among the components of the cytoplasmic membrane are the complete system for energy transduction in the bacterial cell and (where appropriate) for oxidative phosphorylation. These include the aerobic respiratory chain together with ATP-synthesizing systems and (in facultative and anaerobic species) the electron transport system needed for anaerobic growth. As well as the proteins necessary for energy generation, the cytoplasmic membrane contains numerous transport systems. Most substrates enter the cytoplasm using more than one system (see p. 80). The affinities of each system differ and some uptake mechanisms are only detectable in response to specific growth conditions.

Membrane invaginations. Although the bacterial cytoplasm is completely surrounded by the cell membrane and lacks intracellular membrane-bound organelles, electron microscopy may reveal numerous invaginations. These can be seen at the surface or relatively deep in the cytoplasm. Those most commonly seen are termed mesosomes, and are found in both Gram-positive and Gram-negative cells. Their occurrence in the latter is dependent on the growth conditions and they may indeed be artifacts of the techniques needed for preparing specimens for electron microscopy. Mesosomes are located usually in association with the bacterial DNA or with sites of septum formation, and may therefore be regions in the membrane involved in the organization of chromosome segregation and cell division (see p. 233). When protoplasts of *Bacillus subtilis* are formed under slightly hypotonic conditions, mesosomes are evaginated and the nuclear material is dragged to the cell membrane. Mesosomes have variable structures in electron micrographs. This is probably due to changes induced in a basic structure by the fixation and embedding techniques used. Despite their contiguity with the cell membrane they differ from it in their lipid composition and in their content of proteins such as cytochromes and enzymes.

Much more complex membrane investigation systems are found in autotrophs and specialized groups of bacteria such as nitrifying bacteria (e.g. *Nitrocystis* spp.) and photosynthetic bacteria (see p. 104) as well as in the dinitrogen-fixing genus *Azotobacter*, and methylotrophs (methane-utilizing bacteria) (Fig. 1.15). Membrane invaginations in these bacteria provide a greatly increased effective surface area to the cell. This may be of particular importance to those species using gaseous substrates poorly soluble in water—oxygen, nitrogen or methane. They may also facilitate the maintenance of reducing or anaerobic conditions at the site of these reactions (see p. 119).

In photosynthetic bacteria, internal membrane structures called thylakoids are arranged either as sac-like vesicles (green sulphur bacteria) or as tubular or lamellate invaginations of the cell membrane (purple sulphur and purple non-sulphur bacteria, cyano-bacteria). These membranes contain the complete photosynthetic apparatus (chlorophylls, carotenoids, cytochromes, etc.) and their extent within the cell varies inversely with the intensity of light falling on the cells.

Functions of the bacterial membrane

The bacterial membrane has many important functions; some are essential to the maintenance of cell viability, while others are involved in the process of growth and division of the micro-organism.

Maintenance of osmotic gradients and transport of solutes. The cell membrane is selectively permeable, permitting the transport of some ions and low-molecular weight molecules into or out of the cell. Other compounds, including those of higher molecular weight, are almost totally excluded. The specificity of transport is such that two structurally closely related sugars may have very different rates of entry to the cell. The membrane has a definite polarity; while some molecules are taken up, the exit of others is facilitated. This is discussed in more detail in Chapter 3.

Organization of cell envelope synthesis. Enzymes involved in the synthesis of precursors of cell envelope and extracellular poly-saccharides are associated with the membrane. These precursors are transported outward across the cytoplasmic membrane cova-lently bound to an isoprenoid component of the membrane lipid. Since cell envelope synthesis is localized in regions of the cyto-plasmic membrane, such as the periplasmic bays revealed by plasmolysis (see p. 24), it is possible that this series of multi-enzyme complexes reflects organization by the membrane. In addition, *zones of adhesion (Bayer zones)*, where the two mem-branes of the Gram-negative cell envelope are temporarily attached to one another, may be involved in the transfer of polymers from one membrane to another as well as to extracellular locations. Extracellular proteins, outer membrane proteins and lipoproteins in Gram-negative bacteria are exported across the cytoplasmic membrane and signal sequences are removed by specific signal peptidases (p. 174 and Chapter 6).

Attachment and segregation of DNA, cell division. The possible role of mesosomes in these processes has been inferred. Other aspects of this are discussed on p. 232.

Site of oxidative metabolism and energy generation. The bio-chemical processes associated with ATP synthesis in non-photo-synthetic bacteria (oxidative phosphorylation and the respiratory chain, see pp. 98–101), and also ion and solute transport, are organized as multi-enzyme–protein–cofactor complexes. Stalked particles or granules (similar to those found on the inner mito-chondrial membrane) containing the ATPase activity associated with oxidative phosphorylation are scattered randomly over the entire inner surface of the bacterial membrane.

Flagellar attachment. This has already been discussed on pp. 3–6.

Eukaryotic cell wall

Microbial eukaryotes are more diverse in their cell wall structures, ranging from the silica of siliceous diatoms to the various poly-saccharides in fungi. The walls of fungi have been studied in some detail: the entire spectrum of different fungi can be separated into categories on the basis of the chemical nature of their cell walls. These categories follow conventional taxonomic bound-aries closely. Fungal cell walls are composed of polysaccharides (80–90%), including cellulose, chitin, glucans, galactans and mannans. The vast majority of fungi, including all forms with typical septate mycelium, have a wall containing chitin and glucan, whereas yeasts have an increased mannan component. In fungi exhibiting dimorphism (the ability to change from a mycelial to a yeast-like mode of growth), this change is accompanied by a change in the relative amounts of mannan and chitin in the cell walls. The shape of a cell is therefore related to the type of polymer present in the wall—although there is undoubtedly a contribution from the spatial arrangements of sites for wall syn-thesis in the cell membranes. In filamentous fungi, the cell wall grows by deposition mainly at the hyphal tip, whereas in yeasts, new wall material is inserted more diffusely with a concentration of synthesis near the base of the bud. Another indication that the cell wall components play an important part in structural dif-ferentiation is the association of chitin solely with bud scars in *Saccharomyces cerevisiae.*

Electron microscopy shows that the fungal wall is a fabric of interwoven microfibrils embedded in, or cemented by, amorphous components. The microfibrils are usually chitin, a 1,4 β-linked polymer of *N*-acetyl-D-glucosamine, or cellulose, or a highly branched glucan with 1,6 and 1,3 β-linked glucosyl residues. This arrangement is seen by partially digesting the cell wall with specific enzymes. The amorphous components of yeast walls are mannans; these are the immunodeterminant surface constituents. Mannans of two types of yeast are indicated in Fig. 1.16. The mannans are phosphorylated and linked to proteins. In *Schizosaccharomyces pombe* the cell wall is devoid of chitin but contains 50% β-glucan, 30% α-glucan and 10–15% of galactomannan. The galactomannan is located on the cell surface at the periphery of the wall and near the plasmalemma.

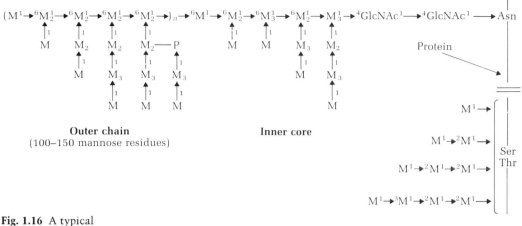

$$(M^1\!\rightarrow^6\!M^1_2\!\rightarrow^6\!M^1_2\!\rightarrow^6\!M^1_2\!\rightarrow^6\!M^1_2\!\rightarrow)_n\!\rightarrow^6\!M^1\!\rightarrow^6\!M^1_2\!\rightarrow^6\!M^1_3\!\rightarrow^6\!M^1_2\!\rightarrow M^1_3\!\rightarrow^4GlcNAc^1\!\longrightarrow^4GlcNAc^1\longrightarrow Asn$$

Fig. 1.16 A typical yeast mannan structure. M = D-mannose; GlcNAc = *N*-acetyl-D-glucosamine; Asn = asparagine; Ser = serine; Thr = threonine.

Eukaryotic plasma membrane

The plasma membranes of eukaryotes do not usually perform as many functions as those of the prokaryotic cell. They are thus not directly concerned with oxidative phosphorylation or organization of DNA, these activities being associated with membranes of organelles, but they function in osmotic regulation, nutrient uptake and product excretion, and in some cases wall biosynthesis. In fungi, growth is restricted to the hyphal tip, and it is not clear to what extent the cytoplasmic membrane is involved. In the cytoplasm below the hyphal tip a large number of membrane-bound vesicles are found. These may contain enzymes and wall precursors which are synthesized within the cytoplasm and are released by fusion of the vesicle with the cell membrane. In eukaryotes the export of macromolecules, including extracellular enzymes, probably occurs by synthesis at the endoplasmic reticulum into vesicles and release by fusion with the external membrane (Fig. 1.17).

Endoplasmic reticulum

This is a vast network of membranes within the eukaryotic cell, and it is continuous with both the cell and nuclear membranes. It is in part covered by closely associated ribosomes and one of its functions may be to organize sites of protein synthesis. Proteins synthesized on the ribosomes of the rough endoplasmic reticulum pass into the lumen of the endoplasmic reticulum. From there, they are transferred to the Golgi apparatus. Synthesis on the endoplasmic reticulum is associated with proteins that will be exported by the secretory pathway or transferred to other organelles such as the vacuole. The endoplasmic reticulum may be involved in the transport of messenger RNA from the nucleus. It is also associated with a number of enzyme activities not directly related to protein

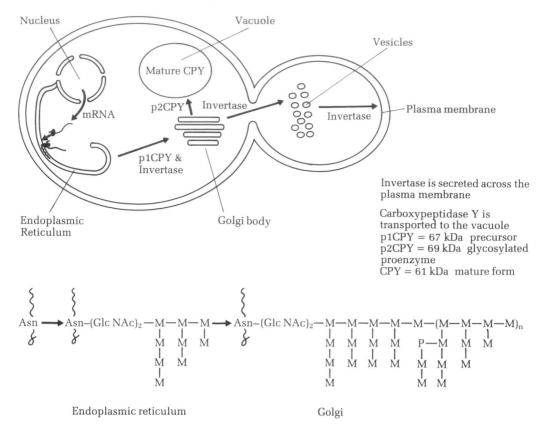

Fig. 1.17 Secretory pathway in yeast. Genes encoding proteins that are targeted for secretion or transport to the vacuole are transcribed in the nucleus. The mature mRNA is transported to the rough endoplasmic reticulum (ER) and proteins for secretion are synthesized across the ER into its lumen, where glycosylation begins. From the ER, the proteins move to the Golgi body where further glycosylation occurs and sorting to the vacuole or to secretion occurs. If the protein contains a particular short sequence of amino acids it is transported to the vacuole. The 'default' pathway in the absence of this signal is secretion via the secretory vesicles. Each of the steps illustrated can be affected by sec mutations of which more than 20 have been identified. The glycosylation steps occurring in yeast during transport are also indicated. Asn = asparagine; Glc(NAc) = *N*-acetylglucosamine; M = D-mannose; P = phosphate. (Redrawn from Schekman (1982). *TIBS* (July) 243–246.)

synthesis. Both rough and smooth (ribosome-free) endoplasmic reticulum membranes are sites of phospholipid synthesis.

Cytoskeletal structures

The eukaryotic cell contains various structural features absent from prokaryotes. *Microtubules* are thin cylinders 20–30 nm in diameter composed of tubulin protein subunits of relative molecular mass 50–60 000. The microtubule provides the structural skeleton of the mitotic spindle and also appears to be involved in maintaining the cell shape. Sets of microtubules are also found within the cilia and flagella, enclosed in an extension of the cell membrane. *Microfilaments*, composed of actin, are found in the peripheral cytoplasm where they may be attached to the cytoplasmic membrane and may effect cytoplasmic streaming, amoeboid movement and cell division. Microfilaments can also occur crosslinked with filaments of actin into a network, thus maintaining the high viscosity of the cytoplasm. A further series of *intermediate filaments* are intermediate in size between microtubules and microfilaments.

Bacterial nucleoid

Thin-section electron micrographs of bacterial cells reveal a region of fibrous material. This is sensitive to DNase and forms the bacterial nucleus or nucleoid. It is a compact structure attached to the cytoplasmic membrane (in Gram-positive cells at the mesosome). Unlike eukaryotic cells there is no nuclear membrane. At high ionic strengths the nucleoid is compact, but the volume increases if the intracellular K^+ pool is lost through damage to the cytoplasmic membrane. Very gentle treatment of the cells, and extraction with detergents and 1 M NaCl, releases the nucleoids to which fragments of the cell envelope may still be attached. Very gentle lysis of [^{3}H]-thymidine labelled cells of *E. coli* has shown that, following autoradiography, the DNA occurs as a single circular (or branched circular) molecule of about 1100 µm (this compares with the length of the *E. coli* cell at 1 to 2 µm). This physical arrangement was predicted from genetic studies which indicated that the *E. coli* chromosome was a single circular molecule of about 4400 kb. The DNA is further organized in the cell into about 100 supercoiled loops. Treatment with RNase, or isolation from cells in which RNA synthesis is inhibited, leads to unfolding of the nucleus, but RNA probably does not function in stabilizing the supercoiled loops *in vivo*. The chromosomal origin is associated with the cell envelope, probably in the case of *E. coli* through two minor inner membrane proteins of 80 and 56 kDa.

So far, most of the prokaryotic organisms which have been studied in sufficient detail genetically (including Gram-positive *B. subtilis*, Gram-negative *S. typhimurium* and filamentous *Streptomyces coelicolor*) conform to this general pattern of having one circular linkage group. However, an exception is *Rhodobacter sphaeroides*, which has two distinct circular chromosomes and this may prove to be true for a range of related photosynthetic bacteria.

Bacteria contain histone-like proteins, some of which have an amino acid composition similar to eukaryotic histone. The histone-like proteins condense the DNA into a nucleosome-like structure with a repeat length of about 150 base pairs. Two of these proteins appear to participate in wrapping, acting as accessory proteins in processes involving the recognition of specific nucleotide sequences. The sequences are recognized during site-specific recombination and during initiation of DNA replication.

One of the proteins is not associated with bulk DNA in the nucleoid but is located in areas of the cell where metabolically active DNA associates with ribosomes. In these areas, single-stranded DNA–RNA polymerase and DNA topoisomerase I are also located. The basic polyamines *putrescine* and *spermidine* are also present in microbial cells and are essential for normal growth, but the specific function of these molecules is not known.

Plasmids

In some bacteria, extrachromosomal DNA is present as plasmids and correlates with cytoplasmic genetic elements. These include sex factors (F) and colicinogenic (Col) and drug resistance transfer factors (R). These are usually circular DNA molecules smaller than the bacterial chromosome, but ranging in size up to 20% of that of the chromosome. They can be separated from nuclear DNA either by virtue of differences in buoyant density or by their inter-action with dyes capable of intercalating between bases in DNA (acridines or ethidium bromide).

The eukaryotic nucleus

The nuclear DNA of eukaryotic microorganisms is enclosed within a nuclear envelope composed of two concentric unit mem-branes (except during meiosis and mitosis). The membranes are fused together at regular intervals to form a series of nuclear pores through which materials are exchanged between the nucleus and the cytoplasm. In a number of microorganisms, including yeasts,

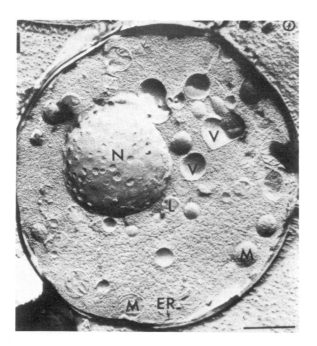

Fig. 1.18 Freeze-etch electron micrograph of a *Saccharomyces cerevisiae* cell. Nuclear pores are prominent. N = nucleus; V = vacuole; M = mitochondria; L = lipid granule; ER = endoplasmic reticulum. (Courtesy of Dr Conti and the *Journal of Bacteriology*.)

meiosis and mitosis occur atypically with no dissolution of this membrane. In some protozoa, i.e. the ciliates (e.g. *Tetrahymena* spp. and *Paramecium* spp.), there are two different types of nuclei in each cell. One, the *macronucleus*, appears to divide amitotically and is concerned with gene expression. The macronucleus is inactive during vegetative growth, but is involved in the sexual process of meiosis. It divides by mitosis during cell division.

The nucleus is surrounded by a double unit membrane structure, each layer with some degree of selective permeability in isolated nuclei. The nuclear membranes are more permeable than those of the cell, possibly due to the presence of relatively large pores (Fig. 1.18).

The DNA of eukaryotes is arranged into a number of chromosomes, which can vary from four per haploid cell of the yeast *Hansenula* through seven in *Neurospora* to 16 in *Saccharomyces*. These chromosomes are seen to be linear from both cytological and genetic studies. At one point on each chromosome there is a *centromere*, which is the point of attachment of the chromosomes to the *spindle apparatus* formed during mitosis and meiosis for segregation of the replicated chromosomes into daughter nuclei. The eukaryotic chromosome usually appears heterogeneous, having regions of highly staining heterochromatin (which is apparently genetically inert) and less densely staining euchromatin. Histones are a group of arginine- or lysine-rich proteins which bind firmly to DNA. They are involved in the structural organization of the chromosome and may also have some role in the control of gene expression. This latter function is also dependent on other non-histone proteins present in the nucleus (see Chapter 7).

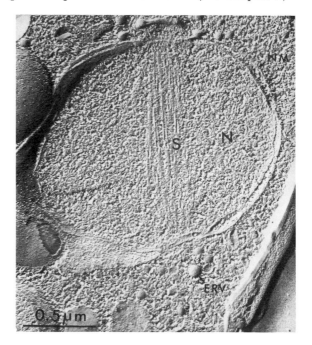

Fig. 1.19 Freeze-etch electron micrograph of the spindle apparatus (S) in *Saccharomyces cerevisiae* in an early stage of meiosis during sporulation. N = nucleus; ERV = endoplasmic reticulum vesicles; NM = nuclear membrane. (Courtesy of Dr Conti and the *Journal of Bacteriology*.)

The nucleus is commonly seen to contain one or more densely staining areas, *nucleoli*. By a combination of autoradiographic, DNA–RNA hybridization and direct electron microscopic studies, the nucleolus can be shown to be the site of synthesis of ribosomal RNA (rRNA) on highly repetitive sequences of rDNA. In larger eukaryotic microorganisms the nucleolus is associated with a particular chromosome, e.g. chromosome 2 in *Neurospora*.

Other RNA is present in the nucleus. This is heterogeneous in size and is presumed to be in part the precursor to the messenger RNA (mRNA) template for protein synthesis in the cytoplasm. Much of this heterogeneous nuclear RNA is, however, degraded in the nucleus.

Segregation of chromosomes during mitosis and meiosis takes place on the spindle apparatus. The structure found during mitosis in *Saccharomyces* is depicted in Fig. 1.19. It is composed of a set of microtubules emanating from a spindle plaque structure located just outside the nuclear membrane. In other eukaryotes, the spindle plaque is replaced by a more conventional centriole structure.

Mitochondria

Mitochondria are found in most, if not all, eukaryotic microorganisms. These organelles are characteristic in electron micrographs, being bounded by two unit membranes. The inner membrane with much greater surface than the outer membrane, is convoluted into folds called *cristae*, which are covered on their internal surface by granular structures. These contain ATPase activity and are the complexes involved in the oxidative metabolism of substrates and generation of ATP (see p. 98 and p. 101). Mitochondria are therefore specialized membranous structures in eukaryotes carrying out one of the functions of the bacterial cell membrane. Transfer of molecules from the cytoplasm of the eukaryotic cell to the intercristal space is by means of a porin resembling those in Gram-negative prokaryotic cells. This is formed from a polypeptide of molecular weight 29 000 in yeast and permits diffusion through the outer membrane. It is the sole protein in the mitochondrion known to function in this manner.

Mitochondria are needed only in microbial eukaryotes which metabolize aerobically. In some organisms capable of anaerobic growth the mitochondrion is repressed under anaerobic conditions or when glucose is present in excess. Such organisms, notably the yeast *S. cerevisiae*, are very useful for studying the interactions between the organelle, the nucleus and the cytoplasm. The *petite* mutations in yeast such as *Saccharomyces* lead to cells which have completely lost mitochondrial activity. These strains are viable provided that they are supplied with a fermentable carbon source.

Mitochondria contain DNA capable of coding for some, but not all, of their proteins. This DNA is usually circular, but it is linear in *Tetrahymena*. They also contain a protein-synthesizing system distinct from that in the eukaryotic cytoplasm. The mitochondrial system is inhibited by chloramphenicol, erythromycin and other inhibitors of bacterial protein synthesis, but not by cycloheximide, which specifically inhibits eukaryotic ribosomes. These inhibition data have been used to support the theory that mitochondria may be highly evolved bacterial endosymbionts, initially taken up by an amoeboid or phagocytic cell that depended on fermentation for its energy production. A number of important features found in mitochondria are normally absent from bacteria, but one bacterial species, *Paracoccus denitrificans*, does possess many of these, including: phosphatidylcholine as a major component of membrane phospholipid; straight-chain saturated and unsaturated fatty acids accounting for nearly all the membrane fatty acids; and a mitochondrion-like respiratory chain (Fig. 4.2). It is interesting to note in this context that the giant amoeba *Pelomyxa palustris* lacks mitochondria but contains endosymbiont bacteria which presumably grow on lactic acid produced by fermentation of glucose by the host. Similarly *Paramecium* species contain different 'species' of endosymbiont bacteria which are associated with killer activity and are incapable of autonomous growth. It should be emphasized that there are other theories for the origin of mitochondria and chloroplasts; one suggestion is that eukaryotes have evolved from phagocytic cyanobacteria.

Chloroplasts

These eukaryotic organelles contain the photosynthetic pigments and enzymes needed for photosynthesis. Those from different groups of algae differ in photosynthetic pigments but have the same general structure. This involves bundles of closely stacked vesicles or lamellae (thylakoids) each made up of a pair of membranes; the sets of lamellae are enclosed in a double unit membrane. The photosynthetic pigments (chlorophylls and carotenoids) are present in the lipid matrix of the thylakoid membranes.

Chloroplasts also contain DNA, and a protein-synthesizing system which is sensitive to inhibitors of bacterial protein synthesis. They also possess pores with a diameter of *c.* 3 nm, allowing solutes of molecular weight 7000–13 000 to pass through the outer membrane into the intramembrane space.

Ribosomes

Ribosomes can be seen as granular background in uranyl acetate-stained thin sections. The prokaryotic ribosome is a nucleic acid–protein complex of M_r *c.* 2.8×10^6, seen as a spherical particle of diameter *c.* 20 nm. The ribosomal proteins and nucleic acids are held together by electrostatic forces. They can be dissociated by changing the ionic environment, then reconstituted to yield active ribosomal particles. Their role in protein synthesis is discussed in Chapter 6. Eukaryotes contain two types of ribosome: the majority are cytoplasmic, either free in the cytoplasm or attached to regions of the endoplasmic reticulum; the others are located in the mitochondria (and chloroplasts if they occur). Cytoplasmic ribosomes differ markedly from mitochondrial and bacterial forms in both size (80S against 70S) and in sensitivity to antibiotics. Cytoplasmic protein synthesis is not inhibited by chloramphenicol, erythromycin and tetracyclines, but is sensitive to cycloheximide, which does not affect bacterial or mitochondrial ribosomes.

Careful extraction under defined ionic conditions yields polysomes—sets of ribosomes arranged linearly along mRNA. Each ribosome is associated with nascent polypeptide chains, and in bacteria the polysomes are formed while mRNA is still being transcribed from DNA (see Fig. 6.18).

Vacuoles

In some prokaryotes specialized gas-filled vacuoles enable the cells to adjust their buoyancy. These gas vacuoles are found mainly in purple photosynthetic bacteria and cyanobacteria, and more rarely in other aquatic non-photosynthetic bacteria. They can occupy up to 40% of the cell volume, and are collapsible when exposed to a sudden increase in pressure. They are surrounded by an unusual proteinaceous membrane which has a structure distinct from that of unit membranes.

In fungi and many algae large membrane-bound vacuoles are often found, particularly in aged cultures. Vacuoles isolated from yeast contain highly active lytic enzymes, including ribonuclease, esterases and proteases; their role may be to separate these enzymes from sensitive substrates within the cytoplasm. They may also act as sites for the storage or accumulation of ions and metabolites.

Protozoa contain a number of different vacuoles. During the phagocytosis of particulate substrates the plasma membrane pinches off to form a *food vacuole*, into which lytic enzymes are released to digest food. Ciliates (the most familiar being *Paramecium* spp.) have an oral region leading into the cell to the site at which food vacuoles are formed. A second type of vacuole found in ciliates (and euglenid algae resembling protozoa) is the *contractile vacuole*, which functions as a pump in media of low osmolarity to excrete water from the cell.

Inclusion granules

In addition to ribosomes and organelles, the microbial cytoplasm often contains other particulate components whose occurrence varies with the species and cultural conditions. Many of these 'inclusion granules' in prokaryotes are storage compounds formed during growth in the presence of excess nutrients. These include: lipids, including poly-β-hydroxybutyric acid (PHB) and other polyhydroxyacids, glycogen and volutin (polymetaphosphate); in some specialized bacteria (photosynthetic purple sulphur bacteria) molecular sulphur can accumulate as large intracellular crystals. These energy storage compounds are discussed in Chapter 4.

In the Gram-positive bacterial genera *Bacillus*, *Clostridium* and *Sporosarcina*, as well as most fungi and many algae, specialized resting stages or endospores are produced within cells facing starvation. These specialized cells are discussed separately in the chapter on morphogenesis (Chapter 9). The *parasporal crystals* associated with sporulation in *Bacillus thuringiensis* and several other *Bacillus* species are particularly interesting; each crystal is composed of protein antigenically related to spore coat protein, and is lethal to certain species of Lepidoptera. These bacteria or their crystals are used in the biological control of several insect pests.

Apart from essential features such as cell walls, cell membranes, nuclei, ribosomes and (in eukaryotes) mitochondria, no single type of prokaryotic or eukaryotic cell possesses all the structures outlined in this chapter. Some structures such as flagella or glycogen granules are widespread in their occurrence. Others, such as pili, have only been identified in a more limited number of bacterial species; generalization is even more difficult in eukaryotes, which do not form PHB or volutin but do (in some species) form starch.

2 Population growth and death

In this chapter, we are concerned with dynamic aspects of microbial physiology: how microorganisms grow, factors influencing their growth, the way they reproduce, the mechanisms of their response to a hostile environment and, ultimately, how they die. Why are we interested in studying these phenomena? Obviously there are many practical reasons; growth of pathogenic microorganisms can be deleterious and it is important to be able to control the growth of such species as much as possible. On the other hand, growth of many microorganisms is used to produce or preserve human and animal food, to synthesize antibiotics and other compounds such as ethanol, vitamins, essential amino acids and enzymes, or in treating and detoxifying waste materials. In addition to these practical interests, there is the fascination of trying to understand how cells reproduce.

What is growth?

The answer to this question depends largely on one's point of view. In terms of a single cell, growth can be seen as increase in its size or mass with time. Once a cell has reached a particular size (or mass), it usually divides; therefore growth can also be considered in terms of an increase in cell numbers.

Thus the microbiologist may sometimes be interested in the growth of individual cells, including the way they increase in size, how they replicate essential structures, and how they divide. Alternatively, interest may focus on the way in which a population increases in numbers or in total mass. These are two quite different aspects of growth and will be discussed separately. This chapter is concerned with populations of cells, and those aspects concerned with the growth of individual cells are discussed later (Chapter 8).

POPULATION GROWTH

Measurement of cell growth

For microorganisms such as bacteria, algae, protozoa and yeasts, which divide by binary fission or budding, it is possible to measure growth in terms of increase in cell numbers, or in cell mass, whereas for fungi growing with a hyphal habit, measurement of cell numbers is clearly not feasible. If a culture is in a state of 'balanced growth', which can be attained if care is taken to ensure that the environmental conditions are maintained in as constant a state as possible, then most of the cell parameters (e.g. mass, numbers, cellular constituents such as DNA, RNA, protein and peptidoglycan) will increase at the same rate. There are, however, occasions when it is necessary to distinguish between mass growth and increase in cell numbers, and techniques for measuring these separately have been developed.

Cell numbers

The number concentration of organisms in a culture can be determined by direct microscopic counting using a specially designed microscope chamber, or by particle counting techniques. The most widely used of the electronic counting devices is the *Coulter Counter*, in which the culture sample is passed at a given rate through a narrow orifice across which a voltage is maintained. As a cell passes through the orifice, it causes a change in the conductance of the suspension and this can be detected and recorded electronically. One advantage of the technique for those studying cell division is that the change in conductance is a function of the cell volume, so it is also possible to determine the distribution of cell sizes in a culture, while counting total cell numbers. This technique is obviously restricted to cultures in which there are no extraneous particles, and the method cannot be used for foods or many other biological samples.

Both of the above procedures only estimate total cell numbers and it is sometimes necessary to distinguish viable cells (those capable of continued reproduction) from non-viable ones, for example, when studying the death of a microbial population due to some treatment such as irradiation. The number of viable cells in a population is usually estimated by plate counting, in which a suitable dilution of the culture is spread on the surface of a growth medium (or is distributed within it using the pour plate technique) and colonies are allowed to develop for counting. After treatments which injure cells (for example when studying the effects of exposure to heat), the ability of a cell to recover depends very much on the composition of the medium, so 'viability' is not necessarily a rigorous concept. Plate counting methods are time consuming and tedious to perform and are used only when it is necessary to estimate viability or in some statutory tests of food or drinking water.

Cell mass

Cell mass can be estimated by a number of methods; some are direct, involving weighing the microorganisms, while others are indirect and are based on some parameter related to cell mass, such as light scattering or protein content.

Direct weight measurements can be of wet weight (although moisture content can be very variable) or more reliably of dry weight, in which cells are filtered or centrifuged, washed free of medium components and dried to constant weight at a given temperature. These procedures are accurate but time consuming and tend to be used only by fermentation technologists concerned with the yield of cells obtained under defined physiological conditions. In the laboratory, there is often a need for a rapid way of estimating cell dry mass to ensure that a culture is growing, to determine how fast it is growing, or to indicate when it is in a particular phase of growth. The most commonly used technique involves light scattering, either in nephelometers, which are designed to detect light that has been scattered at some angle to the incident beam, or in spectrophotometers, which measure the decrease in light transmitted due to scattering and absorption (usually negligible) by the cells. Since light scattering is a function of cell volume (larger cells scatter light more than smaller cells) and wavelength of incident light (more light is scattered at shorter wavelengths), it is necessary to calibrate the instrument separately for each organism at a particular wavelength. Moreover, light scattering by cells is not a linear function of cell mass concentration; at higher cell concentrations less light is scattered per unit cell mass, and hence it is often necessary to dilute cultures so that they fall into a more linear part of the curve.

In some cases, metabolic functions can be used to monitor cell growth: examples include oxygen consumption, CO_2 production, and fermentation products.

Growth kinetics

Organisms growing by binary fission or budding in a particular set of growth conditions do not all have the same individual generation times (i.e. the time from formation of the cell by division of its parent to the time it itself divides) as shown in Fig. 2.1. Nonetheless, for a given set of conditions, there is

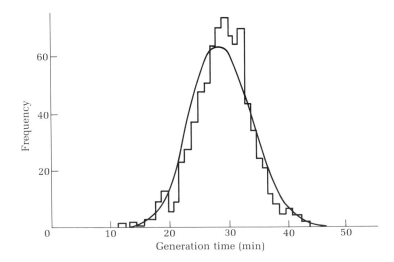

Fig. 2.1 Distribution of generation times for exponentially growing *Escherichia coli* cells. The histogram shows experimental data with a continuous curve fitted according to a theoretical distribution function. (From Powell & Errington (1963) *Journal of General Microbiology* **31**, 315–327.)

a characteristic *mean generation time* which can be used to describe the microbial population. For populations, the term *doubling time* (symbol t_d, units: h) is used as a measure of how long it takes for the population to double in mass or numbers.

In terms of numbers, if there are N_0 cells at zero time, then after one doubling time there will be $2N_0$ cells and these will give rise to 2^2N_0 cells after another doubling time. The series for growth can be represented by:

$$2^0N_0 \rightarrow 2^1N_0 \rightarrow 2^2N_0 \rightarrow 2^3N_0 \rightarrow \ldots \rightarrow 2^nN_0$$

where n is the number of doubling times or (generations). If the culture has been growing for time t, then:

$$n = \frac{t}{t_d}$$

The general equation for growth of cells can then be written:

$$N_t = 2^nN_0$$

where N_t is the number of cells present at time t.

This type of increase is known as *exponential growth* for obvious reasons. Note that if the above equation is expressed in logarithmic form, then:

$$\ln N_t - \ln N_0 = n . \ln 2 = \frac{t}{t_d}\ln 2 = 0.693\frac{t}{t_d}$$

For exponentially growing cells, the plot of the log of cell concentration against incubation time is linear and it is therefore customary in displaying growth curves to use semilog graph paper with cell concentration plotted on the ordinate. From this it is easy to determine the doubling time of a microbial culture by direct inspection of the graph as shown in Fig. 2.2.

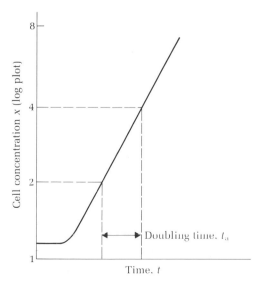

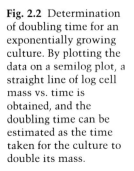

Fig. 2.2 Determination of doubling time for an exponentially growing culture. By plotting the data on a semilog plot, a straight line of log cell mass vs. time is obtained, and the doubling time can be estimated as the time taken for the culture to double its mass.

Specific growth rate

Another way of expressing growth (and one which is important in fermentation technology) is to assume that the rate at which the number, N, or mass, x, of microorganisms per millilitre increases in a culture depends on the number present at any time t, i.e.

$$\frac{dN}{dt} = \gamma N; \quad \frac{dx}{dt} = \mu x$$

where γ and μ are *specific growth rate constants* for number or mass respectively. Under conditions of balanced growth, γ is equivalent to μ. Integration gives the exponential function:

$$x_t = x_0 e^{\mu t}$$

x_t is mass/ml at time t, x_0 is mass/ml at zero time.

The specific growth rate constant can readily be related to the mean generation time for the population, t_d, by substituting $x_t/x_0 = 2$ and $t = t_d$ in the exponential function:

$$t_d = \frac{\ln 2}{\mu} = \frac{0.693}{\mu}$$

Either of these constants can be used in describing the rate of growth of a culture, but the specific growth rate μ is useful in the theoretical analysis of growth, e.g. in continuous culture systems.

The growth rate of a culture is a very important parameter in microbiology, not only for its use in predicting concentrations of organisms at some future time, but also as a sensitive indicator of the status of a microorganism and its response to its environment. Cell composition and metabolism are very dependent on the rate at which an organism grows.

Factors affecting growth rate

The influence of environmental factors on growth rate has been studied extensively, in order to develop and improve methods for preserving perishable commodities and ensure sufficient product formation in fermentation processes. Since growth is a culmination of many chemical reactions, the factors affecting growth are those which affect the rate of chemical reactions in general, including the availability of substrates, presence of products, and physical parameters such as temperature, pH and pressure. Since some reactions require oxygen, while others are inhibited by oxidizing conditions, the concentration of oxygen is also an important parameter. The solvent for most cellular reactions is water; hence conditions reducing the availability of water to the cell will also affect growth.

Each organism needs a particular range of conditions in which it can grow, and for each parameter such as temperature or pH, there will be an optimal value at which growth occurs at a maximal

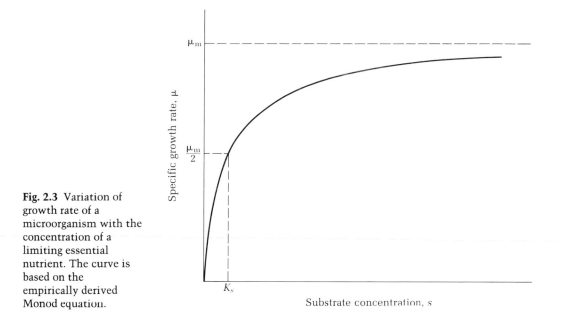

Fig. 2.3 Variation of growth rate of a microorganism with the concentration of a limiting essential nutrient. The curve is based on the empirically derived Monod equation.

rate. Microorganisms are characterized by their very great metabolic diversity and they have evolved to inhabit a vast number of different ecological niches. The microbial physiologist is therefore interested both in the way in which the growth rate is affected by different parameters, and in the mechanisms by which the cell responds or adapts to extremes and, in particular, the specialized aspects of those microorganisms which can resist these extremes.

Availability of nutrients

There are two facets of nutrient effects on growth rate: (i) concentration and (ii) quality. The effect on growth rate of altering the concentration of a particular nutrient *essential* for growth (in the presence of an excess of all other essential components) is illustrated in Fig. 2.3. This curve is hyperbolic and can be represented by the equation derived empirically by Monod on the assumption that the effect of substrate concentration on growth rate followed first-order kinetics:

$$\mu = \mu_m \left(\frac{s}{K_s + s} \right)$$

where μ_m = maximal growth rate obtained in excess nutrient, s = concentration of growth-limiting substrate and K_s = half maximal saturation constant.

From Fig. 2.3 it can be seen that, at saturating substrate levels, the cells grow at a maximum rate. As the substrate concentration is reduced, the specific growth rate decreases. However, this

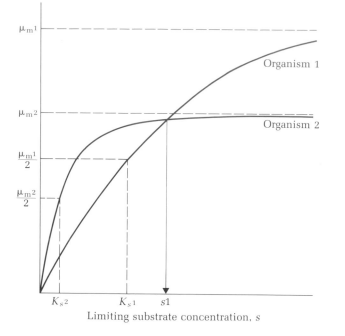

Fig. 2.4 Competition between different organisms may have different outcomes depending on the nutrient concentration. The Monod plots for two organisms differing in μ_m and K_s are shown. Above substrate concentration s_1 indicated, organism no. 1 will grow faster, but below this concentration, organism no. 2 will outgrow the other due to its higher affinity for the substrate.

decrease is not noticeable until relatively low substrate concentrations are reached.

The Monod equation is analogous to the Michaelis–Menten equation for the rate of an enzyme-catalysed reaction. In general the values of K_s encountered for most growth substrates are very low, of the order of $2\,\mu M$ to $20\,\mu M$ for sugars, and $2\,nM$ for amino acids, and reflect the high affinities of the systems for substrate uptake. This means that, in a normal batch culture, the specific growth rate μ approximates to μ_m until the end of the exponential phase of growth, when very little of the growth-limiting substrate remains.

The two parameters μ_m and K_s are important in considering the outcome of growth of mixed cultures. It can be seen from Fig. 2.4 that a situation can arise in which one organism (with a higher μ_m) would outgrow the other at high substrate concentration, whereas the latter would grow faster at low substrate concentration by virtue of having a higher affinity for the substrate (lower K_s).

Quality of the nutrient medium

Even in the presence of an excess of all the medium components, the growth rate of a microorganism can vary over a wide range, depending on the complexity of the medium. From Table 2.1 it can be seen that *Salmonella typhimurium* can grow on a simple medium containing one source of carbon and energy (e.g. lysine or glucose) and a mixture of inorganic salts, which provides the N, P,

Table 2.1 Growth rate as a function of medium composition, *Salmonella typhimurium.*

Medium	Specific growth rate (μ, h^{-1})
Lysine + salts	0.62
Succinate + salts	0.94
Glucose + salts	1.20
Threonine + tyrosine + cysteine + histidine + phenylalanine + isoleucine + hydroxyproline + arginine	1.46
20 amino acids	1.83
Casein amino acids	2.00
Nutrient broth	2.75
Brain–heart infusion broth	2.80

S and trace element requirements. Some single carbon sources support a much higher specific growth rate than others, reflecting the extent to which each compound can provide energy for essential cell reactions and carbon metabolites for growth. On increasing the number of substrates available to a culture (e.g. by adding mixtures of amino acids), the growth rate increases further, since the organisms use preformed precursors of their constituents and can then redirect energy otherwise needed for precursor synthesis into processes essential for growth (e.g. solute uptake, synthesis of protein, RNA, membranes and cell walls, etc.). In the optimal case, obtained with brain–heart infusion broth, the mean generation time can be as low as 15 min.

For laboratory purposes, this method is commonly used to obtain different growth rates. However, care must be taken in interpreting data obtained, since cells grown on one substrate will differ metabolically from those grown on another and the differences observed may have little connection with the differences in growth rate *per se*.

Not all microorganisms respond to high concentrations of nutrients. Bacteria termed oligotrophs (mainly found in aquatic environments) cannot grow above quite low concentrations of organic nutrient in the medium. These bacteria can be overlooked when trying to enumerate the total population present in a particular habitat, as they do not grow on the media usually employed to count bacteria present in food or water. Oligotrophic bacteria have adapted especially to very low nutrient environments such as seawater or stream water and have very efficient systems for concentrating nutrients from the environment.

Temperature

This is one of the most important environmental variables affecting microbial growth. Every microorganism possesses a charac-

teristic range of temperatures over which it can grow. Most
eukaryotic microorganisms fail to grow and are killed above 45°C,
although some fungi can grow up to about 60°C, whereas bacterial
growth is found between extremes of −7°C and 90°C. Considerably higher growth temperatures of about 120°C or more have
been indicated for some specialized bacteria living near deep-sea
thermal vents.

For a particular organism there is a minimum, an optimum
and a maximum temperature for growth. The optimum lies fairly
close to the maximum temperature. Organisms can be classified
according to their temperature dependence into three groups.
These are arbitrarily defined and do not in fact reflect the continuous nature of the microbial response to different temperatures;
they do, however, provide useful categories in practice.

Psychrophiles. Definitions vary to include either those species
capable of growth at 0°C, or those with optimum temperatures
below 20°C. Psychrophiles include many bacterial species (particularly *Pseudomonas, Flavobacterium, Achromobacter, Micrococcus*
and *Serratia* species), yeasts, other fungi and some algae. They
grow, albeit slowly, at temperatures below 0°C, provided that the
water in the medium is not frozen completely (due to solutes
depressing the freezing temperature of water).

Mesophiles. These have temperature optima between 20°C and
37°C, and include many of the commonly encountered microorganisms, including human, animal and plant pathogens.

Thermophiles. These grow at temperatures in excess of 40–50°C,
and include some of the cyanobacteria, actinomycetes and bacterial
species from the genera *Bacillus* and *Clostridium*. Thermophiles
are found in almost any material in contact with soil, or in very
hot environments such as the high-temperature pools adjacent to
sites of thermal activity (geysers, etc.).

How does temperature affect growth rate? The rate of a chemical
reaction varies with temperature according to the Arrhenius
equation:

$$\log v = \frac{-\Delta H}{2.303\ RT} + \text{constant}$$

where v = rate, ΔH = activation energy, R = gas constant and
T = absolute temperature. This gives a linear plot of log rate
versus $1/T$. For most microorganisms the plot obtained resembles
Fig. 2.5. At higher temperatures, the nature of the curve is
often explained in terms of competition between synthetic and
degradative processes—such as protein denaturation leading to a
breakdown of cellular components. At intermediate temperatures,
the Arrhenius relation applies, while at the lower end of the
growth range, there is a more rapid decrease in μ than expected

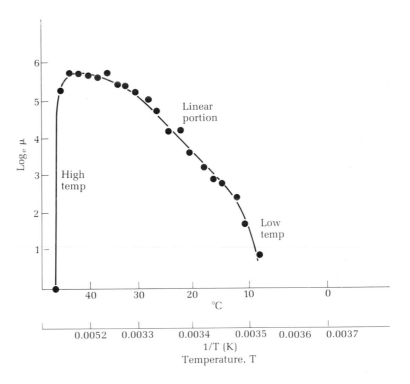

Fig. 2.5 Arrhenius plot of the relationship between growth rate and temperature for a mesophilic microorganism (*Escherichia coli*).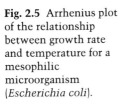

from reaction rate theory. This could be due either to the breakdown of control mechanisms at low temperature (explicable if one considers the nature of allosteric enzymes (p. 221) or to changes in membrane fluidity as a result of crystallization of some lipid components.

pH

As with temperature, every organism has a range of pH over which growth is possible, and an optimal pH. In general, bacteria are less tolerant of either pH extreme than fungi, but some acidophilic bacteria can grow at lower pH values, including those producing acids such as lactic acid (*Lactobacillus* species), acetic acid (*Acetobacter xylinum*) and sulphuric acid (*Thiobacillus thiooxidans*). Most fungi have a minimum pH for growth of between 1.5 and 2.0, but some species (*Acontium velatim* and *Demiataceae* species) have been reported to grow in 2.5 N H_2SO_4 saturated with $CuSO_4$.

At the other end of the pH range are the alkalophiles which can grow at pH values of up to 10.5. Most alkalophiles identified to date are archaebacteria but *Vibrio cholerae*, the causal agent of cholera, will also grow at relatively high pH values.

The microorganism accommodates extremes of pH by expending energy to maintain the internal pH much closer to neutrality than the environment. Resistant organisms have evolved external structures which are resistant to the external pH.

Water activity (a_w)

In most microorganisms, water is the major component of the cell (*c.* 80%) and is the solvent for many of the cellular reactions. There are a number of ways of effectively restricting the water available to the cell, including:

1 Dissolving salts or sugars to increase the osmotic pressure of the environment.

2 Physically removing water by evaporation or sublimation.

3 Freezing, which if done rapidly leads to crystallization of ice within the microbes; slow freezing leads to the formation of ice crystals external to the cell and to damaging concentrations of its internal solutes.

None of these treatments is necessarily lethal to the microorganism; in fact, rapid freezing or freeze-drying (lyophilization) is often used to preserve cultures almost indefinitely.

The availability of water to an organism is indicated by the water activity, a_w. This is the ratio of the vapour pressure of water in the solution under study (ρ soln) to the vapour pressure of pure water (ρ H$_2$O) at the same temperature and pressure:

$$a_w = \frac{\rho \text{ soln}}{\rho \text{ H}_2\text{O}}$$

The range of minimum water activities for growth of a number of microorganisms is given in Table 2.2. Most bacteria cannot grow below an a_w of 0.9. An exception is *Staphylococcus aureus* (0.86) which can cause food poisoning, and the halophilic bacteria (*Halobacterium* species) which can grow at $a_w = 0.75$ (equivalent to 5.5 M NaCl). The osmophilic yeast *Zygosaccharomyces rouxii* and a number of xerophilic fungi can grow in high concentrations of sugars at an a_w of 0.6 (by comparison a saturated sucrose solution or 70% fructose has $a_w = 0.76$). Note that some organisms which are resistant to high sugar concentrations may not be so resistant to high salt concentrations. This is due to differences in the way they respond to ions rather than to uncharged organic molecules.

Table 2.2 Limiting values of water activity (a_w) for growth of various microorganisms.

Bacteria		Yeasts		Other fungi	
Bacillus mycoides	0.99	*Saccharomyces*	0.94	*Mucor spinosa*	0.93
Bacillus subtilis	0.95	cerevisiae		*Penicillium* species	0.8–0.9
Serratia marcescens	0.94	*Torula utilis*	0.94	*Aspergillus flavus*	0.90
Escherichia coli	0.93			*Aspergillus niger*	0.84
Sarcina species	0.92	Osmophilic yeasts:			
		Zygosaccharomyces	0.65	Xerophilic fungi:	
Salt-tolerant bacteria:		rouxii		*Xeromyces*	0.60
Staphylococcus aureus	0.87			bisporus	
Halophilic bacteria:					
Halobacterium species	0.75				

Oxygen tension and redox potential (Eh)

Some organisms require oxygen for growth (*strict aerobes*) while *obligate anaerobes* are killed in the presence of oxygen and need care in the preparation of their culture medium (e.g. addition of reducing agents such as ascorbate or thioglycollate, boiling to remove oxygen). The anaerobes can then be maintained in an oxygen-free atmosphere by growing them in special anaerobic jars or under a stream of oxygen-free nitrogen. There are also many organisms which can tolerate either condition (*facultative anaerobes*). Some organisms, termed *microaerophiles*, can grow in the presence of oxygen but only at concentrations less than the 20% v/v found in the atmosphere.

Oxygen is potentially toxic to all actively metabolizing cells, since there are some enzyme-catalysed side-reactions which produce peroxides and toxic free radicals in the presence of oxygen. One of the most toxic of the side-products is the superoxide free radical $O_2 \cdot^-$. Those organisms which need molecular oxygen to grow (usually as a terminal electron acceptor in aerobic respiration) possess enzymes which can detoxify these reactive oxidants, e.g. superoxide dismutase, which catalyses the reaction:

$$2 H^+ + 2 O_2 \cdot^- \rightarrow H_2O_2 + O_2$$

and catalase which converts hydrogen peroxide to water:

$$2 H_2O_2 \rightarrow 2 H_2O + O_2$$

Of these, the superoxide dismutase appears to be essential for aerobic growth, since mutants of the normally facultative anaerobe *Escherichia coli* that lack this enzyme are strict anaerobes.

In the case of those organisms that do require oxygen, care must be taken that it is supplied to the culture at an adequate rate. Molecular oxygen is poorly soluble in water; hence it is necessary to aerate cultures by growing them in vessels with a large surface area to volume ratio, by shaking flasks to improve the oxygen transfer, or by using spargers and mechanical agitation to introduce fine bubbles of air into the culture.

CELL CULTIVATION

Growth yield

An important growth parameter is the yield of organisms that can be grown for the consumption of a given amount of a specific substrate. When growing an organism for commercial purposes, it is necessary to minimize the cost of substrates and a knowledge of the yield constant for each substrate is vital:

$$Y = \frac{\text{mass of bacteria formed}}{\text{mass of substrate used}} = \frac{x}{s}$$

The yield constant Y for a given substrate can be estimated in batch growth experiments. When cells enter the stationary phase, they have usually exhausted a compound that is essential for growth, the limiting component. Varying the initial concentration of this compound gives a plot of total growth versus substrate concentration which is usually linear and, from the slope, Y can be estimated. Y is a constant only for a particular organism under a given set of cultural conditions, and varying pH or temperature (or any other parameter affecting the growth rate of the organism) can lead to changes in the yield constant.

For heterotrophic organisms, the yield for carbon substrates is not directly related to the mass of carbon available to the cell, but depends on two factors. The first is the pathway by which the carbon substrate is metabolized to produce energy and metabolites needed for biosynthesis (discussed in Chapter 5). Secondly, when the carbon source on which the yield constants are estimated is also the energy source, the yield is much more dependent on how efficiently the cell converts the chemical energy in the substrate to ATP, and how much ATP is expended in withstanding the adverse effects of the environment. For this reason, there have been a number of attempts to estimate Y_{ATP}, to determine how much ATP is required for growth. This value is difficult to estimate, since the rate of ATP production cannot be measured directly and has to be estimated using assumptions about the metabolic pathways operating in the cell.

Batch culture

The traditional method of studying microbial growth has been batch culture, in which a volume of medium is inoculated with a small number of organisms and their growth followed with time. This procedure has a number of disadvantages over other methods of growing cells, since the culture medium is in a state of continuous change. It does, however, have the advantage of convenience.

The nature of the growth curve obtained in batch cultivation is illustrated in Fig. 2.6. After an initial *lag phase* during which the organisms adjust to their new environment, cells begin to grow and divide at the exponential rate characteristic of the medium and experimental conditions. If there is a single source of carbon (often glucose), the population will continue to grow at virtually the same rate until they have almost exhausted this substrate. This is the *exponential* or *log phase*. Note that in such a medium, the substrate concentration will fall at an ever increasing rate, since the rate of consumption is a function of the mass of cells in the culture. This means that if growth ceases due to exhaustion of a single substrate, there is a fairly sharp decline in the growth rate at the *late log phase*.

In more complex media, containing mixtures of substrates, the

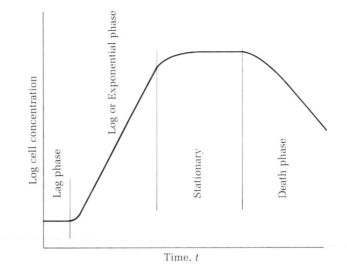

Fig. 2.6 The phases of growth in batch cultivation.

organisms can control their utilization of substrates so that one is consumed first, then another, until all are exhausted. Under these conditions, the slope of the growth curve is not constant and, in some cases, there is a brief interval as the cells adapt from one growth substrate to another. This phenomenon of *diauxic growth* is discussed in Chapter 7.

Eventually, the organisms cease to grow and enter the *stationary phase*. They are not metabolically inert during this phase, but adapt to survival. Unnecessary components are slowly degraded to provide the energy needed for maintaining the cells. Some micro-organisms can survive extensive periods (weeks or more) without loss of viability, while others begin to die almost as soon as they have entered the stationary phase. There are many reasons for death of the cells, due to either the accumulation of toxic metabolites, or the activity of lytic enzymes. There are some organisms in which starvation triggers the development of defective viruses. The various phases of growth and their significance are summarized in Table 2.3.

Phased batch culture

In some cases, there is a need to grow cells in a vessel of nearly constant volume, as in batch culture, but to alter the nutritional conditions as growth proceeds. This type of phased culture is illustrated by the way in which bakers' yeast is produced. Even in the presence of air, *S. cerevisiae* grows on moderate concentrations of glucose or sucrose by fermentation, producing ethanol and some CO_2. This is in part due to the repression by sugars, such as glucose, of the mitochondrial activity of yeast. Since fermentation results in a much lower yield of cell mass than that obtained by aerobic respiration via the citric acid cycle (p. 102), steps must be taken to encourage the yeast to respire the sugar substrate (usually

Table 2.3 Growth phases in batch culture.

Growth phase	Cell activity
Lag	Adaptation to new environment, synthesis of new enzymes. Also seen when large proportion of inoculum is composed of dead cells. Longer lag for starved cells or when fresh medium is not 'rich'
Log or exponential	Unhindered multiplication; all nutrients present in excess. Rate of growth determined by the composition of the medium and environmental factors
Late log	Concentration of one (or more) nutrients becomes limiting and falls to a low level with concomitant decline in growth rate
Stationary*	Can be due to nutrient deprivation or accumulation of inhibitory products of metabolism. Organisms still viable and using endogenous reserves for maintenance
Death	Occurs at a variable time after onset of stationary phase. Due to cell lysis by autolytic enzymes or effects of toxic metabolites

* In some Gram-positive bacteria and many eukaryotes a process of sporulation is initiated at the end of log phase and is maintained by endogenous reserves accumulated during log phase.

sucrose in molasses). This can be achieved by keeping the concentration of the sugar in the medium low at all stages of the fermentation, so that mitochondrial activity is not repressed. As the cell density increases, the sugar is fed into the culture at a rate which keeps pace with its consumption by the cells, so that its concentration does not rise high enough to encourage fermentation at the expense of respiration.

Continuous culture

In batch culture, microorganisms are subject to a continuously changing environment as substrates are consumed and products of metabolism accumulate. Exponential growth cannot be maintained indefinitely. There are, however, a number of ways of maintaining continuous growth and these are finding increasing application in research and in industry. The advantages of continuous over batch culture can be summarized as follows:
1 Smaller fermenter vessels are required and continuous operation reduces cleaning times and costs.
2 Growth occurs at a constant rate in a constant environment and it is easier to control such parameters as temperature, pH and oxygen concentration.
3 In some continuous systems, growth rate can be varied in a controlled way, thus enabling study of the effect of growth rate on cell size and composition.

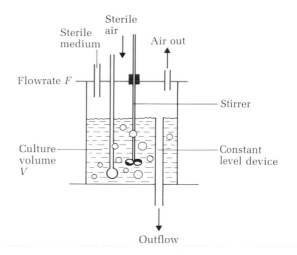

Fig. 2.7 Diagrammatic representation of the chemostat. To this basic design can be added systems to control temperature, pH, dissolved oxygen concentration and foaming.

There are also problems with continuous cultures. The main difficulty arises from the need to maintain a high degree of sterility of inflowing substrates, and to prevent contamination from other sources, due to the long periods during which the culture will be maintained. This is not very difficult on the laboratory scale, but becomes more of a problem as the size (and complexity) of the culture vessel is increased to commercial scales.

The chemostat

The simplest continuous culture arrangement, the chemostat, is depicted in Fig. 2.7. Fresh medium is pumped into the culture vessel at constant flowrate, F, and mixed as efficiently as possible. The culture volume, V, is maintained constant by a weir or syphon device so that excess culture is removed at the same rate as fresh medium flows in. For extremely accurate control of inflow and outflow, vessels mounted on balances may be employed.

An important parameter in this system is the dilution rate, D, which indicates how fast the culture contents are diluted:

$$D = \frac{F}{V}$$

For a pure culture of an organism, the rate of increase of cell mass *in the culture vessel* will be given by:

rate of change of cell concentration =
rate of growth of cells − washout of cells to effluent

$$\frac{\mathrm{d}x}{\mathrm{d}t} = \mu x - Dx$$
$$= (\mu - D)x$$

where x = cell concentration in vessel; μ = growth rate.

We have seen previously that μ is a function of the concentration of the limiting substrate according to the Monod equation (p. 43). If D exceeds μ_m, the maximal growth rate constant for the organism, washout of the culture will occur. If, however, $D < \mu_m$, the culture will adjust to a steady state; i.e. for $dx/dt = 0$, $\bar{\mu} = 0$, where $\bar{\mu}$ is the steady state growth rate.

This system is self-adjusting. From a low inoculum, organisms will grow at μ_m and the population will increase, since there is an excess of substrate, s. As the population grows, the rate of consumption of substrate increases. For organisms in the culture, the rate is given from the differential form of the yield equation:

$$-\frac{ds}{dt} = \frac{1}{Y} \cdot \frac{dx}{dt} = \frac{\mu x}{Y}$$

Eventually, the population will consume the substrate at such a rate that the concentration in the vessel will decrease and with it the growth rate, μ, until a balance is reached.

The balance equation for substrate utilization is given by:

rate of change of substrate concentration =
    input from the reservoir − output in effluent −
    consumption by microorganisms

$$\frac{ds}{dt} = D s_R - D_s - \frac{\mu x}{Y}$$

$$= D(S_R - s) - \frac{\mu x}{Y}$$

where S_R is the concentration of the limiting substrate in the inflowing medium. At steady state, $ds/dt = 0$, and therefore:

$$D(S_R - \bar{s}) = \frac{\mu \bar{x}}{Y}$$

By substituting for μ from the Monod equation and solving the two balance equations, it is possible to calculate the steady state values of substrate concentration, $\bar{s}$, and cell mass, $\bar{x}$, for any given dilution rate, D, in terms of the measurable constants K_s, μ_m, S_R and Y:

$$\bar{s} = K_s \cdot \frac{D}{\mu_m - D}$$

$$\bar{x} = Y(S_R - \bar{s})$$

The theoretical variations of $\bar{x}$ and $\bar{s}$ are plotted in Fig. 2.8, together with some deviations from this theoretical curve obtained in practice. Note that Fig. 2.8 represents an infinite number of steady state conditions obtained by setting the dilution rate. Also, that the cell mass concentration at the critical value of $D = \mu_m$ is zero. This is sometimes difficult to understand at first sight, but not if one remembers that for cells to grow at μ_m they will

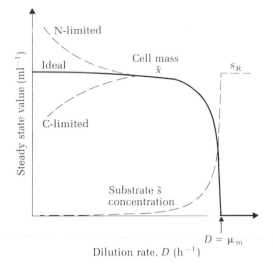

Fig. 2.8 Theoretical curves for steady state values of substrate concentration and cell concentration in a chemostat as a function of dilution rate. Deviations from the ideal curve for cell concentration are indicated.

need to have the substrate concentration in the vessel at the highest value, i.e. S_R. There can therefore be no consumption of substrate by cells for this condition to be attained. In practice, it is difficult to maintain a chemostat stably at D values near $D = \mu_m$.

If one wants very rapidly growing cells, then the chemostat can be modified by imposing an external control circuit on it: by measuring the cell concentration in the vessel and using the value to adjust the flow rate of medium into the vessel. In this arrangement, the turbidostat, the same theoretical curve will apply but the operator is imposing the control on the system. From Fig. 2.8 it can be seen that the turbidostat will operate in the region in which $\bar{x}$ changes most with D, i.e. at higher D values. Turbidostats are in principle more difficult to operate, mainly due to problems associated with measuring cell density in a continuous way. Usually, turbidity measurements are used and growth of organisms on the surfaces of optical cells needs to be avoided.

At all growth rates under *glucose limitation*, some of the energy obtained from the metabolism of the limiting substrate is consumed in maintenance processes (e.g. maintaining osmotic potential) and is not used for growth and cell division. This *maintenance energy* (that is energy not used for cell growth and division, but to maintain existing cells in a viable state) becomes significant at low dilution rates and this has been used to modify the theoretical equation to explain the decrease in $\bar{x}$ seen at low growth rates under carbon limitation.

At low growth rates under *nitrogen source limitation*, the opposite situation sometimes applies and excess mass is obtained because glucose or other carbon substrate (which is not limiting) is diverted to production of large amounts of glycogen (or PHB) and extracellular polysaccharide.

Applications and limitations of continuous culture

Chemostat systems operate over a wide range of growth rates but provide conditions approximating to those found in batch culture approaching the stationary phase. If one is interested in a metabolite produced by a microorganism in full exponential growth or under strict starvation conditions, a simple chemostat is inadequate, although multistage systems overcoming these limitations have been devised.

Technical problems are also posed by organisms which adhere to surfaces or grow as filaments. In both these states, the microorganisms are in a different physiological status from cells in suspension. Thus, cells adhering to the surfaces of the fermenter vessel lead to departures from the theoretical performance of the chemostat.

Mutation is a potential problem in a continuous system. For a neutral mutation, such as resistance to bacteriophage, which does not affect the kinetics of substrate utilization, the concentration of mutant cells increases in a chemostat linearly with time (initially). If, however, a mutant can use the limiting substrate more efficiently than the desired cell type, it will rapidly take over the culture. For example, amino acid-overproducing strains are used for producing biologically active (L-) amino acids by fermentation; these are, however, usually at a disadvantage with respect to non-overproducers which can easily arise by mutation.

In some cases, chemostats are useful in selecting mutants; by growing a continuous culture under limitation for a compound metabolized by inducible enzymes, *constitutive mutants* are rapidly selected (see Chapter 7).

Chemostats are very useful tools for studying many aspects of physiology related to growth, such as energetics, nutrient uptake and product formation. Moreover, they have application in studying physiological changes induced by varying the concentration of a single component in the growth medium. For example, bacterial sporulation and the synthesis of many degradative enzymes are subject to repression by carbon and nitrogen sources and chemostats are used in research on these phenomena. Multistage systems have also been used to study simple interactions between different microorganisms, as a first step towards analysing symbiotic, competitive and predatory interactions in mixed populations.

SURVIVAL, INHIBITION AND DEATH

Of significant concern to many microbiologists are methods for either inhibiting or delaying growth, or for killing microorganisms. There are many physical and chemical treatments which can inhibit or kill microorganisms (Table 2.4). Each has an application

Table 2.4 Effects on microorganisms of various extreme treatments, and the resistance and response to damage induced by the extreme condition.

Extreme treatment	Damage to cells	Resistant organisms	Adaptation or response to extreme condition
Heat	Enzyme denaturation	Thermophiles	Synthesis of more heat-stable proteins
Cold	Loss of regulation; decreased membrane fluidity	Psychrophiles	Synthesis of higher proportion of unsaturated fatty acids
Low a_w	Dehydration and inhibition of enzyme activity	Osmophiles, Xerophiles, Halophiles	Accumulation of compensating solute or possession of enzymes adapted to high ionic strength
Low pH	Protein denaturation; inhibition of enzymes	Acidophiles	Active exclusion of protons, adaptation of surface appendages
Ionizing radiation	Free radical or photon-induced damage to DNA and proteins	Radiotolerant	Enzymatic DNA repair

in medicine, in the preservation of perishable goods or in sterilization processes. In each of these areas, the range of methods available is limited. In medicine, for example, the problem is one of selective destruction of microbes with minimal damage to the host; in food preservation, physical treatments alter flavour, texture and aroma, and legislation restricts the use of chemical additives. The microbiologist is interested in studying methods which kill or inhibit microorganisms; also of interest are the factors which influence survival and death, the organisms which are most resistant to the treatments used, and the mechanism by which they survive exposure to stress.

Response of microorganisms to environmental extremes

There are a number of ways of looking at the response of an organism to adverse conditions. These include study of:

1 The physiology of those organisms which show considerable resistance, including naturally resistant species (*Deinococcus radiodurans* to gamma irradiation, *Bacillus stearothermophilus* to heat) and resistant mutants of more sensitive organisms.

2 Sensitive mutants, e.g. temperature-sensitive, radiation-sensitive.

3 Physiological changes in those microorganisms exposed to near-lethal extremes.

Usually, there are many cellular processes which are impaired by a sublethal treatment and it is often difficult to determine which is most important to the survival of the cell. If we take as an example the effects of high temperature on bacteria, the following changes are induced: damage to the cytoplasmic membrane;

breakdown of ribosomes; irreversible enzyme denaturation; and DNA strand breakage. Obviously any of these effects will lead to a reduction in the growth rate of a cell. However, the extent to which each change contributes to growth inhibition or death is less obvious.

There are several ways by which an organism can survive and grow under conditions lethal to most others. These are considered below.

Possession of more stable cell components. Many enzymes from the thermophilic bacterium, *B. stearothermophilus*, are less susceptible to heat denaturation than their counterparts in mesophilic *Bacillus* species. Halophilic bacteria have a cell membrane made of acidic proteins which is so adapted to high salt concentrations that it dissolves at low ionic strength. These organisms avoid desiccation by being permeable to the salt in their environment, and their enzymes have been adapted to function at high ionic strength.

Certain genera of Gram-positive bacteria, notably *Bacillus* and *Clostridium*, produce extremely resistant spores as the cells face starvation conditions. These spores are metabolically almost completely dormant and can survive to a remarkable extent at high temperatures, under desiccation or at high concentrations of organic solvents. These specialized cells are discussed in more detail in Chapter 9.

Effective repair mechanisms. This applies particularly to radiation damage. There are at least six systems for repairing radiation-induced damage in both *E. coli* and *S. cerevisiae*.

Rapid resynthesis of damaged structures. One explanation sometimes given for the resistance of thermophiles to heat, is that they can resynthesize protein at a rate which matches the rate of denaturation.

Compensation. One of the best examples of physiological compensation is the way fungi and some salt-tolerant bacteria (*Staphylococcus* species) adapt to low a_w environments. Some fungi, including osmophilic yeast and the halotolerant alga *Dunaliella* synthesize large amounts of intracellular polyols such as glycerol, to raise the internal osmotic pressure to that of the environment. The disaccharide trehalose may also be used for the same purpose. In bacteria, the accumulated solute is usually an amino acid, commonly proline, glutamate or glycine betaine.

Table 2.4 summarizes the damage to, and response of, micro-organisms to various environmental extremes. Some of these responses apply to all species, whereas others represent a specific evolutionary adaptation and are restricted to resistant species. Excluded from this table are bacterial spores, which are in general more resistant to physical and chemical extremes than are vegetative cells. This resistance can be attributed to many factors, including the low permeability of dormant spores to non-aqueous solvents, modification of some enzymes during sporulation to increase heat resistance, stabilization of structures by high concentrations of calcium dipicolinate (see Chapter 9), the arrangement of DNA in a different physical state from that found in vegetative bacteria, and the possession of highly efficient DNA repair enzymes activated after germination of the spore.

Stress responses

All organisms, whether they are resistant or sensitive to a condition causing stress, possess mechanisms to avoid the damaging effects. The best studied of these include the *SOS response* of coliform bacteria to accumulation of single-stranded DNA, due to damage caused by agents such as radiation, and the *heat shock response* of cells of all organisms (prokaryotic and eukaryotic) exposed to heat or osmotic stress (or other damage causing accumulation of denatured proteins in the cell). Both of these systems involve a coordinated regulation of many functions in the cell. They are thought to involve changes in DNA structure and supercoiling, and are discussed in detail in Chapter 7. The physiological aspects of the osmotic stress response are discussed on p. 210.

Death

Death of a microbial cell is usually defined as the loss of reproductive ability. Measuring death can present practical problems, since the extent of survival of a population largely depends on the way in which the culture is treated after exposure to a lethal agent. This is particularly true of the medium used to detect survivors. In general, richer media enable a higher degree of resuscitation. Survivors vary greatly in the times taken for their recovery; some cells only begin to divide many days after inoculation into the recovery medium.

Kinetics of death

Cells in a population do not all die at once on exposure to lethal conditions. The kinetics of their death usually follows an exponential function as illustrated by the curves obtained for survivors against dose for a particular treatment (Fig. 2.9).

There is one important parameter obtained from dose/survivor curves. The dose (time at a given intensity) required to inactivate by tenfold is the *D value*, and it is a measure of the resistance of an organism to a particular treatment.

Exponential loss of viability is often explained in terms of target

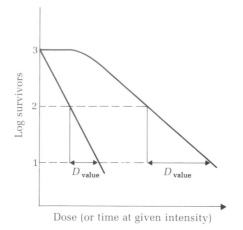

Fig. 2.9 Exposure of a microbial population to lethal conditions. Two common examples of survival curves for populations exposed to lethal agents. Note the shoulder on one of the curves and the way to estimate the D value for each organism.

theory, most easily understood for radiation-induced death. In every cell there is a function (or functions) sensitive to the lethal agent. For a given dose (a given number of bullets), the probability of cell survival depends on the proportion of targets which are not hit by these randomly sprayed 'bullets'. An approximate mathematical treatment of this simple model leads to an exponential function. A shoulder on the survival curve is often seen at low doses, particularly for radiation-induced damage, and is interpreted in terms of either the need for multiple hits, or the existence of systems repairing damage after the lethal treatment.

This model is probably an over-simplification, since cells within a population have a range of susceptibilities and there are likely to be a number of different targets, each with different susceptibilities to a given dose. It does, however, focus attention on what might constitute target sites within cells. When damage is induced by ionizing radiation, the primary target is quite clearly seen as DNA, since mutants lacking enzymes involved in DNA repair are much more sensitive to various forms of radiation. In microorganisms subjected to heat treatment, moreover, we have seen that there are more candidates for targets, since many functions are damaged by heat. There is, however, fairly strong evidence that death is ultimately the result of irreversible damage to membranes since:

1 Leakage of cell constituents through membranes occurs after heat injury.

2 Mutants with temperature-sensitive lesions or an auxotrophic requirement can usually recover after return to permissive growth conditions. Those which lose viability under the non-permissive condition are defective in membrane synthesis or function. It is interesting to note that these 'suicide' mutants can be prevented from losing viability under the restrictive condition by inhibiting protein synthesis. Death in these mutants (and possibly in other organisms) therefore appears to be the result of unbalanced growth due to defective membrane function and a loss of coordination between membrane and macromolecular synthesis.

Sterilization

Many techniques for killing microorganisms are available and the choice of method of achieving sterility depends on the medium that is to be sterilized. In order to achieve sterility, it is necessary to kill *all* organisms in the sample without destroying vital ingredients of the medium; in most cases, the organisms most resistant to the treatment used will be endospores of *Bacillus* or *Clostridium*. The most widely used method of sterilization in the food and fermentation industries is steam sterilization, since heat in the presence of moisture is more effective than dry heat. Since spores survive treatment at 100°C for long periods, it is necessary to use steam under pressure (in an autoclave) to obtain temperatures of 120°C. Laboratory media are commonly sterilized by exposure to steam at 15 psi (pounds/sq. inch) for 15 min.

Other treatments can be used. Liquids free of particulate or colloidal material can be sterilized by filtration, usually through nylon or cellulose acetate membranes of controlled pore size of around 0.22 µm. This is used for solutions containing compounds sensitive to heat. Medical products such as syringes, wound dressings, sutures, swabs and plastic ware can be sterilized by irradiation from X-ray or gamma-ray sources (radioactive cobalt). Other surfaces can be exposed to ethylene oxide; this is a gas requiring considerable care in handling since it is a potent mutagen. Solutions of glutaraldehyde are effective against bacterial spores.

Cells in a population do not all die at once on exposure to the lethal treatment, so one must be aware of the statistical nature of the sterilization process. Since death is an exponential function, complete sterility cannot be guaranteed. It is, however, possible to calculate the chance that one or more microorganisms will survive to spoil the product. The treatment is thus arranged to reduce this chance to an acceptable level.

For example, in the canning of low acid foods, the main organism of concern is the anaerobic spore-former *Clostridium botulinum*, since it produces an extremely potent exotoxin. Such foods are usually treated to reduce the concentration of *C. botulinum* spores by a factor of 10^{12}, i.e. a $12 D$ dose. Since spores are not likely to be present at a level of more than about 10^6 per can, this means that only about one can in a million will have at least one surviving spore of *C. botulinum*. To ensure that even these are not sold to an unsuspecting consumer, all sterilized cans are stored for 6 months to let any surviving spores germinate and grow, causing the can to blow and ensuring its rejection.

ANTIMICROBIAL AGENTS

Antibiotics are compounds synthesized by microorganisms which kill or inhibit the growth of other microbial species, whereas antimetabolites are synthetic chemical agents active against microorganisms. For any antimicrobial agent to be useful in chemotherapy, it must have: (i) *selective toxicity* against the pathogen and not the host; (ii) solubility in aqueous systems; and (iii) the ability to penetrate from the site of application to the site of infection, and hence to its target on or in the microbial cell. There are many compounds with antimicrobial activity, but relatively few of them meet these criteria. This is particularly true for antibiotics active against eukaryotic pathogens (e.g. fungi and protozoa), since in these cells there are fewer sites for selective toxicity than in bacteria with their differences in ribosomal composition and in the structure of the wall or cell envelope.

Antibiotics, including many which have no clinical application, can be very useful laboratory tools since they are often specific inhibitors of particular metabolic functions. Some which were originally manufactured as products of fermentation are now synthesized in whole or in part by chemical processes. Others are semisynthetic compounds resulting from the chemical modification of natural products.

Antimetabolites

Ehrlich, from studies on histological stains, conceived the idea of finding a dye with selective affinity for a parasite and attaching to it an active group lethal for the microorganism. In this way, he hoped to obtain selectivity against pathogens. The first compounds tried were organic derivatives of arsenic, and eventually one, salvarsan, was found to be active against the causative organism of syphilis, *Treponema pallidum*.

The most successful antimicrobial agents, however, are the sulphonamides, all derivatives of sulphanilamide:

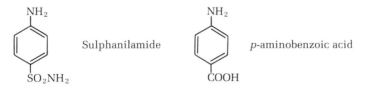

These compounds are bacteriostatic in their action, the effect *in vitro* being an inhibition of growth directly related to drug concentration. This inhibition is reversed competitively by the addition of *p*-aminobenzoic acid (PAB), a growth factor for some bacterial species. PAB is a component of folates, which are central to one-carbon metabolism, and sulphonamides inhibit the first enzymic stage in synthesis. Thus, these drugs are active against both microorganisms which can synthesize PAB and those which must be supplied with PAB for growth, but not against humans, who obtain folate directly from the diet.

Antibiotics

Antibiotics are synthesized by a wide range of microorganisms, many from *Streptomyces* species. Penicillin and cephalosporin are produced by fungi, while bacitracin and polymyxin are from *Bacillus* species. Chloramphenicol, although originally isolated from *Streptomyces venezuelae*, is now manufactured by chemical synthesis. There are many poorly characterized antibiotics recorded in the literature; rather than list large numbers of these, we will consider those best known in terms of their sites of action, and illustrate a few of the mechanisms of action. Structures of three of these antibiotics are indicated in Figs 2.10 and 2.11.

Compounds affecting synthesis of the cell envelope

Inhibition of synthesis of the prokaryotic cell envelope can be effected at various points in the process. *Fosfomycin* (phosphonomycin), an analogue of phosphoenolpyruvate (PEP), inhibits formation of UDP-*N*-acetyl-D-muramic acid, the first in the

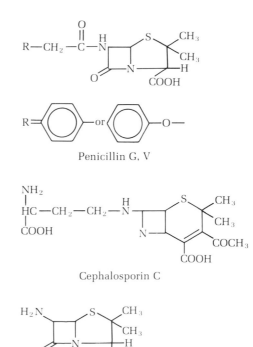

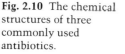
Fig. 2.10 The chemical structures of three commonly used antibiotics.

sequence of 'Park Nucleotides' (p. 184). D-*cycloserine* is a structural analogue of D-alanine (Fig. 2.11); it competitively inhibits both the formation of D-alanine and its subsequent conversion to the dipeptide D-alanyl-D-alanine. UDP-*N*-acetylmuramic acid tripeptide accumulates and osmotically fragile spheroplasts are formed.

Tunicamycin affects synthesis of the peptidoglycan layer of the bacterial cell by inhibiting translocase reactions in which the carrier lipid *undecaprenyl phosphate* participates (p. 185).

UDP-MurNAc-pentapeptide + C_{55}-lipid-P $\leftrightarrow$
$$C_{55}\text{-lipid-P-P-MurNAc-pentapeptide} + \text{UMP}$$

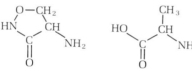

Chloramphenicol

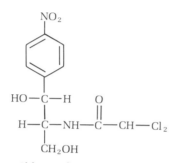

D-*cycloserine*   D-*alanine*

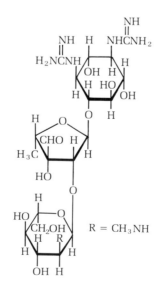

R = CH_3NH

Streptomycin

Fig. 2.11 Some common antibiotics. Where the antibiotic is an analogue of a cell metabolite, that compound is also shown.

It also inhibits the analogous transfer of GlcNAc-1-P from UDP-*N*-acetylglucosamine to undecaprenyl phosphate in biosynthesis of the linkage group of teichoic and teichuronic acids (p. 17). Tunicamycin differs from other cell envelope-inhibiting antibiotics in also inhibiting addition of GlcNAc-1-P to dolichol-P in eukaryotic walls, and is a useful aid in the study of the biosynthesis of such systems.

Penicillins and *cephalosporins* are β-lactam antibiotics that inhibit prokaryotic cell envelope synthesis, causing an accumulation of precursors, including the 'Park Nucleotides (p. 184). A further effect is to prevent the crosslinking of peptides on adjacent peptidoglycan chains (p. 185). These antibiotics bind to a number of *penicillin-binding proteins* (PBPs), in some of which carboxypeptidase or (rarely) transpeptidase activity (or both) can be demonstrated. The target of penicillin is the D-alanyl-D-alanine peptide bond; L-alanyl-D-alanine bonds are insensitive. The PBPs are located on the periplasmic face of the cytoplasmic membrane in Gram-negative cells. The effects of the antibiotics on cell envelope synthesis are complex and various morphological changes are observed due to interaction with distinct penicillin-binding proteins. Growth ceases as a result of the inhibition of peptidoglycan synthesis. Thereafter, cell viability decreases and the bacteria lyse.

Vancomycin, like penicillin, causes accumulation of peptidoglycan precursors; it inhibits incorporation of amino acids into peptidoglycan. The antibiotic prevents transfer of the amino sugar disaccharide-pentapeptide (the repeating unit of the peptidoglycan) from the lipid carrier to nascent peptidoglycan by combining with the substrate of the enzyme involved. It will combine with either of the two lipid intermediates terminating in the ... D-alanyl-D-alanine pentapeptide or with the Park Nucleotide, UDP-MurNAc-pentapeptide. Because of the molecular mass (*c.* 1400 Da), it cannot penetrate to the periplasm of Gram-negative bacteria and they are consequently resistant to the antibiotic. As it binds to a substrate rather than an enzyme, a large number of vancomycin molecules (10^7) are bound to each susceptible Gram-positive cell.

Bacitracin prevents dephosphorylation of the isoprenoid lipid pyrophosphate after transfer of the repeating unit to nascent peptidoglycan. It also inhibits other systems in which the carrier

Fig. 2.12 The structures of antimicrobial agents which bind to *penicillinases.* (a) Thienamycin: binds to and inactivates β-lactamases; (b) clavulanic acid: binds, but not hydrolysed. Mixed with amoxycillin → augmentin.

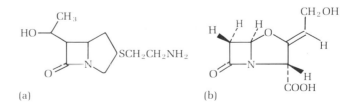

(a)   (b)

lipid pyrophosphate is produced, such as lipopolysaccharide and extracellular polysaccharide biosynthesis.

Clavulanic acid is of little value on its own. It is, however, a strong inhibitor of periplasmic β-lactamase enzymes and is used clinically with *amoxycillin* to treat infections caused by bacteria carrying β-lactamase activity (Fig. 2.12).

Antibiotics active against cell membranes

Antibiotics may act against cell membranes by any one of five mechanisms:

1 They may cause major disorganization of the membrane with resultant loss of its barrier function.

2 A channel may be formed through the membrane allowing substances to pass in or out.

3 Changes in the membrane may result in specific ionic permeability.

4 Enzymes in the membrane involved in transport processes may be inhibited.

5 Enzymes involved in the synthesis of membrane components may be inhibited.

Several antibiotics of this group are produced by sporulating bacilli: *tyrocidin* and *gramicidin* by *Bacillus brevis*, and *polymyxin* by *Bacillus polymyxa*.

Tyrocidins and *gramicidin* are decapeptides consisting primarily of L-amino acids. They are classified as *ionophores*, since they lead to an increased permeability of prokaryotic and eukaryotic membranes to ions, usually K^+, Na^+ or H^+ (see p. 88). Their mode of action can best be understood by considering their structure, outlined for gramicidin A in Fig. 2.13. This molecule forms a helix which is left-handed and lipophilic; the amino acid

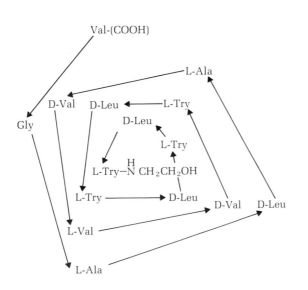

Fig. 2.13 The structure of gramicidin A viewed along axis of peptide from C to N terminal end.

side-chains extend radially from the axis of the helix and become embedded in the lipid of the membrane. The C=O groups are arranged in such a way that hydrogen-bonded head-to-head antibiotic dimer formation can occur; in the membrane, this is sufficiently long to form a channel or hole across the membrane lipid bilayer and allows leakage of ions. Valinomycin also forms pores in the membrane with similar results.

Polymyxins are decapeptides in which the last seven residues form a cyclic heptapeptide and a branched-chain fatty acid (6-methylheptanoate or 6-methyloctanoate) is linked to the first residue. This structure has a cationic detergent property which may account for some of its lethal effects on sensitive cells,

Table 2.5 Inhibitors of macromolecular synthesis.

Synthesis	Inhibitor	Effective against:	Site of inhibition
Protein	Chloramphenicol	70S ribosomes; 50S subunits	Inhibits peptide bond formation
	Erythromycin	70S ribosomes; 50S subunits	Inhibits translocation
	Tetracylines	70S/80S ribosomes; 30S/50S subunits or 40S/60S subunits	Inhibits mRNA binding by the ribosomal subunits
	Streptomycin	70S ribosomes; 30S subunits	Causes misreading of mRNA during translation
	Neomycin and aminoglycosides	70S ribosomes; 30S/50S subunits	Mistranslation of mRNA
	Puromycin	70S/80S ribosomes; 50S or 60S subunits	Premature termination of polypeptide chain
	Cycloheximide	80S ribosomes; 60S subunit	
	Cryptopleurine	80S ribosomes; 40S subunit	Inhibits translocation from 40S ribosomal subunits
RNA	Rifamycins	Prokaryotes	β Subunit of RNA polymerase
	Lomofungin	Eukaryotes	Mg^{2+} chelator affects nuclear RNA synthesis
	α-Amanitin	Eukaryotes	Nuclear DNA-dependent RNA polymerase synthesizing mRNA
	Actinomycin D	Prokaryotes/eukaryotes	Binds to DNA, inhibiting transcription
DNA	Nalidixic acid (quinolones)	Prokaryotes, especially Gram-negative bacteria	DNA replication (gyrase subunit A)
	Mitomycin	Prokaryotes/eukaryotes	Crosslinks DNA
	Novobiocin	Prokaryotes	Energy transduction of DNA replication (gyrase subunit B)
	Streptonigrin, bleomycin	Eukaryotes/prokaryotes	Cause single-stranded breaks in DNA

although cationic detergents including quaternary ammonium compounds can also lead to precipitation of acidic molecules in the cell. Addition of the antibiotic causes rapid loss of nucleotides and other small molecules from the microorganisms.

The *polyenes*, produced by some *Streptomyces* species, act only on eukaryotic membranes. They form complexes with membrane sterols and cause leakage of ions, solutes and even proteins. Some polyenes have specific ionophoric activity and uncouple oxidative phosphorylation in mitochondria. This group includes *nystatin*, which is used to treat fungal infections.

Globomycin mimics the signal sequence of the outer membrane protein precursors of certain Gram-negative bacteria, preventing their export from the cytoplasmic membrane.

Antibiotics active against DNA, RNA and protein synthesis

Many antibiotics of diverse structure and function belong to this group (Table 2.5). Some are inhibitors of nucleic acid synthesis, either at the level of nucleotide metabolism or at that of polymerization. Many are inhibitors of bacterial protein synthesis; selectivity is mainly due to the marked differences between eukaryotic and prokaryotic ribosomes. Some of the selective inhibitors of ribosome function are used clinically. Other antimicrobial agents inhibit the growth of both prokaryotes and eukaryotes. The processes affected in protein synthesis are initiation, elongation and release. The majority of antibiotics which inhibit protein synthesis do so by inhibiting ribosomal function. The antibiotics may be specific inhibitors of the ribosomal subunits (Table 2.5). A further target is the bacterial enzyme *DNA*

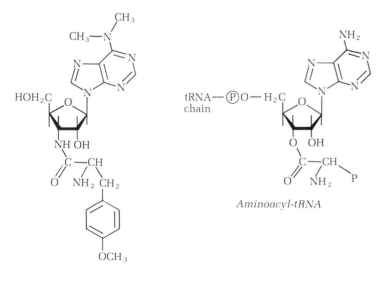

Aminoacyl-tRNA

Puromycin

Fig. 2.14 The structure of puromycin and aminoacyl-tRNA.

gyrase, which is inhibited by a group of synthetic antibacterial agents, the *quinolones*, of which *nalidixic acid* is the prototype. Other possible targets for selective inhibition of bacteria include DNA-dependent RNA polymerases and DNA polymerases, as the enzymes are quite different in eukaryotic and prokaryotic systems (see Chapter 7).

Puromycin inhibits protein synthesis in eukaryotes, being a structural analogue of aminoacyl tRNA (Fig. 2.14). It is incorporated into growing polypeptide chains. As it lacks a free carboxyl group to accept another aminoacyl group, puromycin causes premature termination of the polypeptide chain. It inhibits protein synthesis in cell-free systems from any source, the reaction inhibited being catalysed by the 50S ribosomal subunit in bacteria.

It has to be remembered that, for activity against the intact microorganism, the antimicrobial agent must be able to gain access to its site of action. This is usually accomplished through uptake mechanisms used for normal microbial metabolites (Table 2.6).

Resistance to antimicrobial agents

The use of many antimicrobial agents is to some extent becoming restricted through the emergence of bacteria carrying resistance plasmids, in part due to widespread abuse in the application of antibiotics. Resistance to a number of commonly used antibiotics, including penicillin, erythromycin and tetracyclines, can be coded on extrachromosomal plasmids, *resistance transfer factors*, which are transferable between bacterial species.

Bacterial cells become resistant to antibiotics in a number of ways:
1 Bypassing the metabolic step affected.
2 Overproducing an inhibited enzyme or product.

Table 2.6 Mechanisms of entry of antimicrobial agents.

Compound	Passage through outer membrane	Mechanism	Passage through inner membrane	Mechanism
Quinolones	+	Porins/self-promotion	+	Energy dependent?
Chloramphenicol	+	Porins	+	?
Tetracyclines	+	Porins	+	Energy dependent
Allophosphin	+	Porins	+	Tripeptide permease
Cycloserine	+	?	+	Alanine/glycine permease
Fosfomycin	+	Porins	+	Glycerophosphate permease
Streptozotocin	+	?	+	Group translocation
β-Lactams	+	Porins/facilitated diffusion	−	−

? = Not known.

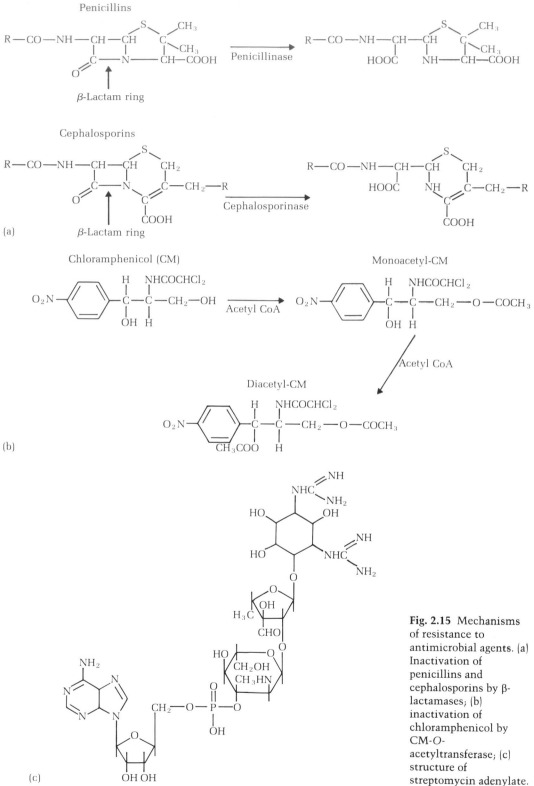

(a)

(b)

(c)

Fig. 2.15 Mechanisms of resistance to antimicrobial agents. (a) Inactivation of penicillins and cephalosporins by β-lactamases; (b) inactivation of chloramphenicol by CM-*O*-acetyltransferase; (c) structure of streptomycin adenylate.

3 Altering the structure of a target enzyme or other protein so that it still functions but no longer recognizes the inhibitor. This is one form of resistance to antibiotics affecting ribosomal functions; in the extreme case with streptomycin, it is possible to isolate strains which are *dependent* on the antibiotic for growth. Nalidixic acid resistance generally results from mutation in the *gyrA* gene encoding the A subunit of the DNA gyrase.

4 By alteration of the membrane or its uptake systems so that the cell is no longer permeable to the drug. This is commonly seen when the drug is a competitive inhibitor of a low molecular weight metabolite (e.g. resistance to canavanine, an analogue of arginine, is usually acquired through the mutational loss of an arginine permease) (Chapter 3).

5 Destruction of the antimicrobial agent, as happens with enzymes such as β-lactamases (e.g. penicillinase and cephalosporinase).

6 Modification of the antibiotic to prevent it binding at the target site (e.g. adenylation or phosphorylation of streptomycin; acetylation of chloramphenicol) (Fig. 2.15).

Resistant mutants are very useful laboratory tools. Where the site of action of an antibiotic is known, mutations to resistance provide a way of specifically affecting the function concerned. An example of the usefulness of this approach is the study of ribosome function using inhibitors of protein synthesis. Often, mutation for resistance to an antibiotic affects a particular ribosomal protein and with knowledge of the step in protein synthesis inhibited by that antibiotic, it is possible to identify which ribosomal subunit is involved in the step. Since it is convenient to select for resistance mutations, the plasmids carrying antibiotic resistance markers have become widely used as vectors in *in vitro* genetic manipulation and biotechnology.

3 Substrate uptake and entry to the cell

Growth is a highly dynamic process requiring considerable amounts of energy and substrates for the synthesis of components of the microbial cell. The source of the substrates is the extra-cellular environment; thus the first essential steps in growth of a microorganism are the location of substrates in the environment and their transport into the cell. These processes in themselves require the expenditure of some energy by the cell. This energy is derived from the coupling of intracellular metabolism to the transport mechanisms. The actual mechanism of coupling the energy to membrane transport is not always clear. For the uptake of ions (e.g. H^+ and Ca^{2+}) by mitochondria and for ions and some solutes by respiring bacteria, the energy derives from the oxidation of substrates via the respiratory chain (p. 99). Some inhibitors of the respiratory chain, in particular uncouplers of oxidative phosphorylation such as dinitrophenol, inhibit transport. In other cases, especially in microorganisms growing anaerobically without a respiratory chain (e.g. *Streptococcus faecalis*), other energy sources are important.

Chemotaxis

In their natural environments, most microbes are surrounded by very dilute concentrations of ions and nutrients; it is thus possibly an advantage to a cell to be able to locate and bind considerable amounts of specific nutrients. Chemotaxis, the ability to move along a concentration gradient of a compound in the nutrient environment, has been shown to occur in several motile species. Attractants include amino acids (seven for *Escherichia coli*, 20 for *Bacillus subtilis*) and many sugars (Table 3.1). Many aspects of chemotaxis are possibly analogous to processes found in higher organisms. The attractants or chemo-effectors are bound to chemoreceptors, proteins which specifically bind the attractant and are frequently involved in nutrient transport. In *E. coli*, the chemoreceptors fall into three categories: (i) soluble, periplasmic substrate-binding proteins, as in the maltose system (see p. 81); (ii) cytoplasmic membrane transport components such as the enzyme II of the phosphotransferase system (p. 83); or (iii) primary chemotactic signal transducers themselves, located in the cytoplasmic membrane. On binding of the attractant, the information is conveyed to the flagella, the motor apparatus of the cell, altering their direction of rotation and causing the bacteria to swim smoothly (Fig. 3.1). This is achieved by methylation of methyl-accepting proteins (MCPs), using S-adenosylmethionine as methyl donor. In *E. coli*, the MCPs are the receptors for the amino

Table 3.1 Chemotactic stimuli.

Compounds	Examples	Effect
Amino acids	Serine, aspartate	Strong attractants
Carboxylic acids	Malate, citrate	Attractants
Sugars	Glucose, galactose, ribose	Attractants
Hydrophobic amino acids	Leucine, isoleucine, valine	Repellants
Aliphatic alcohols	Ethanol, isopropanol	Repellants
Inorganic ions	Co^{2+}, Ni^{2+}	Repellants

acids, whereas sugars bind to binding proteins which, in turn, bind to the MCPs. A single monomeric enzyme of relative molecular mass $28-30 \times 10^3$ methylates the MCPs. A *methylesterase* demethylates the protein, yielding methanol as product. As both enzymes from *B. subtilis* are very active on *E. coli* membranes, there appears to be considerable conservation of the methylation-accepting regions of MCPs in both species.

UTILIZATION OF LOW-MOLECULAR WEIGHT SUBSTRATES

Iron uptake and transport

Iron is essential for all microorganisms. Although it is present in considerable quantities in the environment, its availability to the microbial cell is limited by its solubility. Moreover, in the human or animal body, iron is very tightly complexed in the form of haemoproteins. At pH 7.0, the concentration of soluble ferric ion in natural environments is likely to be about 10^{-14} mM. Many

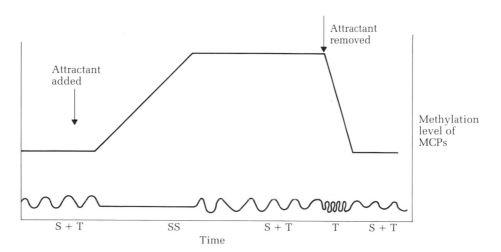

Fig. 3.1 Methylation of MCPs and swimming behaviour of *Escherichia coli*. S + T = smooth swimming and tumbling; SS = smooth swimming; T = tumbling.

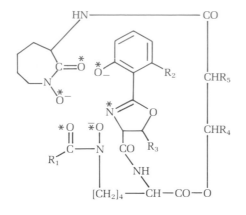

(a)

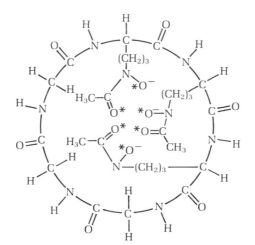

(b)

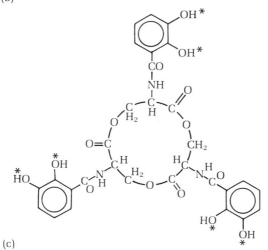

(c)

Fig. 3.2 Siderophore structures. (a) General structure of the mycobactins (deferri). Variations occur at R_{1-5}; (b) structure of ferrichrome (deferri); (c) structure of enterochelin (enterobactin) (deferri). Iron-chelation sites are indicated by asterisks.

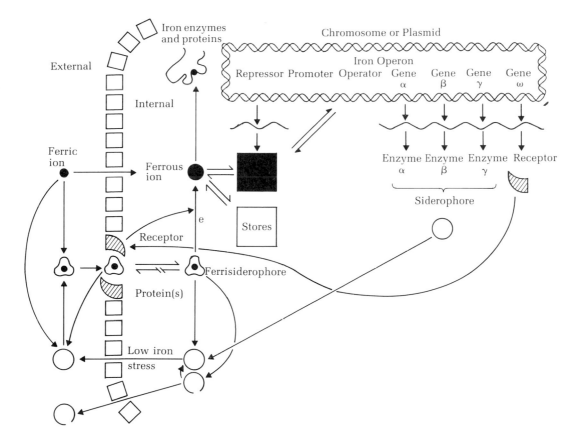

Fig. 3.3 Schematic model of low- and high-affinity iron assimilation pathways in aerobic and facultative anaerobic microorganisms.

assimilatory systems exist for the uptake of this essential ion and, as with uptake of most other ions, these can be divided into 'high' and 'low' affinity systems. High-affinity systems, found in virtually all aerobic and facultatively anaerobic microbial cells, normally utilize siderophores, low-molecular weight iron-specific ligands, for the solubilization and transport of ferric ions. In laboratory media, in which excess iron is generally available, the high-affinity iron transport systems are repressed. However, in pathogenic bacteria growing in the human or animal body, very little iron is readily available to the microorganisms and iron-regulated outer membrane proteins are induced together with siderophores. The siderophores are of various chemical types (Fig. 3.2), which may either provide iron at the cell surface or be transported intact into the cell (Fig. 3.3), the ligand then being recycled or degraded. The siderophores possess extremely high affinity for ferric ion. Typically, the microbial cell excretes siderophore, which complexes with extracellular iron. The size of the complex exceeds the limit of porins in Gram-negative bacteria, and requires specific receptors in the cell envelope for recognition and transport. The intracellular iron concentration regulates the uptake and utilization of the siderophore–iron complex. As the outer membrane receptors for the iron-chelate in the Gram-negative bacteria are frequently also capable of acting as receptors for bacteriophage and colicins, their synthesis and properties under various physiological conditions can be readily studied. After transport into the cytoplasm, the iron is released from the chelate by a specific esterase, under coordinate control with other components necessary for iron chelation. In bacteria such as *E. coli*, there are several high-affinity iron uptake systems, not all of which are well characterized. In addition, in *E. coli* but not in *Salmonella typhimurium*, growth in the presence of citrate induces a ferric citrate uptake mechanism.

Siderophores are not always utilized. In such pathogenic bacteria as *Neisseria* species, they are not produced. Instead, iron bound to lactoferrin is utilized.

Ammonia uptake and utilization

Bacteria possess two mechanisms for ammonia assimilation, in both of which glutamate is formed from ammonia and 2-oxoglutarate. At high ammonia concentrations, the *glutamate dehydrogenase* (GDH) pathway operates in a reversible reaction which does not require any additional energy source:

$$\text{2-oxoglutarate} + NH_4^+ + NAD(P)H \leftrightarrow$$
$$2 \text{ L-glutamate} + NAD(P)^+ + H_2O$$

An alternative mechanism is present in most bacteria studied, although for some species, such as methanol-utilizing bacteria, it may be the *only* mechanism present. It involves two enzymes, *glutamine synthetase* (GS) and *glutamate synthase* (GOGAT). The two enzymes catalyse the amination of 2-oxoglutarate to glutamate with glutamine as an intermediate:

$$NH_3 + \text{L-glutamate} + ATP \rightarrow \text{L-glutamine} + ADP + P_i$$

$$\text{L-glutamine} + \text{2-oxoglutarate} + NAD(P)H \rightarrow$$
$$2 \text{ L-glutamate} + NAD(P)^+ + H_2O$$

This reaction is irreversible and, unlike the GDH pathway, consumes one mole of ATP for each mole of ammonia assimilated. GS has a very high affinity for ammonia, enabling the bacteria to obtain it at very low concentrations. Because of its key role in nitrogen metabolism, both synthesis and activity of glutamine synthetase are controlled. In some eukaryotes such as *Saccharomyces cerevisiae*, this pathway has a role, although glutamate is synthesized by GDH and glutamine by GS when NH_4^+ concentrations are not limiting.

UTILIZATION OF HIGH-MOLECULAR WEIGHT SUBSTRATES

Some microorganisms have adapted to efficient use of particulate or macromolecular substrates by producing structures for attaching their cells to surfaces. These include holdfasts, pili or fimbriae (in prokaryotes only) and stalks as in *Caulobacter* species. Some eukaryotic microorganisms, including ciliate and amoeboid protozoa and slime moulds, ingest particles into membrane-bound food vacuoles prior to digesting them to smaller molecular weight compounds. Others, which are surrounded by rigid cell walls, cannot ingest particulate matter directly.

Microorganisms thus use two initial mechanisms for assimilating larger substrates: engulfment and subsequent degradation by intracellular enzymes, and secretion of enzymes to hydrolyse the substrates into smaller molecules. These two processes are not as different as they may at first appear, since engulfment occurs into membrane-bound vacuoles; in both processes, there is the same problem of transporting enzymes across membranes. Engulfment is the more efficient process since the substrates and the enzymes needed to degrade them are confined within a vacuole and neither enzymes nor hydrolysis products are lost to the cell.

In microorganisms with rigid walls, hydrolytic enzymes are secreted into the culture medium. Enzymes found in the supernatant after removing cells from a culture by centrifugation can have different origins:

1 Intracellular enzymes released from the cytoplasm of dead or leaking cells.

2 Extracellular enzymes which are synthesized at and extruded through the cell membrane in prokaryotes, or into vesicles which fuse with the membrane in eukaryotes. In Gram-positive bacteria, these enzymes appear in the culture fluid, whereas in Gram-negative bacteria, the enzyme may either appear in the culture fluid or, as in the case of ribonuclease or alkaline phosphatase, may be retained in the periplasm (the region between the outer and cytoplasmic membranes). Many bacteria produce a wide range of extracellular enzymes for hydrolysing a variety of substrates; other bacteria may produce a more limited range of enzymes (Table 3.2). Eukaryotes also produce extracellular enzymes, including amylases, cellulases and proteases. Some of the enzymes from *Aspergillus* and *Trichoderma* species are used industrially, as are a number from *Bacillus* species.

Table 3.2 Some microbial extracellular enzymes.

Microorganism	Enzymes	Substrates
Bacillus licheniformis	α-Amylase	Starch
Aspergillus oryzae	α-Amylase	Starch
Trichoderma reesei	Cellulase	Cellulose
Bacillus subtilis	β-Glucanase	β-Glucans
Aspergillus niger	Pectinase	Pectins
Klebsiella pneumoniae	Pullulanase	Starch
Bacillus megaterium	Penicillin amidase	Penicillin
Bacillus licheniformis	Alkaline protease	Proteins, peptides
Bacillus amyloliquifaciens	Neutral protease	Proteins, peptides

In most microorganisms, the synthesis of extracellular enzymes is tightly regulated. Low-molecular weight substrates are usually utilized preferentially; extracellular enzymes are not usually synthesized until the cells face starvation (e.g. amylases, ribonucleases and proteases in *Bacillus* species). The mechanism of this control is not fully understood, but it is probably analogous to catabolite repression of the synthesis of intracellular enzymes (p. 215). In some cases, an extracellular enzyme degrades a polymer into oligomers, which act as inducers of further specific hydrolases needed to complete the hydrolysis to compounds which can be taken up by the cell.

MECHANISMS OF NUTRIENT UPTAKE AND TRANSPORT

At this point, we should recall the structure of the cytoplasmic membrane (p. 20): a lipid bilayer containing proteins embedded in, on, or across the hydrophobic matrix. Polar or ionic species cannot therefore pass freely across the membrane, but lipid-soluble substrates such as urea can enter the cell by free diffusion. This process is known as *passive transport*. The rate of entry of these compounds into the cell depends on the difference in concentration between the inside and outside of the membrane, and such a solute will enter the cell only if its external concentration exceeds that inside. For passive entry, the rate of uptake of related compounds is greatly affected by the size and charge of the molecule concerned. In the case of the Gram-negative bacterium, the molecules must first traverse the outer membrane, generally through the porins (pp. 22–23).

A variety of mechanisms are used in bacteria to enable substrates to enter the cytoplasm. These mechanisms are generally closely regulated and related to the control of metabolic processes involving the same substrates. Carbohydrates provide an excellent example of the diverse mechanisms available, as five distinct processes are known whereby carbohydrates and related compounds are taken into the Gram-negative bacterium.

Facilitated diffusion

Glycerol enters the cells of prokaryotes and eukaryotes by facilitated diffusion. In eukaryotes, the transport of glycerol probably involves a carrier-type mechanism. In prokaryotes, the glycerol traverses through a non-stereospecific protein pore or facilitator coded by a gene forming part of an operon containing the glycerokinase gene. The pore is a transmembrane channel of diameter *c.* 0.4 nm allowing glycerol to diffuse into the cytoplasm down a concentration gradient without any requirement for linkage to energy-providing systems. In addition to glycerol, the *E.*

coli system permits entry of erythritol, pentitols and hexitols, the rate of transport depending on the structure and size of the carbohydrate. Efflux is prevented by phosphorylation of the substrates in the cytoplasm.

Chemiosmotic systems

The respiratory chain is orientated across the membrane (which must be impermeable to H^+ and OH^- ions), such that the oxidation of a substrate leads to translocation of proteins from the inner side of the membrane to the outer (see Fig. 3.4). This generates an ion gradient, creating a chemical and electrical potential capable of driving a reaction requiring energy. For example, the uptake of Ca^{2+} ions by mitochondria is driven by the membrane potential generated by H^+ translocation. On the other hand, phosphate ion transport is thought to occur via a co-transport of protons and phosphate, and is driven by the pH gradient established by respiration. In other systems, the energy may be derived from hydrolysis of ATP.

Evidence in support of the chemiosmotic mechanism acting in the uptake of certain ions and metabolites includes the following:
1 Reactions coupled to respiration (e.g. oxidative phosphorylation) do not occur in membranes or vesicles which are not intact (closed).
2 The mitochondrial and bacterial membranes are inherently impermeable to ions, including H^+ and OH^-, and all transport systems examined so far function to maintain osmotic, pH and ion equilibrium.

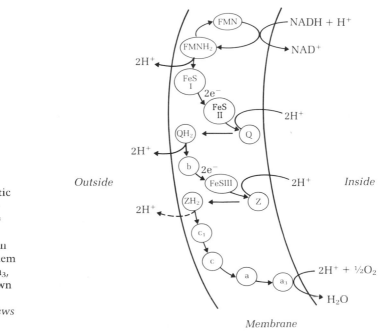

Fig. 3.4 Chemiosmotic theory of respiration-linked transport. Q = coenzyme Q; Z = hypothetical hydrogen carrier; FeS = non-haem iron proteins b, c, a, a_3, cytochromes. (Redrawn from Harold (1972) *Bacteriological Reviews* **36**, 177–230.)

3 A number of antibiotics and antimetabolites affect membrane function by allowing the specific conduction of H^+ or K^+ ions across the membrane. These ionophores uncouple oxidative phosphorylation and inhibit active transport. Included in the ionophores are the group of antibiotics known as the macrolides (valinomycin, gramicidin, nigericin), which are large molecules forming a hydrophobic shell around a central 'pore' region. In the pore region, ions can form clathrate compounds; for some macrolides, this is specific to one ion; others are less selective.

Symports are systems in which a single carrier functions in the simultaneous transport of two substrates. When one flows down a concentration gradient, the other flows with it. If the driving force is a proton gradient, it can be used to allow an oppositely charged ion or a neutral molecule into the microbial cell.

Two examples of chemiosmotic processes involving carbo-hydrate uptake have been well studied. *Melibiose transport* proceeds by a Na^+ symport, the accumulation of the disaccharide being driven both by membrane potential and the Na^+ concentration gradient. The balance of Na^+ within the cells is maintained by a sodium/proton antiport. *Lactose transport* is achieved by the β-galactosidase permease system functioning as a proton symport. The translocation of lactose or other β-galactoside is coupled to translocation of protons. The flow of protons *down* the electro-chemical gradient permits the accumulation of lactose *against* the concentration gradient. The specificity of this has been widely studied and the effect for various β-galactosides can be seen in Table 3.3. Each of the β-galactosides competes for binding with other substrates, the permease showing an enzyme-like affinity for the molecules which are transported. Carrier-type mechanisms, such as that for lactose, involve proteins possessing a single sugar-binding site and a distinct proton-binding site. As the protein can only be extracted from the membrane with difficulty, using detergent treatments, it is assumed to be firmly attached to the membrane.

Melibiose and lactose permeases exhibit some common pro-perties, including cation co-transport and broad and slightly overlapping substrate specificities; each is encoded by a single

Table 3.3 Specificity of the *E. coli* β-galactoside permease.

Substrate	K_m binding of substrate (mM)	% Displacement of TDG from complex with permease protein
Lactose	0.07	—
Thiomethylgalactoside	0.5	1
Thiodigalactoside (TDG)	0.02	(100)
Melibiose	0.2	95
α-Methylglucoside	—	0
Galactose	—	0
Glucose	—	0

structural gene and both systems are regulated by the PEP-dependent phosphotransferase system by similar mechanisms.

Maltose transport

Unlike the previous two systems, uptake of maltose involves a functional complex enabling the substrate to traverse both outer and inner membranes of Gram-negative bacteria. An outer membrane protein, LamB (which is also the receptor for bacteriophage lambda), functions as a porin with very high specificity for maltose, maltotriose and related maltodextrins (oligosaccharides in the α-D-glucosyl 1,4 α-D-glucose series). This protein binds and transports the oligosaccharides across the outer membrane, then interacts with the *malE* gene product, a periplasmic maltose-binding protein. A further more complex system involving three further proteins carries maltose across the cytoplasmic membrane. Two of the proteins, malF and malG are membrane proteins, the former being hydrophilic, while the third protein, malK, appears to interact with the malG protein at the internal face of the cytoplasmic membrane to provide energy for transfer of the substrate. It may indeed possess ATPase activity. In *E. coli*, the regulation of these proteins is through two regions of the chromosome. The *malB* region consists of two operons coding for the proteins involved in permeation. The *malA* region, also consisting of two operons, codes for the enzymes maltodextrin phosphorylase and amylomaltase as well as an activator protein of the *mal* regulon.

The source of the energy required by the maltose transport system is probably ATP and the system can accumulate maltose more than 105-fold against a concentration gradient. The various mechanisms of the carbohydrate uptake systems discussed so far are illustrated in Fig. 3.5.

The phosphotransferase (PTS) or group translocation system

A feature restricted to certain prokaryotic species is a carbohydrate transport system capable of *translocation* and *phosphorylation* of a range of substrates. This system is found in both Gram-positive and Gram-negative facultatively anaerobic bacteria, primarily in species using the Embden–Meyerhof scheme for hexose catabolism. Such species include members of the Enterobacteriaceae, *Streptococcus* and some photosynthetic species. The system comprises a number of cytoplasmic and membrane-bound proteins which can exist either in a phosphorylated or non-phosphorylated state. In addition to their role in carbohydrate transport, they are involved in regulation of uptake of carbohydrates which are not substrates of the PTS scheme. Two components, 'enzyme I' and a low-molecular weight (9100 Da in *E. coli*) heat-stable protein (HPr), are required for the initial transport and phosphorylation of

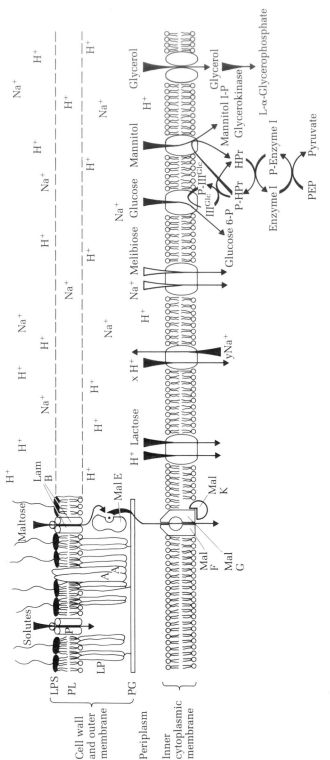

Fig. 3.5 A schematic outline of the Gram-negative bacterial wall–membrane complex indicating the various mechanisms by which carbohydrates and related compounds enter the cell. (Reproduced from Mitchell (1985) *Microbiological Sciences* **2**, 330–334.)

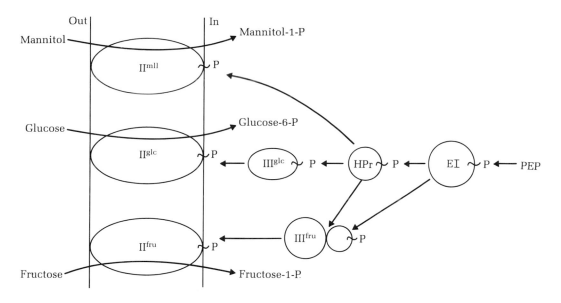

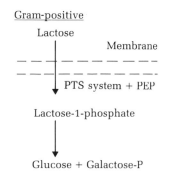

Fig. 3.6 The
phosphotransferase
(PTS) system. The
diagram indicates the
enzymes responsible for
the transport and
phosphorylation of
sugars such as
mannitol, glucose and
fructose. EI = enzyme I;
HPr = heat-stable
phosphocarrier protein;
III^{glc} = glucose-specific
enzyme III, etc. The
sugar-specific enzyme
IIs are membrane
proteins functioning as
sugar permeases.

all PTS carbohydrates. A phosphoryl group from PEP is donated to
enzyme I and is then transferred to HPr and hence via a specific
membrane-bound 'enzyme II' to the carbohydrate. Each enzyme II
recognizes a series of structurally related carbohydrates (a further
soluble cytoplasmic protein, 'enzyme III', may interact with the
enzyme II). The PTS scheme can be represented as shown by Fig.
3.6. In the Enterobacteriaceae, a range of hexoses, hexitols and
some oligosaccharides are transported by the PTS system, the
enzyme II components varying in their specificity. In streptococci,
oligosaccharides including lactose are also assimilated and phosphorylated by a PTS system (Fig. 3.7).

Enzyme III^{glc} has a key role in the regulation of carbohydrate
uptake, the *glucose effect*, in which glucose is metabolized in
preference to other carbohydrates. The dephosphorylated protein
appears to be an inhibitor of non-PTS systems for carbohydrate
transport, while the phosphorylated enzyme III^{glc} activates adenyl
cyclase. Thus the PTS system at the metabolic level controls both
the cyclic adenosine monophosphate (cAMP) concentration and

Fig. 3.7 Lactose uptake
in Gram-positive
bacteria.

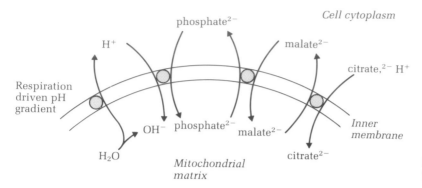

Fig. 3.8 Solute uptake by mitochondria.

the inducers of non-PTS operons. The presence of glucose results both in dephosphorylation of the enzyme III^{glc} and consequently in deactivation of cAMP synthesis, and inhibits uptake of an inducer. The net effect is to repress inducible enzyme systems such as those for metabolism of glycerol, lactose, maltose and melibiose.

Solute transport in the mitochondrion

Transport of solutes into the mitochondrion does not involve direct coupling to respiration. For malate, the uptake system involves a specific exchange at the membrane of phosphate for malate, energy being supplied by the previous accumulation of phosphate ions. For citrate, the link is even less direct since citrate is specifically exchanged for malate (Fig. 3.8). The prime mover in all solute transport, however, appears to be the generation by respiration of a membrane potential across the membrane.

Transport in bacterial vesicles

In order to study transport across the bacterial membrane, it is necessary to have an intact closed structure. The bacterial cell is such a closed form, but is much too complicated to use in studying the interaction of components during transport. Considerable progress has been made by the development of methods for preparing closed membrane vesicles from bacteria. Spheroplasts can be lysed under very carefully controlled conditions to give vesicles with the original membrane polarity preserved (ATPase stalks inward, Fig. 3.9) and with very little contamination by cytoplasmic enzymes and cofactors. These vesicles can transport ions and solutes against a concentration gradient provided that a suitable energy source is added. Vesicles have been prepared from both Gram-positive and Gram-negative bacteria, including *E. coli*, *B. subtilis*, *Staphylococcus aureus* and *Mycobacterium phlei*. They have been very useful tools since in them transport is still coupled to respiration and, by using different oxidation substrates, it is possible to explore the site of energy coupling in the respiratory chain (see p. 99) during respiration-linked uptake.

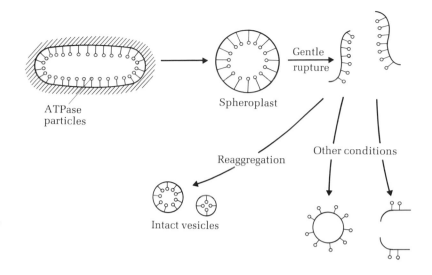

Fig. 3.9 Preparation of membrane vesicles from bacteria.

Osmotic stress

Most bacteria exposed to osmotic stress accumulate in their cytoplasm organic solutes together with K^+. This increases the osmotic strength of the cell and prevents osmotic dehydration. Simultaneously, in Gram-negative bacteria, the pattern of the outer membrane porins is altered, although the overall number of porin molecules in the outer membrane remains relatively constant. The organic osmolytes utilized by bacteria comprise amino acids such as proline and glutamate, betaines (*N*-methylated amino acid derivatives), trehalose and other sugar derivatives.

$$CH_3-{}^+\overset{\displaystyle CH_3}{\underset{\displaystyle CH_3}{N}}-CH_2-COO^-$$

betaine

Synthesis of glutamate or trehalose provides an endogenous mechanism for achieving a low level of osmotic tolerance, but these compounds have no detectable osmoprotective effect when supplied exogenously. High-level osmotic tolerance involves the uptake and synthesis of betaines. Decrease in the turgor pressure, the osmotic differential between the cell and the environment, appears to give a signal for the transcription of several osmotically regulated genes. In moderately halophilic bacteria, the cell envelope appears to be involved in regulating the ionic environment of the cytoplasm by binding and transporting ions. In eukaryotes, the osmoprotectant normally found is glycerol.

4 Energy production

All living systems must expend energy, not only for growth, but also to allow survival of the non-growing cell. Energy is needed to perform mechanical work during propulsion by flagella, during cytoplasmic streaming, or when separating chromosomes during cell or nuclear division. Energy is also needed for chemical work to drive highly endergonic reactions such as those involved in the synthesis of macromolecules and their subunit monomers from the substrate available to the cell. They need to do work to maintain osmotic differentials and to transport ions and molecules across membranes against concentration gradients. A number of microorganisms are even capable of coupling their energy-producing systems to the emission of light.

What is the source of this energy? Ultimately, it is derived from the energy of sunlight, either directly by transfer of photon energy to chemical bond energy, as in photosynthetic bacteria and algae, or through chemical transformations of organic molecules derived from photosynthesis. There is one exception: *chemolithotrophic bacteria* can obtain energy from reactions involving inorganic compounds. The manner in which energy is obtained from chemical sources varies with the type of microorganism. Some processes are limited to a very few species, while others are of widespread occurrence. Usually exotic substrates, including the xenobiotic compounds, are metabolized by a restricted number of organisms to intermediates which are then metabolized by enzyme systems common to many microorganisms.

Nutritional categories

On the basis of the energy sources used, microbes can be subdivided into two major groups. Those utilizing light directly are phototrophs, while those oxidizing either organic or inorganic compounds are termed chemotrophs. There is also subdivision based on the nature of the carbon source: in lithotrophs, the carbon requirements for synthesis of cell components can be satisfied by reduction of CO_2; in organotrophs, organic compounds provide the main source of carbon. All microorganisms can therefore be subdivided into four major groups on the basis of their modes of nutrition and their sources of energy (Table 4.1) (see also pp. 89–99).

The majority of reactions producing energy are oxidations. How is the energy released in these reactions coupled to do useful work? If an oxidation–reduction couple occurs with direct electron transfer, then the energy produced is dissipated as heat and lost to the organism. If the two half-cell reactions are separated, but

Table 4.1 Nutritional categories of microorganisms.

Nutritional type	Principal energy source	Principal carbon source	Found in
Photolithotrophic	Light	CO_2	Plants, many algae, some bacteria
Photo-organotrophic	Light	Organic compounds	Algae, bacteria
Chemolithotrophic	Oxidation of inorganic compounds	CO_2	Bacteria
Chemo-organotrophic	Oxidation of organic compounds	Organic compounds	Animals, fungi, protozoa, many bacteria

connected electrically so that the electron or ion transfer occurs through a circuit, useful work can then be done. This type of coupling can be made in a number of ways:

Direct chemical coupling

Direct chemical coupling to the synthesis of an energy-rich bond can occur. The example illustrated is an important reaction from the fermentation pathway and is an example of the *substrate-level phosphorylation* of ADP.

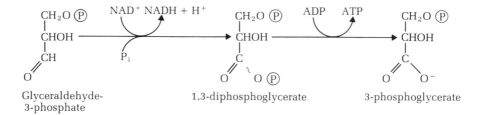

Glyceraldehyde-3-phosphate   1,3-diphosphoglycerate   3-phosphoglycerate

The oxidation of glyceraldehyde-3-phosphate to 3-phosphoglyceric acid occurs via an intermediate which permits the phosphorylation of ADP to ATP. Some of the free energy change in this oxidation–reduction reaction is conserved in the phosphoryl bond of ATP.

Electrical coupling

We have already discussed in the previous chapter (see Fig. 3.4) how a series of redox reactions can be coupled into proton or ion translocation across membranes. Both potential difference and the pH gradient formed, collectively termed the *membrane potential*, can be used to transport ions, or as we shall see later (p. 101) to synthesize energy-rich bonds by reversing energetically-unfavourable reactions such as the phosphorylation of ADP.

ATP and related high-energy molecules are formed during catabolic reactions that involve the oxidation of substrates (or during photosynthesis in the coupled transport of electrons ejected from chlorophyll by absorption of photons). There are a number of ways in which they provide energy for the endergonic reactions of biosynthesis. These can involve coupling in the opposite direction to that found in substrate-level phosphorylation, so that the intermediate is activated by phosphorylation. Another important mechanism seen commonly in the activation of monomers during polysaccharide synthesis, is the formation of nucleoside diphospho intermediates; e.g. in bacterial glycogen synthesis:

glucose-1-phosphate → ADP-glucose → glycogen primer

There are other possibilities, one system being protein synthesis, in which ATP and GTP participate in activation and translocation reactions in a number of ways (see p. 163).

Coupling of reducing equivalents

Since the breakdown of energy-yielding substrates usually involves their oxidation, an acceptor of reducing equivalents (an electron acceptor) is needed. On the other hand, there are many biosynthetic processes which require reduction steps. In order to couple oxidations to reductions in a general way, several important coenzymes act as electron (and hydrogen) acceptors and donors. Thus, although most enzymes are quite specific in the reactions that they catalyse, a common redox coupling mechanism allows one oxidation reaction to provide reducing equivalents to many other reactions.

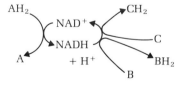

The two commonest coenzymes fulfilling this function are nicotinamide adenine dinucleotide (NAD^+) and its phosphorylated derivative $NADP^+$. As the NADH can be reoxidized by the respiratory chain (p. 99), which is the major site of energy generation in many microbial systems, the cofactor therefore acts also as a common link between many oxidative reactions and the respiratory chain. Catabolism generally requires oxidized pyridine nucleotides, while the reduced forms are needed for biosynthesis. The intracellular pool of the two coenzymes normally comprises NAD^+ and NADPH, but the equilibrium can be altered by the enzyme *transhydrogenase*:

$$NADP^+ + H^+ + NADH \leftrightarrow NADPH + H^+ + NAD^+$$

This membrane-bound enzyme is present in many chemoheterotrophs and facultative phototrophs.

MAIN ENERGY PATHWAYS

Heterotrophic organisms can use a wide variety of carbon substrates as energy sources. These include carbohydrates, amino acids, fatty acids, alkanes, purines and pyrimidines. In general, a few substrates are preferred and these support the highest growth rates (see catabolite repression, p. 215). For many microorganisms, the preferred substrates are carbohydrates, usually glucose, although there are some bacterial species, including *Myxococcus xanthus*, which are not able to use glucose as a source of energy.

Two terms describe different types of energy-yielding systems. *Fermentation* is widely used in industrial terminology, but in its formal sense is used for those pathways in which organic compounds serve as both electron donors and electron acceptors. *Respiration* is applied when oxygen, or some other inorganic compound or ion, acts as the terminal electron acceptor.

Fermentation

A variety of fermentative pathways are available to microorganisms. The fermentable substrates include carbohydrates, organic acids and amino acids.

Glucose metabolism has received considerable attention from biochemists, not only because of energy requirements, but also since it contributes many precursors for biosynthetic reactions. Three pathways are known in prokaryotic microorganisms; these differ in their initial steps but share common later reactions leading to the conversion of 3-carbon (triose) sugar phosphates to pyruvate. Pyruvate is not the end product of most fermentations, but is the common precursor to most end products.

Hexose diphosphate pathway (Embden–Meyerhof–Parnas scheme)

Louis Pasteur first showed that a balance existed between the amount of glucose fermented by yeast and the alcohol and carbon dioxide formed. The reaction sequence in yeast, outlined in Fig. 4.1, was the first major pathway to be elucidated by biochemists and occurs in many prokaryotic and eukaryotic microorganisms. It is one of three pathways common to respiratory and fermentative metabolism, by which sugars are converted to the key intermediary product, *pyruvic acid*. The essential features of the pathway are:

1 Glucose is activated by phosphorylation (either during or after entry to the cell, see p. 81), in a step requiring the expenditure of

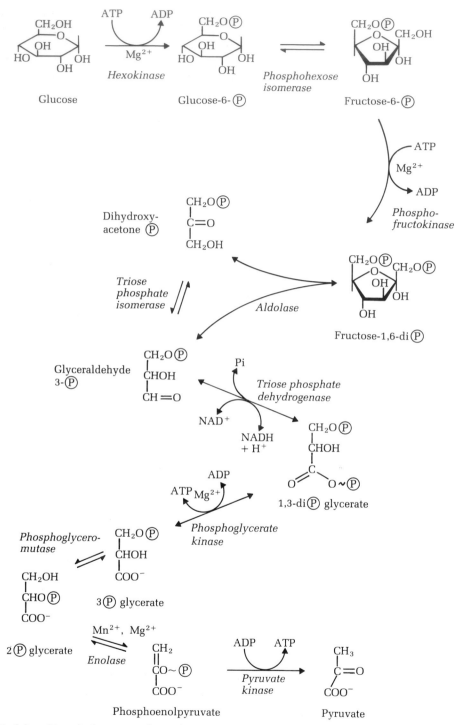

Fig. 4.1 Embden–Meyerhof–Parnas scheme for glucose fermentation.

ATP. A second phosphorylation forming fructose-1,6-diphosphate uses a second molecule of ATP. There is, however, net synthesis of two ATP molecules per molecule of glucose oxidized, since two 3-carbon sugar fragments are formed in the step catalysed by *aldolase,* and the conversion of each of these to pyruvate leads to the phosphorylation of two ADP molecules.

2 The phosphorylation steps involve substrate-level coupling of the energy of oxidation to ATP synthesis, at a thermodynamic efficiency of about 30%.

3 During conversion of glucose to pyruvate, NAD^+ is reduced to NADH. Since NAD^+ is in limited supply in the cell, the metabolism of glucose would cease unless the NADH so formed was re-oxidized. There are many reactions found in different microorganisms for converting pyruvate to final fermentation products with the balanced re-oxidation of NADH. The same organism may produce different compounds when grown in different environments; e.g. under anaerobic conditions or in glucose excess, yeast cytoplasmic enzymes ferment glucose to ethanol, but in the presence of bisulphite, forming an addition product with acetaldehyde, they convert glucose to glycerol by the NADH-linked reduction of glyceraldehyde to glycerol-1-phosphate.

In several bacteria, e.g. *Lactobacillus* spp., *Bacillus* spp., *Streptococcus* spp. and *Clostridium* spp., the homolactic fermentation converts all the pyruvate to lactate:

$$CH_3.CO.COO^- + H^+ \underset{\text{Lactate dehydrogenase}}{\overset{\text{NADH} \quad \text{NAD}^+}{\rightleftharpoons}} CH_3.CHOH.COO^-$$

Thus lactate is the major product of the fermentation of hexose in these bacteria and the process can be represented by the equation:

$$C_6H_{12}O_6 + 2\ P_i + 2\ ADP \rightarrow$$
$$2\ CH_3.CHOH.COOH + 2\ ATP + 2\ H_2O$$

The enzymes involved are mainly soluble proteins found in the microbial cytoplasm or associated with the cytoplasmic membrane. Bacteria such as *Escherichia coli* and related facultative anaerobes perform a *mixed acid fermentation* which yields ethanol (in small amounts) along with other products:

$$2\ (C_6H_{12}O_6) + H_2O \rightarrow C_2H_5OH$$
hexose $\qquad\qquad$ ethanol
$$+\ 2\ CH_3CHOHCOOH + CH_3COOH + 2\ CO_2 + 2\ H_2$$
$\qquad\qquad$ lactate $\qquad\qquad$ acetate

The difference in the end products in these microorganisms reflects the fate of pyruvate and not a fundamental difference in the hexose diphosphate pathway. Some enteric bacteria are anaerogenic, i.e. no gas is evolved from the degradation of the carbohydrate substrate. These species, including *Shigella dysenteriae*, produce a 2-carbon fragment (as acetyl CoA) and formate from pyruvic acid. The enzyme *hydrogenlyase* is absent from *Shigella* and the formate is not further degraded to carbon dioxide and hydrogen as in *E. coli*:

$$H^+ + H.COO^- \rightarrow H_2 + CO_2$$

Another group of closely related bacteria, comprising the genera *Klebsiella*, *Serratia* and *Erwinia*, produces a neutral compound,

Table 4.2 Products derived from the hexose diphosphate pathway.

Fermentation	Products	Microorganisms
Homolactic	Lactate	*Streptococcus*, *Lactobacillus*
Mixed acid	Lactate, acetate,* succinate, formate, ethanol	*Escherichia*, *Proteus*, *Shigella*, *Salmonella*
Butanediol	As in 'mixed acid', butanediol[†]	*Klebsiella*, *Serratia*, *Erwinia*
Butanol	Acetate, butyrate, butanol, acetone, ethanol, i-propanol	*Clostridium* species
Butyric acid	Acetate, butyrate*	*Clostridium*, *Butyribacterium*
Propionic acid	Acetate, propionate, succinate[†]	*Propionibacterium*, *Veillonella*

* Also CO_2 and H_2.
[†] Also CO_2.

butane-2,3-diol. This characteristic product is used in the diagnostic differentiation of these genera. Further variations in the final products from the hexose diphosphate pathway are found in other microbial groups (see Table 4.2).

Phosphoketolase pathway (Warburg–Dickens pathway)

The hexose phosphate pathway does not enable microorganisms to form pentoses or to use them as sources of energy. In some bacteria, e.g. *Leuconostoc* species and some *Lactobacillus* species, the phosphorylation of glucose is followed by its oxidation to 6-phosphogluconate. Further oxidation and decarboxylation of this intermediate yields a pentose phosphate which is split by the enzyme *phosphoketolase* to give a 2-carbon fragment (acetyl phosphate) and triose phosphate. Subsequently, these products are converted to ethanol and lactate respectively; the overall reaction scheme is shown in Fig. 4.2 and can be represented by the equations:

$$\text{glucose} \rightarrow \text{lactate} + \text{ethanol} + CO_2 + \text{ATP}$$

and

$$\text{ribose} \rightarrow \text{lactate} + \text{acetate} + 2\text{ ATP}$$

Organisms which carry out this fermentation lack *aldolase*, needed to cleave hexose phosphates into 3-carbon fragments. A characteristic of this pathway is that the yield of one mole of ATP per molecule of pyruvate formed from glucose is half that obtained in the Embden–Meyerhof pathway. Another feature is that roughly equal amounts of lactic acid, ethanol and carbon dioxide are produced (other compounds such as glycerol and formate are formed in separate reactions). This type of fermentation is often called the *heterolactic fermentation* and is readily distinguished from homolactic fermentation since carbon dioxide is not produced in the latter, and the ATP yield of heterofermentative organisms for a given amount of glucose is less. The pathway is found in many microbial species, including both prokaryotes and eukaryotes.

Entner–Doudoroff pathway

Isotopic studies on *Pseudomonas* (*Zymomonas*) *lindneri* showed that pyruvate could not have been formed by the reactions of the hexose diphosphate pathway, although the initial reaction, the formation of glucose-6-phosphate, is the same. The existence of this third pathway is confined to prokaryotes and is a feature of the metabolism of *Pseudomonas*, *Rhizobium* and *Xanthomonas* species. The remaining reactions are shown in Fig. 4.4.

The characteristics of this modified pathway are:
1 The formation of 3-deoxy-2-oxo-6-phosphogluconate.
2 The labelling pattern in which the carboxyl group of one mole of pyruvate is derived from C1 of the hexose and that of the second pyruvate from C4.
3 The lower energy yield of one mole of ATP per mole of glucose—due to the oxidation of a single mole of triose phosphate as opposed to the two moles available in the hexose diphosphate pathway.

The process is much less widely used by microorganisms than is the hexose diphosphate pathway, but occurs in a number of *Pseudomonas* species and a few other Gram-negative bacteria. In *Zymomonas lindneri*, the major products of glucose catabolism are ethanol and CO_2, which are produced from pyruvate by the same mechanism as in *Saccharomyces cerevisiae*.

Fermentation of nitrogenous compounds

Fermentation of amino acids and other nitrogenous compounds is also important. The microorganisms mainly responsible are either anaerobic sporing rods (*Clostridium* spp.) or anaerobic cocci (*Micrococcus* spp.). The catabolism of glutamate by *Clostridium tetanomorphum* is one typical example of many fermentations; the rate resembles that of glucose breakdown by other microorganisms. The major products of glutamate fermentation are shown in Fig. 4.5. From this it can be seen that:
1 An initial rearrangement of glutamate occurs. Isotopic labelling has shown that this involves the carbon atom at the three position.
2 Pyruvate and acetate are formed as cleavage products. The pyruvate can be oxidized or it can be converted to a number of

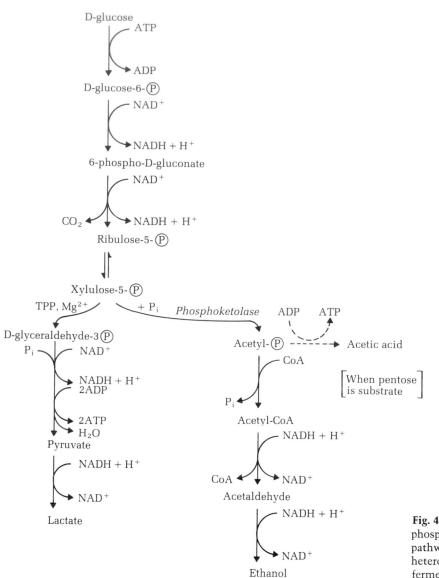

Fig. 4.2 The phosphoketolase pathway for heterolactic fermentation.

products in a series of transformations which provide energy, either as ATP or as acyl CoA derivatives.

Respiration

Fermentation is a relatively inefficient process since glucose is not completely oxidized. Much more energy is available if it can be converted to CO_2 and water. In aerobic respiration, oxygen is ultimately reduced, but the coupling of this reaction to substrate oxidation is indirect. Electrons are transferred from substrates to NAD^+ and subsequently proceed via a series of intermediate carriers (the respiratory chain) to the step involving oxygen. Most of the energy obtained during respiration is derived from the

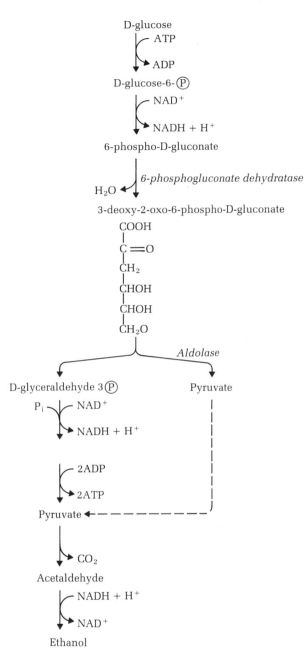

Fig. 4.3 The Entner–Doudoroff pathway.

oxidation of NADH by the respiratory chain and can be used to do work in solute and ion transport (p. 79) or can be coupled to the biosynthesis of ATP.

Respiration can therefore be studied from two angles—one dealing with the flow of carbon compounds to CO_2 and the reduction of NAD^+, the other with electron transport and oxidative phosphorylation in the respiratory chain.

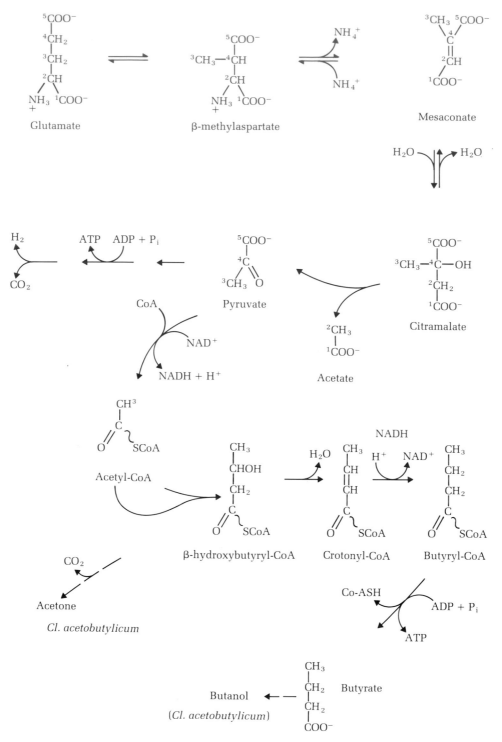

Fig. 4.4 Fermentation of glutamate by *Clostridium* species.

Citric acid cycle (CAC or Krebs cycle)

In most aerobic organisms, the citric acid cycle (CAC) is present, serving a dual role in energy metabolism and in yielding metabolic intermediates. In such groups as the cyanobacteria an incomplete cycle is found. The principal intermediate of hexose metabolism during glycolysis is pyruvate; it is also derived from the oxidation of many amino acids and lipids. Under aerobic conditions, pyruvate is initially converted to acetyl CoA by an oxidative decarboxylation reaction sequence involving the participation of several cofactors and catalysed by a multi-enzyme complex.

Acetyl CoA is the substrate for the citric acid cycle, which is set out in Fig. 4.5. The important features of this cycle can be summarized:

1 Acetyl CoA condenses with oxaloacetate to form citrate. Completing the cycle once results in the oxidation of the acetyl group to two CO_2 molecules and the regeneration of oxaloacetate. Thus the intermediates of the citric acid cycle are effectively catalysts and are not generated in substrate amounts.

2 There are four oxidation–reduction steps. At three of these, NAD^+ is reduced to NADH (in some microbial systems, $NADP^+$ acts as substrate for isocitrate dehydrogenase), while at the succinate to fumarate step, the flavin prosthetic group (fp) of *succinate dehydrogenase* is reduced.

3 The oxidative decarboxylation of 2-oxoglutarate follows the same mechanism as the oxidation of pyruvate to acetyl CoA. At the end of this sequence, there is one substrate-level phosphorylation of ATP coupled to the hydrolysis of succinyl CoA.

Central role of the CAC

The citric acid cycle occurs in almost all organisms and performs the dual function of generating energy and providing precursors in the biosynthesis of important metabolites, including amino acids, purines and pyrimidines. They are also produced by the catabolism of many metabolites, and the enzymes of the CAC therefore assist in the interconversion of compounds, such as the formation of aspartate from glutamate during sporulation in *Bacillus subtilis*. If, during these reactions, intermediates of the citric acid cycle are drained off into biosynthesis, replenishment reactions known as *anaplerotic sequences*, must operate (see Chapter 5).

The citric acid cycle provides much more energy than fermentation. Facultatively anaerobic bacterial species can alternate between aerobic and anaerobic metabolic pathways. Thus they can generate energy either by fermentative or respiratory mechanisms. When growing anaerobically, all the CAC enzymes are to some extent repressed. Two key enzyme activities, *succinate dehydrogenase* and the *2-oxoglutarate dehydrogenase* complex,

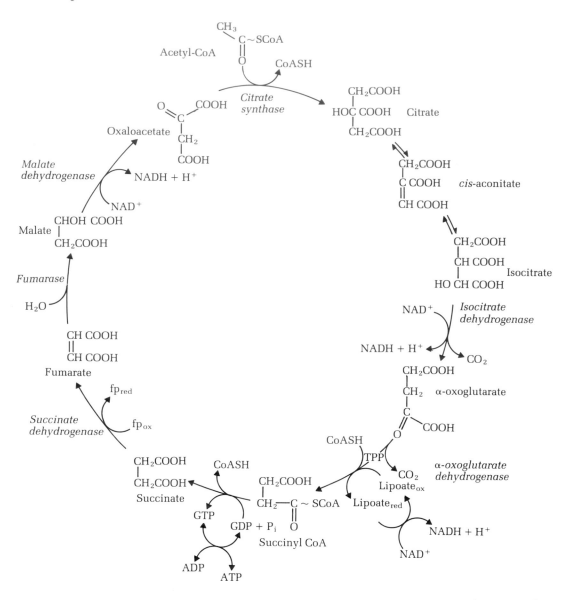

Fig. 4.5 The citric acid cycle (CAC).

are almost totally repressed. Under these circumstances, other enzymes of the CAC function as two separate pathways in cells growing in minimal medium. This allows synthesis of amino acids and other metabolites requiring CAC intermediates. Under these conditions, an alternative *fumarate reductase* is derepressed to allow reduction of fumarate to succinate.

Electron transfer, respiratory chain and oxidative phosphorylation

We have seen that NAD^+, lipoate and the flavin prosthetic group of succinate dehydrogenase are reduced during the fermentation of glucose to pyruvate and its oxidation to CO_2 via pyruvate

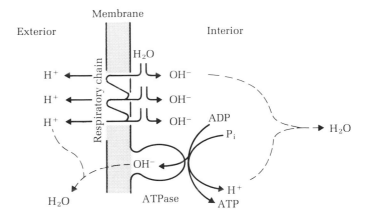

Fig. 4.6 Diagrammatic representation of the coupled phosphorylation of ADP.

decarboxylase and the CAC. These steps are summarized in Table 4.3. Under aerobic conditions, the electrons produced in the re-oxidation of NADH and flavins are transferred to oxygen:

$$O_2 + 4\,H^+ + 4\,e^- \rightarrow 2\,H_2O$$

This electron transfer occurs via a sequence of intermediate electron carriers in such a way that there are discrete steps of energy release. At three of these, the free energy change is sufficiently great for coupling to the phosphorylation of ADP (Fig. 4.6). However, in bacterial systems the complete respiratory chain is not always present and oxidative phosphorylation rarely yields three molecules of ATP per molecule of NADH oxidized or atom of oxygen reduced.

The characteristic electron transport chain of eukaryotes is located in the mitochondrial inner membrane. In bacteria, the respiratory chain forms part of the cell membrane and is in general terms similar to that found in the mitochondrion: i.e. it contains various redox carriers including flavoproteins, iron–sulphur

Table 4.3 ATP yield in aerobic respiration via the CAC.

Reaction step	ATP yield
GLYCOLYSIS	
Glucose + 2 NAD$^+$ → 2 pyruvate + 2 NADH	8
CAC	
Pyruvate + NAD$^+$ → acetyl CoA + NADH	3
Isocitrate + NAD$^+$ → 2-oxoglutarate + NADH	3
2-Oxoglutarate + NAD$^+$ → succinyl CoA + NADH	3
Succinyl CoA → succinate	1
Succinate + flavin → fumarate + flavin H$_2$	2
Malate + NAD$^+$ → oxaloacetate + NADH	3
SUMMARY	
Pyruvate → CO$_2$	15
Glucose → CO$_2$	38

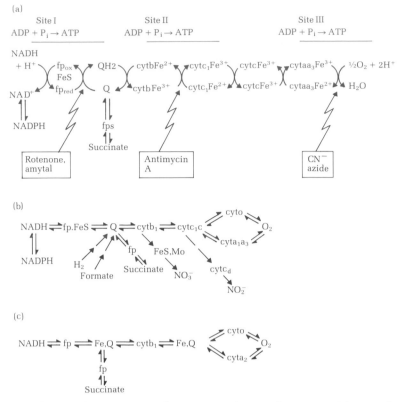

Fig. 4.7 Respiratory chains (a) *Mitochondrial*; (b) *Paracoccus denitrificans*; (c) *Escherichia coli*.

proteins, quinones, cytochromes and cytochrome oxidases. As indicated in Fig. 4.7, it varies from species to species in the nature and number of components present.

The major components of the electron transport chain are flavoproteins, quinones and cytochromes. Flavoproteins contain a prosthetic group, either FAD or FMN, which is firmly bound to the apoprotein and acts as an acceptor of reducing equivalents from NADH. FAD is usually covalently bound to a histidinyl residue, whereas FMN is normally bound ionically through its phosphate groups. The respective redox potentials are $>0\,mV$ and $<-100\,mV$.

Iron–sulphur proteins are relatively small proteins ($M_r = c.$ $30\,000$) in which two, four or eight iron atoms are present together with the same amount of labile sulphur. The nature of the redox centre varies and their potential ranges from -600 to $+350\,mV$. The quininoid compounds can be of two types: *ubiquinones* are derivatives of 2,2-dimethoxy-5-methylbenzoquinone with isoprenoid chains 6–10 units long attached to each C6; the *vitamin K* (menoquinone) groups are derivatives of 2-methyl-1,4-naphthaquinone, again attached to an isoprenoid chain. Gram-positive bacteria contain mainly naphthaquinones, facultatively anaerobic Gram-negative bacteria have both, while in others ubiquinones form the major constituents.

The cytochromes reveal the diversity of bacterial systems as opposed to those of other microorganisms. Identical cytochrome types are found in all eukaryotic mitochondria, whereas bacteria contain a wide variety of cytochromes, few of which correspond directly to those in mitochondria.

Energy coupling to ATP formation

We have already discussed the coupling of energy released in electron transport to ion or solute transport and the theories proposed for the mechanism (p. 79). As with ion transport, oxidative phosphorylation is susceptible to uncoupling agents, including ionophore antibiotics, and can only occur in intact preparations. Associated with all preparations capable of coupled ATP biosynthesis, and intimately associated with the process, is an ATPase activity. This activity is a complex composed of a number of polypeptides located in granules found on the inner surface of the mitochondrial inner membrane or of the bacterial cell membrane. The ATPase activity in mitochondria has been studied in some detail using a number of specific inhibitors and techniques for reversibly dissociating the complex. In eukaryotes, mutations conferring resistance to the inhibitors show mitochondrial inheritance, indicating that some of the components of the ATPase complex are coded by the mitochondrion genome. The synthesis of others is inhibited by cycloheximide (an inhibitor of cytoplasmic protein synthesis) and these are coded by the nucleus.

Chemiosmotic hypothesis

According to this hypothesis, the respiratory chain is organized across the membrane in such a way that electron transport causes excretion of protons. This generates a pH and electrical gradient across the membrane and can be used to reverse the ATPase reaction (Fig. 4.6). The ATPase complex functions so that the proton movement inwards with the pH gradient drives the reaction to the synthesis of ATP. This can be visualized as an enzyme complex located in the membrane such that ATP, ADP, phosphate and H^+ have access to the active site from the inner side only and OH^- from the outside only. Synthesis of ATP is favoured by a pH gradient since the condensation of ADP and phosphates to ATP would, in turn, be favoured by the outward transfer of OH^- and the inward transfer of H^+, tending to neutralize the gradient.

Anaerobic respiration

Some facultatively anaerobic bacteria, including *E. coli, Enterobacter aerogenes* and some *Pseudomonas* species, use an oxidative type of metabolism under anaerobic conditions. This process is anaerobic respiration. The pathways for the catabolic degradation of the carbon and energy sources are identical to those in aerobic respiration, and electron transport occurs via a respiratory chain similar to that in aerobically grown cells. However, oxygen is replaced as terminal electron acceptor by another inorganic compound or ion, frequently nitrate or sulphate. In this role, metabolism of the inorganic compound is *dissimilatory*; nitrate is reduced to nitrite without incorporation of the inorganic nitrogen into cell components. The enzyme *nitrate reductase* is a membrane-bound iron–sulphur protein containing molybdenum. It is composed of two non-identical subunits and is closely associated with a *b*-type cytochrome. The cytochrome is specific to nitrate reduction and is located in the membrane of bacteria using anaerobic respiration. It is induced by nitrate and repressed by oxygen. Nitrite is toxic to most bacteria and is normally expelled from the cytoplasmic membrane in *E. coli*, but some species can use it as an electron acceptor and the molecular nitrogen formed is lost to the environment. In a few bacterial species, nitrate is successively reduced to nitrite then nitrogen; this process of *denitrification* is found in several genera, including *Pseudomonas*. Inorganic electron acceptors such as nitrate have a lower redox potential than oxygen and the amount of ATP produced in systems with nitrate reductase is therefore usually less than in aerobic metabolism with cytochrome oxidase.

Fermentation versus respiration

We have seen that for every molecule of glucose fermented, there are two molecules of ATP formed. In aerobic respiration, the ATP yield is considerably greater, as indicated in Table 4.3; up to 38 molecules of ATP are produced from every molecule of glucose which is completely oxidized. In terms of total free energy avail-

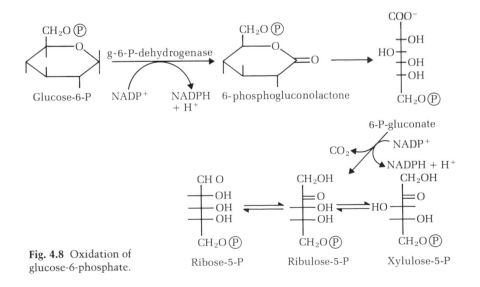

Fig. 4.8 Oxidation of glucose-6-phosphate.

able from the complete oxidation of glucose, about 30% is re-covered in the aerobic pathway, the rest is released as heat. This heat must be removed in large-scale industrial growth of micro-organisms, where cooling of the system can be expensive.

Pentose phosphate cycle

This cycle is found in many bacteria and in most eukaryotic organisms. It can serve several functions in cells:

1 There is conversion of 6-carbon sugars to others, including 5-carbon sugars (pentoses) needed for nucleic acid synthesis and 7-carbon sugars (heptoses) for the formation of aromatic amino acids as well as components of lipopolysaccharides in Gram-negative bacterial walls.

2 It is extremely important for autotrophic organisms since it enables products of CO_2 fixation to be converted to central metabolites.

3 It serves as a source of NADPH, supplying reducing equivalents to biosynthetic reactions.

4 It can provide energy to the cell as an alternative pathway for the oxidation of glucose and a mechanism for obtaining energy from pentoses.

The initial steps in this 'cycle' involve the oxidation of glucose-6-phosphate (Fig. 4.8).

Figure 4.9 shows how six pentoses can be converted to five 6-carbon sugars (hexoses) by the combined activity of the enzymes

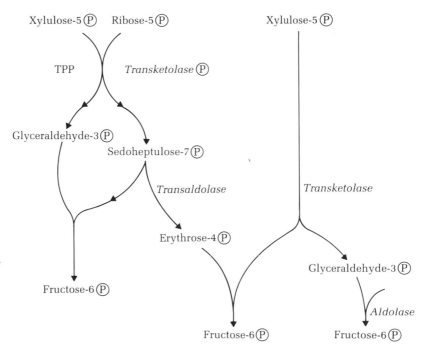

Fig. 4.9 The pentose phosphate cycle. The fate of three pentose phosphates only is shown. If three others react in the same way, the net result is the conversion of six pentose phosphates to five hexose phosphates. Aldolase catalyses formation of one fructose-6-phosphate from two glyceraldehyde-3-phosphate molecules.

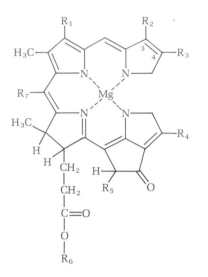

Fig. 4.10 The structure of bacteriochlorophyll. The structure shown is common to different chlorophylls with the R groups varying—R_2 is commonly methyl; R_3 ethyl; R_4 ethyl or methyl; R_6 phytyl, geranyl or farnesyl; and R_7 is either -H or -CH_3.

transketolase, transaldolase and *aldolase*. This means that the overall reaction for six glucose-6-phosphate molecules is:

$$Glc\text{-}6\text{-}P + 12\ NADP^+ \rightarrow 5\ Glc\text{-}6\text{-}P + CO_2 + 12\ NADPH + 12\ H^+$$

The NADPH can be re-oxidized by the respiratory chain providing 36 ATP molecules (or 35 starting from glucose). It is important to consider, however, that the primary role of the pentose phosphate cycle may well be in biosynthesis and not oxidative energy metabolism.

PHOTOSYNTHESIS

Photosynthesis is one of the most important biological processes since it harnesses energy from sunlight and uses it for the fixation of carbon dioxide into organic compounds. It occurs in all green plants, algae and in several bacterial genera. In bacteria three forms of photosynthesis are known to occur. In the cyanobacteria the system utilizes chlorophyll, whereas in the purple sulphur bacteria (Thiorhodaceae), purple non-sulphur bacteria (Athiorhodaceae) and green bacteria (Chlorobacteriaceae), bacteriochlorophyll is used. The halobacteria do not use a chlorophyll type of light-harvesting pigment; it is replaced by bacteriorhodopsin.

In all the eubacteria which use bacteriochlorophyll, the light-dependent cyclic electron transfer systems are composed of similar photopigments and redox carriers. These include bacteriophytins, carotenoids, quinones, cytochromes and iron–sulphur proteins. The photopigments are organized into photosynthetic units within the intracytoplasmic membrane. Each photosynthetic unit is composed of a reaction centre and a light-harvesting complex containing bacteriochlorophyll and carotenoids. The reaction centre contains bacteriochlorophylls (Fig. 4.10) and bacteriophytins.

Fig. 4.11 Cyclic photophosphorylation, chlorophyll (Chl) is excited by a photon to produce an excited molecule Chl*. This can ionize by transfer of an electron to form the chlorophyll ion (Chl$^+$). Chl = bacteriochlorophyll; Pheo = bacteriopheophytin.

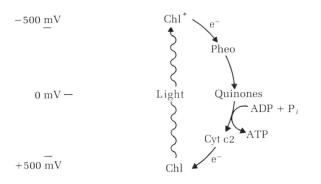

The third essential constituent of the photosynthetic apparatus is the electron transport chain.

The major difference between photosynthesis in the cyano-bacteria and in other eubacterial species is the identity of the final electron donor for the system. Cyanobacteria (together with algae and green plants) use water as the electron donor. Consequently, oxygen is released, the overall process being represented by the equation:

$$CO_2 + 2\ H_2O \xrightarrow{\text{light}} (CH_2O) + O_2 + H_2O$$

The other eubacterial species use reduced sulphur compounds, organic molecules, or molecular hydrogen as electron donors. In these bacteria, the reaction is anaerobic and only *one* photosystem is involved. The reactions can be considered as:

$$CO_2 + 2\ H_2S \xrightarrow{\text{light}} (CH_2O) + H_2O + 2\ S$$

$$CO_2 + 2\ H_2 \xrightarrow{\text{light}} (CH_2O) + H_2O$$

$$CO_2 + 2\ CH_3.CHOH.CH_3 \xrightarrow{\text{light}} (CH_2O) + H_2O + 2\ CH_3.CO.CH_3$$

Differences occur in the light absorption patterns of photosyn-thetic organisms. As the purple bacteria absorb at higher wave-lengths than other groups, this can be used in their isolation by appropriate use of light filters.

The photosynthetic process can be characterized by two groups of reactions: in the *light reactions*, light energy is converted into chemical energy; the *dark reactions*, which can occur in the absence of light, utilize the chemical energy to reduce carbon dioxide to organic compounds.

Light reactions

In bacterial systems other than the cyanobacteria, there is a single photochemically active system which functions in light of wavelengths ranging from the visible spectrum up to 920 nm in the infra-red. The reaction pathway in this case involves a cyclic photophosphorylation of ATP as indicated in Fig. 4.11. The key features are:

1 Absorption of a photon of light excites the chlorophyll molecule and an electron is ejected at a high redox potential. The electron is transferred to a reactive site from which it proceeds through a cyclic transport system coupled to the phosphorylation of ADP in a process similar to oxidative phosphorylation.

2 No NADPH is produced by this electron flow.

3 Light of higher energy than that absorbed by bacteriochlorophylls can contribute to photosynthesis, since there are carotenoids and other accessory pigments which absorb at shorter wavelengths and transmit energy to the bacteriochlorophylls.

Photosynthesis in the cyanobacteria (and in all photosynthetic eukaryotes) is characterized by the presence of two coupled photosystems. The cyanobacteria are mainly obligate photoautotrophs, although a few species can also grow photoheterotrophically. Photosynthesis in the cyanobacteria resembles the process found in algae and in green plants, although in all other aspects of their physiology they resemble other prokaryotes. The cells possess both photosystem I and photosystem II, and oxygen is evolved. Cyclic electron transfer is mediated by photosystem I containing chlorophyll *a* and β-carotene. A chlorophyll *a*–protein complex harvests light of wavelength >600 nm and transfers the energy to a reaction centre complex, the reactions occurring within the thylakoid membrane. Iron–sulphur proteins act as secondary acceptors and the cyclic electron transfer between the final acceptor and the oxidized primary donor utilizes plastoquinones, cytochromes and plastocyanin.

Non-cyclic electron transfer. Photosystems I and II are involved in non-cyclic electron transfer from water to $NADP^+$. Plastoquinone is probably the primary electron acceptor for photosystem II. Subsequently, electrons are transferred via quinones, part of the cyclic system and photosystem I, to iron–sulphur protein. Electrons are then transferred to ferredoxin and ferredoxin-$NADP^+$ reductase to $NADP^+$.

Bacteriorhodopsin

The halobacteria, including *Halobacterium* species, can use photosynthetic electron transfer in a photosystem lacking bacteriochlorophyll or conventional redox carriers. The cells contain carotenoids, but these may serve to protect the bacteria against injurious effects of excess radiation rather than participating in light harvesting. When grown in illuminated culture, *Halobacterium* spp. contain purple patches on up to 50% of the plasma membrane due to the presence of the pigmented protein bacteriorhodopsin. The protein contains *retinal* bound to an apo-protein of molecular weight 25 000 and strongly resembles the pigment rhodopsin that occurs in the visual system of vertebrates. Bacteriorhodopsin absorbs light strongly at about 565 nm. Following light absorption, the retinal chromophore is converted from the *trans* to the *cis* configuration and protons are transferred to the *outside* surface of the membrane. The pigment returns to the *trans* form following proton uptake from the cytoplasm. The accumulation of protons on the outer surface of the membrane then induces ATP synthesis. The light-stimulated proton pump also drives Na^+ from the bacterial cell by an Na^+/H^+ antiport.

Dark reactions

Most photoautotrophs share with chemotrophs the ability to fix carbon dioxide by addition of the CO_2 to ribulose-1,5-bisphosphate to yield two molecules of 2-glyceric acid 3-phosphate. The reaction is catalysed by *ribulose bisphosphate carboxylase.* The glyceric acid 3-phosphate then serves as the precursor for synthesis of a range of different metabolites but it must also be used to ensure an adequate supply of ribulose bisphosphate. Only the fixation of the carbon dioxide and the regeneration of the acceptor from ribulose-5-phosphate catalysed by *phosphoribulokinase* are specific to the reductive pentose phosphate pathway (Calvin–Benson pathway) illustrated in Fig. 4.12. The other reactions are common to reactions found in other non-photosynthetic organisms. The use of this pathway to synthesize hexose (fructose-6-phosphate) from CO_2 constitutes the dark reactions of photosynthesis.

A feature of many carbon dioxide-fixing prokaryotes growing on CO_2 as the principal carbon source, is the presence of *carboxysomes*, polyhedral bodies containing ribulose bisphosphate carboxylase activity together with other Calvin cycle enzymes. The functions of the carboxysomes are unknown and they are clearly not essential for carbon dioxide fixation, as they are absent from the purple photosynthetic bacteria and from the hydrogen bacteria. They are also absent from eukaryotes and from all non-carbon dioxide-fixing prokaryotes.

LITHOTROPHIC ENERGY PRODUCTION—OXIDATION OF ORGANIC COMPOUNDS

Some bacteria, the lithotrophs, can obtain their energy from the oxidation of inorganic compounds. Most are also able to use carbon dioxide as a carbon source and to reduce it to organic compounds. They are therefore also autotrophs. Some of the bacteria are obligate autotrophs, others are facultatively heterotrophic and can vary between both modes of life.

Examples of such bacterial species are found in the genus *Nitro-*

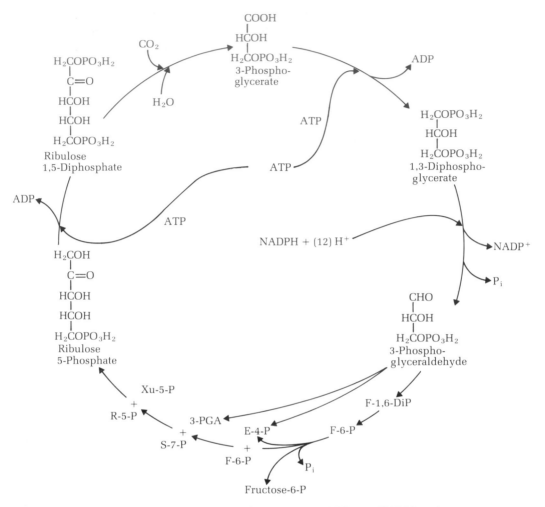

$$(6 CO_2 + 6 H_2O + 18 ATP + 12 NADPH + 12H^+ \rightarrow F\text{-}6\text{-}P + 18 ADP + 12 NADP^+ 17 P_i)$$

Fig. 4.12 The Calvin–Benson (reductive pentose phosphate) pathway. This constitutes the 'dark' reactions of photosynthesis; light energy is not required and chemical energy in the form of ATP is derived from prior photophosphorylation.

bacter, one of several genera forming the nitrifying bacteria. These are soil bacteria which are obligate aerobes and chemolithotrophs; they are also obligately autotrophic. *Nitrobacter* species oxidize nitrite to nitrate, whereas *Nitrosomonas* spp. oxidize ammonia via hydroxylamine to nitrite. As the ATP yield from nitrite oxidation is low and these lithotrophs must synthesize all cell material from CO_2, large amounts of substrate must be oxidized to yield cell material and the *molar growth yield* is low. Within the cells are complex polar stacks of lamellar membranes with highly efficient ATP-synthesizing capability. The respiratory chains of *Nitrobacter* contain a number of high redox potential components, including cytochromes, cytochrome oxidase and iron–sulphur proteins.

The combined actions of *Nitrosomonas* and *Nitrobacter* oxidize ammonia first to nitrite, then to nitrate. A mono-oxygenase oxidizes ammonia to hydroxylamine, using cytochrome P_{450} as the electron donor. During oxidation of hydroxylamine to nitrite, the oxidized cytochrome is reduced.

Hydrogen bacteria

Hydrogen bacteria are mainly facultative chemolithotrophs which can grow readily on organic substrates. They grow either heterotrophically on organic compounds or by aerobic oxidation of hydrogen. The hydrogen is used to provide energy and reducing power for growth and CO_2 fixation.

In *Hydrogenomonas* there are two enzyme systems capable of metabolizing hydrogen. A membrane-bound *hydrogenase* catalyses:

$$H_2 \rightleftharpoons 2 H^+ + 2 e^-$$

The reducing equivalents are passed on to NAD^+; the other enzyme is a soluble *hydrogen dehydrogenase* catalysing:

$$H_2 + NAD^+ \rightleftharpoons NADH + H^+$$

It is not at all clear why two hydrogenases are present, although the soluble hydrogenase may reflect adaptation to growth at higher partial pressures of hydrogen. In most hydrogen bacteria, only the membrane-bound enzyme is present. The NADH formed by either mechanism is then available to reduce $NADP^+$ for the assimilation of carbon dioxide. When these bacteria are grown chemolithotrophically, the presence of hydrogen suppresses the utilization of organic substrates such as fructose in a manner analogous to catabolite repression by glucose in other bacteria; enzymes of the Entner–Doudoroff pathway are not synthesized. Mutants lacking hydrogenase, unable to grow chemolithotrophically, do not show this effect and use fructose equally well in an atmosphere of air or hydrogen; the repression is therefore due to the *products* of hydrogenase and not hydrogenase *per se*. The hydrogen bacteria are unusual in that they can undergo *mixotrophic* growth in the presence of hydrogen, oxygen and organic substrates. This involves the simultaneous assimilation of CO_2 (p. 109) and organic substrates. The genes specifying hydrogen utilization are plasmid-borne in many hydrogen bacteria, whereas those for CO_2 fixation are chromosomal.

Table 4.4 indicates a few of the types of chemolithotrophic organism found and the nature of the inorganic electron donors and acceptors which they employ. In some heterotrophic *Thiobacillus* species, ATP is probably generated in a substrate-level phosphorylation. This involves the formation of the sulphur-containing nucleotide adenosine-5′-phosphosulphate (APS) from sulphite and AMP, catalysed by an Fe^{3+}-containing flavoprotein:

Table 4.4   Metabolism of inorganic compounds by chemolithotrophs.

Bacteria	Electron donor	Electron acceptor	Metabolic products
Nitrobacter	NO_2^-	Oxygen	NO_3^-, H_2O
Nitrosomonas	NH_4^+	Oxygen	NO_2^-, H_2O
Hydrogenomonas	H_2	Oxygen	H_2O
Desulphovibrio	H_2	Sulphate	H_2O, S^{2-}, SO_3^{2-}
Micrococcus denitrificans	H_2	Nitrate	NO_2^-, H_2O
Thiobacillus denitrificans	S	Nitrate	SO_4^{2-}, N_2
T. thiooxidans	S	Oxygen	SO_4^{2-}, H_2O
T. ferrooxidans	Fe^{2+}	Oxygen	Fe^{3+}, H_2O

$$2\ SO_3^{2-} + 2\ AMP \xrightarrow{\textit{APS reductase}} 2\ APS + 4e^-$$

$$2\ APS + 2\ P_i \xrightarrow{\textit{ADP sulphurylase}} 2\ ADP + 2\ SO_4^{2-}$$

$$2\ ADP \xrightarrow{\textit{adenylate kinase}} ATP + AMP$$

One-carbon compounds

One group of mainly prokaryotic microorganisms, the *methylotrophs*, metabolize 1-carbon compounds such as methane, methylamine, methanol and formate as their main energy source. They also assimilate these substrates into organic compounds required for biosynthesis (Table 4.5). Some of the bacteria, such as *Methylomonas* and *Methylococcus*, are obligate methylotrophs, while *Methylobacterium* and some yeasts are facultative methylotrophs. A third group containing both eukaryotes and prokaryotes are facultative methylotrophs but are unable to use methane.

Oxidation of methane to methanol and formaldehyde is a preliminary to assimilation of the substrate. In bacteria, three mechanisms exist for the conversion of C_1 compounds to C_3 compounds—the *Calvin cycle*, the *ribulose monophosphate (RuMP) pathway* and the *serine pathway*. While the Calvin cycle is well known as the mechanism for carbon dioxide fixation by prokaryotes, methylotrophs—microorganisms growing on 1-carbon compounds as their *sole* source of carbon and energy—use one of the other pathways for their assimilation of reduced 1-carbon compounds. So-called Type I organisms use the RuMP pathway, while Type II bacteria use the serine pathway.

Ribulose monophosphate (RuMP) pathway. This operates in methylotrophic bacteria yielding carbon fixation at the oxidation level of formaldehyde, after initial oxidation of methane, methanol or methylated amines. Three moles of formaldehyde yield a net one mole of pyruvate or dihydroxyacetone phosphate. The sequence involves:
1 *Fixation*, in which the formaldehyde (3 moles) is condensed to

Table 4.5 Microbial utilization of one-carbon compounds.

Compound	Used by:	Growth conditions	Energy source
CH_4	*Methylococcus*, etc.	Aerobic	$CH_4 + 2\,O_2 \rightarrow CO_2 + 2\,H_2O$
CH_3OH	*Pseudomonas, Vibrio, Hyphomicrobium*	Aerobic	$2\,CH_3OH + 3\,O_2 \rightarrow 2\,CO_2 + 4\,H_2O$
	Methanosarcina	Anaerobic	$4\,CH_3OH \rightarrow 3\,CH_4 + CO_2 + 2\,H_2O$
CH_3NH_2	*Pseudomonas, Vibrio*	Aerobic	$2\,CH_3NH_2 + 3\,O_2 \rightarrow 2\,CO_2 + 2\,NH_3 + 2\,H_2O$
HCOOH	*Pseudomonas*, etc.	Aerobic	$2\,HCOOH + O_2 \rightarrow 2\,CO_2 + 2\,H_2O$
	Rhodopseudomonas palustris	Anaerobic	Photosynthesis
	Methanobacterium	Anaerobic	$4\,HCOOH \rightarrow 3\,CO_2 + CH_4 + 2\,H_2O$
CO	*Hydrogenomonas*	Aerobic	$2\,CO + O_2 \rightarrow 2\,CO_2$
CO_2	*Hydrogenomonas*	Aerobic	$2\,H_2 + O_2 \rightarrow 2\,H_2O$
	Beggiatoa	Aerobic	$H_2S + 2\,O_2 \rightarrow H_2SO_4$
	Thiobacillus	Aerobic	$H_2S_2O_3 + H_2O + 2\,O_2 \rightarrow 2\,H_2SO_4$
	Ferrobacillus	Aerobic	$4\,Fe^{2+} + 4\,H^+ + O_2 \rightarrow 4\,Fe^{3+} + 2\,H_2O$
	Chlorobium	Aerobic	Photosynthesis
	Purple sulphur and non-sulphur bacteria	Anaerobic	Photosynthesis
	Thiobacillus denitrificans	Anaerobic	$5\,S + 6\,NO_3^- + 2\,H_2O \rightarrow 5\,SO_4^{2-} + 3\,N_2 + 4\,H^+$

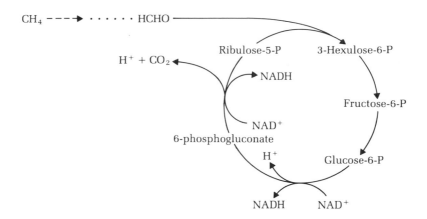

Fig. 4.13 Ribulose monophosphate pathway.

produce hexulose-P. This is isomerized to give fructose-6-phosphate.
2 *Cleavage* of fructose-1,6-bisphosphate or of 6-phosphogluconate to glyceraldehyde-3-phosphate and either pyruvate or dihydroxyacetone phosphate.
3 *Rearrangement* of the remaining molecules of fructose monophosphate together with glyceraldehyde-phosphate leading to the regeneration of 3 moles of ribulose-5-phosphate.

The cleavage of hexose phosphate can involve conversion of fructose-6-phosphate to gluconate-6-phosphate and 2-keto-3-deoxy-6-phosphogluconate by enzymes of the Entner–Doudoroff pathway. The products are then glyceraldehyde-phosphate and pyruvate. Alternatively, fructose-6-phosphate is converted to

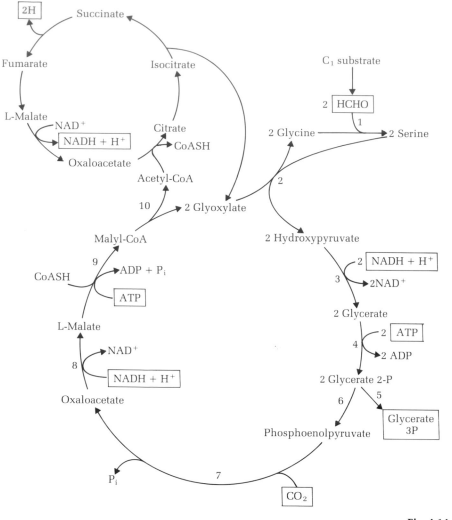

Fig. 4.14 The serine pathway of assimilation of C_1 compounds. The enzymes involved are: 1, serine hydroxmethyltransferase; 2, serine-glyoxylate aminotransferase; 3, hydroxymethyltransferase; 2, serine-glyoxylate kinase; 5, phosphoglycerate mutase; 6, phosphoenolpyruvate hydratase; 7, phosphoenolpyruvate carboxylase; 8, malate dehydrogenase; 9, malyl CoA synthetase; and 10, malyl CoA lyase.

fructose-1,6-bisphosphate by *phosphofructokinase*, then cleaved to glyceraldehyde-phosphate and phosphoglycerate (Fig. 4.13).

The *serine pathway* utilizes carboxylic acids and amino acids rather than carbohydrates for the assimilation of formaldehyde. The key enzyme in the assimilation process is *serine transhydroxymethylase* catalysing the addition of formaldehyde to glycine.

ENERGY STORAGE

In the presence of excess nutrients, microorganisms usually divert some of their metabolism to synthesize compounds which can be degraded during periods of starvation to release energy. These reserves supply the 'maintenance energy' required by nonproliferating cells to maintain their viability, or for spore formation in sporulating microorganisms. The reserve compounds are usually not tapped until intracellular pools of amino acids and nucleotides can no longer be maintained. Large amounts of reserve carbon compounds are also formed when nitrogen sources or other essential ions are limiting, but carbon and energy substrates are still available.

Carbohydrate reserves

Trehalose, a non-reducing disaccharide, is found in fungi and in bacteria, including some cyanobacteria. Although it may function as a storage compound, it is also involved in osmoprotection (see p. 85). In yeasts and slime moulds it is present along with glycogen and is accumulated during vegetative phases of growth. During development leading to sporulation these reserves are used to supply energy. *Glycogen* (see p. 179) is found in a large number of microorganisms and considerable amounts accumulate (up to 50% of the cell dry weight), especially when there is nutrient imbalance in energy-rich conditions. The mechanisms of glycogen synthesis and regulation in prokaryotes differ from those in eukaryotes. In prokaryotes, ADP-glucose is the activated glucosyl donor rather than UDP-glucose, while various primary products of metabolism are involved in regulation and synthesis (see p. 180).

Lipid reserves

Poly-β-hydroxybutyrate (PHB) is the most common lipid storage compound in prokaryotes, accumulating in large amounts in photosynthetic bacteria, cyanobacteria, *Azotobacter vinelandii*, methylotrophs and many other species. In the larger *Bacillus* species, including the *B. megaterium* and *B. cereus* groups, PHB is the main storage compound supporting sporulation. PHB is not found in eukaryotes, where neutral lipids accumulate.

PHB, like glycogen, accumulates under growth conditions where excess carbon source is available and other nutrients are limiting. The amounts accumulated can again be large—up to 60% of the cell dry matter. The key enzyme is *acetyl CoA acyltransferase*. Under balanced growth this enzyme is inhibited by high concentrations of free CoA, and PHB is not synthesized. When excess carbon source is available, the enzyme citrate synthase is inhibited by high concentrations of NADH. The high levels of acetyl CoA accumulated overcome the inhibition, acetoacetyl CoA is produced and converted to PHB:

$$\text{acetoacetyl CoA} \rightarrow \text{3-hydroxybutyryl CoA} \rightarrow \text{PHB}$$
acetoacetyl CoA reductase   *PHB synthetase*

PHB is a linear polymer; its breakdown in cell-free systems requires proteolytic activation of the PHB granules, followed by hydrolysis of the polymer by PHB depolymerase to a dimer, subsequently hydrolysed to β-hydroxybutyric acid.

Polyphosphates

Polymetaphosphates are found in *volutin* granules in many micro-organisms, both eukaryotes and prokaryotes. This polymer acts as both a phosphate reserve and an energy reserve since the phosphoanhydride bond has a high free energy of hydrolysis. Volutin is formed from ATP and undergoes breakdown in the presence of ADP.

Sulphur

Some sulphur bacteria such as *Thiothrix* and *Beggiatoa* store sulphur produced by the oxidation of H_2S. When sulphide in the medium is exhausted, the intracellular sulphur granules are further oxidized to sulphate, supplying the reducing equivalents for photosynthesis or for oxidative phosphorylation.

5 Monomer synthesis

In the previous chapter, we examined the various pathways by which carbon substrates are oxidized to produce energy and, in some cases, reduced pyridine nucleotides. These pathways are also important since they provide intermediates at a variety of oxidation levels for the biosynthesis of all other molecules in the cell. For this reason, they are often referred to as *central pathways*.

Many of the remaining biosynthetic pathways are directed towards forming the precursors of lipids and of the three main groups of polymers: nucleic acids, proteins and polysaccharides. These precursors include approximately five purines and pyrimidines, 20 amino acids, 20 carbohydrates and about 20 fatty acids. In addition, there are pathways for other nucleotides, flavines, quinones and porphyrins, coenzyme A, thiamine pyrophosphate, biotin and other cofactors.

Microorganisms vary in their ability to synthesize these low-molecular weight precursors and cofactors. Some, including autotrophic species and many commonly used laboratory organisms, can synthesize their total requirements from a simple medium containing a single carbon substrate (frequently D-glucose) and inorganic sources of N, P, S and ions needed in smaller amounts. At the other extreme are those microorganisms with a very restricted biosynthetic capacity. *Leuconostoc mesenteroides* is one such, which requires virtually all the amino acids, purines, pyrimidines and cofactors. Where microorganisms are capable of synthesizing these compounds, they usually use the same sequence as other organisms and in only a few cases has there been evolution of distinct pathways. Many pathways, particularly those for amino acids, are branched, with early intermediates common to the synthesis of several metabolites. The control of these complex systems is discussed in Chapter 7.

Methods for investigating biosynthetic pathways

The earliest biochemical pathways to be elucidated were those concerned with carbohydrate breakdown and energy metabolism. These were gradually elucidated by the chemical identification of intermediates, often using metabolic inhibitors to cause their accumulation. As each intermediate was identified, enzymes were isolated which could act on it and eventually the overall sequence was determined. This is now more easily done due to the availability of isotopic methods for labelling. These show which compounds act as precursors to others and from which portion of the molecule the product is derived. Other information comes from pulse-labelling studies with rapid sampling after labelling to

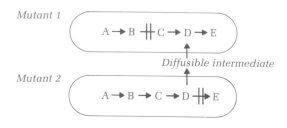

Mutant 1

A → B ┤├ C → D → E

Diffusible intermediate

Mutant 2

A → B → C → D ┤├ E

Fig. 5.1 Determining the reaction sequence of a metabolic pathway by mutant crossfeeding. Mutant 2 can crossfeed mutant 1, but mutant 1 cannot crossfeed mutant 2.

give some details of the reaction sequence. Mutation provides a convenient way of specifically affecting each of the enzymes of a reaction pathway.

Auxotrophic mutants (those unable to synthesize a particular essential metabolite) can be isolated provided that the end product of the pathway can be supplied and used exogenously. These mutants can be defective in any one of the enzymic steps unique to the biosynthesis of the particular metabolite. In some of these, intermediates accumulate and may be excreted into the medium. By 'crossfeeding' tests, it is possible to learn the order of the sequence of intermediates in the biosynthetic pathway, since it is only possible to crossfeed an earlier-blocked mutant with a later-blocked one as indicated in Fig. 5.1.

REPLENISHMENT (ANAPLEROTIC) PATHWAYS

A number of the central metabolites involved in energy metabolism are not synthesized in substrate amounts by the energy-yielding pathways. The most important examples are the citric acid cycle (CAC) intermediates. Several of these are, however, also starting points in the biosynthesis of nearly half the amino acids and pyrimidines. Several mechanisms therefore exist for the conversion of other central intermediates formed in substrate amounts to CAC intermediates; these depend on the organisms and the nature of the carbon substrates used for growth.

In aerobic organisms growing on acetate, the main mechanism is the *glyoxylate cycle*; this is found in many bacteria, fungi, algae and protozoa, and is summarized in Fig. 5.2. It is characterized by the presence of two enzymes: *isocitrate lyase*, catalysing the cleavage of isocitrate to succinate and glyoxylate, and *malate synthase*, which catalyses the condensation of acetyl CoA and glyoxylate to form malate. The net result of these reactions taken with the CAC is the conversion of two molecules of acetyl CoA to one dicarboxylic acid of the CAC.

For organisms growing on 3-carbon compounds (pyruvate or lactate) or substrates leading to these (sugars or glycerol), another system operates, involving the fixation of carbon dioxide. In most microorganisms, there are a number of enzymes for fixing carbon dioxide to either pyruvate or phosphoenolpyruvate, with the syn-

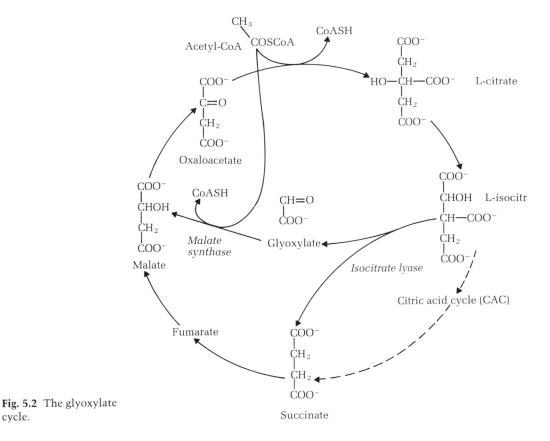

Fig. 5.2 The glyoxylate cycle.

thesis of either malate or 'oxaloacetate. In yeast and *Arthrobacter globiformis*, the anaplerotic role appears to be fulfilled by the enzyme *pyruvate carboxylase* catalysing:

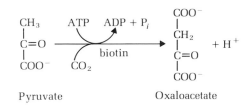

In enterobacteria, however, studies with mutants have shown that another enzyme, *phosphoenolpyruvate carboxylase*, operates in this role:

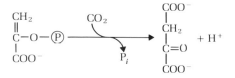

ASSIMILATION OF NITROGEN AND SULPHUR

Many organic metabolites contain N, S and P. These are generally obtained from inorganic sources and their assimilation to an organic form is an essential step in the biosynthesis of many monomers. Phosphorus is usually taken up as phosphate in the medium and converted into organic phosphate in familiar reactions.

Nitrogen can be assimilated as organic nitrogen, or from inorganic sources such as NH_4^+, NO_2^- (rarely), or NO_3^-. A number of specialized bacteria, including cyanobacteria, can utilize molecular N_2, i.e. they can fix atmospheric nitrogen. Ammonia is usually directly incorporated in a reductive addition to α-oxoglutarate to yield glutamate. A second molecule of ammonia can then be used in the conversion of glutamate to glutamine:

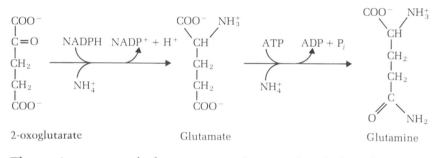

2-oxoglutarate   Glutamate   Glutamine

The amine group of glutamate can be transferred directly to other 2-oxo acids (e.g. pyruvate) to form other amino acids by transamination.

Some microorganisms reduce nitrate not by dissimilatory mechanisms as terminal electron acceptor in energy metabolism, but by assimilatory reactions to NH_4^+ for biosynthesis. This is carried out in a series of reductive steps for which only the first reaction has been characterized. This is catalysed by *nitrate reductase*, the reducing equivalents being transferred from NADPH:

$$NO_3^- \xrightarrow[\text{NADPH}\quad\text{NADP}^+ + H^+]{\text{fp; Mo}} NO_2^- \longrightarrow ? \longrightarrow [NH_2OH] \longrightarrow NH_4^+$$

Fixation of atmospheric nitrogen (dinitrogen) is a feature unique to prokaryotes, in which two distinct groups are found. The genus *Rhizobium* is found in close symbiotic association with leguminous plants, and nitrogen fixation normally only occurs in the root nodules of the legumes. Other nitrogen-fixing bacteria are free living. These include heterotrophs and phototrophs, and they range from aerobic through facultatively anaerobic to strictly anaerobic species (Table 5.1). The facultative species, including *Klebsiella aerogenes* and *Bacillus polymyxa*, only fix nitrogen when they grow under strictly anaerobic conditions. All prepara-

Table 5.1 Examples of nitrogen-fixing (diazotrophic) bacteria.

Bacterium	Type
Azotobacter vinelandii	Heterotroph; aerobe
Methylosinus trichosporium	Heterotroph; microaerophilic
Rhizobium trifolii	Heterotroph; microaerophilic
Klebsiella aerogenes	Heterotroph; facultative anaerobe
Bacillus polymyxa	Heterotroph; facultative anaerobe
Clostridium pasteurianum	Heterotroph; anaerobe
Desulphovibrio desulphuricans	Heterotroph; anaerobe
Rhodospirillum rubrum	Phototroph
Chromatium vinosum	Phototroph
Chlorobium thiosulphatophilum	Phototroph
Cyanobacteria	Phototrophs (includes aerobic and microaerophilic species; unicellular, filamentous and heterocystous types)

tions of the enzyme *nitrogenase* are inactivated by oxygen. The enzyme system, or *nitrogenase complex*, catalysing nitrogen fixation is composed of two proteins. One, of molecular mass $2-2.5 \times 10^5$, contains iron and molybdenum (Protein 1, nitrogenase); the second, smaller protein, of molecular mass $5-6 \times 10^4$, contains iron only (Protein 2, dinitrogen reductase). Both are formed from subunits and are oxygen labile. The Fe-protein is the primary electron donor for reduction of the substrate, which is then passed to Protein 1, where it binds and is reduced. The natural reductant for Protein 2 is ferredoxin, a non-haem iron protein. In *Azotobacter chroococcum*, ferredoxin is replaced by a flavoprotein, flavodoxin. It can also substitute for ferredoxin in *Clostridium pasteurianum* grown under iron limitation. A second type of nitrogenase, discovered fairly recently in *Azotobacter* species, but apparently absent from *Rhizobium*, contains the element vanadium in place of molybdenum. It too is an enzyme with equal amounts of two subunits of M_r 50 000 and 55 000. A third system in *Azotobacter*, containing iron only, has also been discovered, however, *K. aerogenes* only produces one nitrogenase of the iron/molybdenum type.

The energy required for nitrogen fixation is either derived chemotrophically from fermentation or respiration or, in the case of the cyanobacteria and other photosynthetic species, phototrophically. ATP, as the Mg salt, binds to the Fe-protein, altering its configuration and allowing electron transfer to Fe atoms in Protein 1. At least one ATP molecule is hydrolysed for each electron transferred. Protein 1 binds the substrate while electrons are added. The process is highly endergonic, requiring about 16 molecules of ATP to fix each molecule of N_2. The evolution of hydrogen found at the same time as nitrogen fixation may assist in respiratory protection of the nitrogenase complex. In aerobic, nitrogen-fixing bacteria, a membrane-bound hydrogen uptake mechanism normally recycles the hydrogen produced and re-generates ATP through H_2-linked respiration.

The process of nitrogen fixation can be regarded as a series of reactions:

1 Reduction of Fe-protein (Protein 2) by reduced ferredoxin.

2 Activation of Fe-protein by ATP, which binds to the protein and alters its configuration. Mg^{2+} is needed for this binding, which is at a second binding site distinct from that for electrons.

3 Electron transfer between the nitrogenase Protein 2 and Protein 1, leaving Protein 1 reduced by the ATP-activated Protein 2.

4 Binding of substrate (involving the transition metal ion) to Protein 1.

5 Electron transfer to the substrate from the Mo−Fe Protein 1.

6 Release of the products—ammonia, hydrogen and ADP.

$$\text{The net reaction is: } N_2 + 3\ XH_2 \rightarrow 2\ NH_3 + X$$

where X is the low potential electron carrier. The product of nitrogenase, ammonia, is rapidly assimilated into cell material being taken up by the GS-GOGAT pathway (p. 76). This requires a further two molecules of ATP for each molecule of dinitrogen fixed.

All nitrogenase preparations evolve hydrogen and can reduce a number of substrates containing triple bonds. These include acetylene, cyanide, nitrous oxide and azide; for example:

$$HC\equiv CH \rightarrow H_2C=CH_2$$
$$HC\equiv N \rightarrow CH_4 + NH_3$$

All inhibit evolution of hydrogen and fixation of nitrogen. Acetylene, azide and cyanide are all usually very toxic for biological systems due to their high affinity for transition metal ions. The production of ethylene from acetylene is used to measure nitrogenase activity. The scheme for nitrogen fixation is shown in Fig. 5.3. When sufficient fixed nitrogen is present, nitrogen fixation is repressed through dephosphorylation of an activator; the molecular basis of this, through regulation of the *nif* genes, is not yet fully understood.

In those species which are strictly aerobic, such as *Azotobacter vinelandii*, nitrogenase is maintained in an oxygen-free micro-environment by respiratory protection, but in certain of the cyanobacteria, in which oxygen is evolved during photosynthesis, nitrogen fixation is confined to heterocysts. These specialized cells are capable of restricting oxygen entry and lack photosystem II and oxygen evolution. The ammonia formed is incorporated into glutamine by glutamine synthetase, then exported from the heterocyst to the vegetative cell. Energy for nitrogen fixation, in the form of ATP, is obtained from the photosynthetic and respiratory electron transfer chains, which also provide a pathway for re-utilizing the hydrogen evolved by the nitrogenase. Other non-

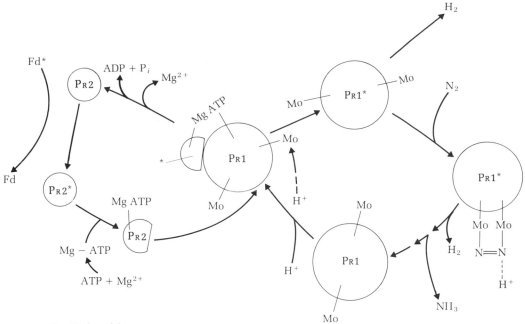

* = Reduced form

Fig. 5.3 Scheme for nitrogenase action in dinitrogen fixation.

In *Klebsiella pneumoniae*, 20 contiguous genes in a 23 kb region close to the *his* operon, have been shown to be required for the synthesis and activity of nitrogenase. Many of these genes are involved in processing the two proteins of nitrogenase and their subunits. It was earlier thought that the *nif* genes were subject to negative control through repressor genes, but the glutamine synthase protein appears to have a positive role in a cascade system of regulation of the nitrogenase operons (see Chapter 7).

Sulphur is usually taken up as sulphate. Studies of cysteine-requiring mutants of various bacterial and fungal species have shown that sulphate is first activated by adenylation to form the nucleotide adenylylsulphate (APS) (Fig. 5.4), then phosphorylated and reduced to sulphite and sulphide in a series of steps:

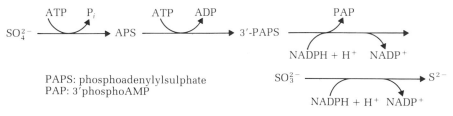

PAPS: phosphoadenylylsulphate
PAP: 3'phosphoAMP

In yeasts and other fungal systems, the final reaction is the condensation of serine and sulphide to form cysteine:

$$H_2S + \begin{array}{c} CH_2OH \\ | \\ CHNH_2 \\ | \\ COOH \\ \text{serine} \end{array} \rightarrow \begin{array}{c} CH_2SH \\ | \\ CHNH_2 \\ | \\ COOH \\ \text{cysteine} \end{array} + H_2O$$

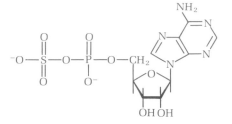

Fig. 5.4 The structure of adenylylsulphate (APS).

In the Enterobacteriaceae, a different reaction occurs, involving the *O*-acetylation of serine and subsequent reduction with sulphide:

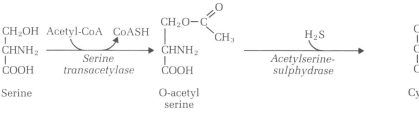

BIOSYNTHETIC PATHWAYS

In this book, we do not intend to describe in detail the biochemical pathways leading to the synthesis of all low-molecular weight metabolites. In most cases, these reactions are common to many organisms and extensive descriptions are available in general biochemistry textbooks. Here, we are more interested in general patterns of the flow of central metabolites to various important compounds, and the synthesis of some metabolites which are unique to microorganisms. A general scheme for the position of central metabolism in biosynthesis is outlined in Fig. 5.5.

Nucleotide synthesis

Nucleotide precursors of nucleic acids are composed of a purine or pyrimidine base glycosidically linked to ribose or to deoxyribose phosphates:

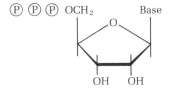

The ribose phosphate moiety is derived from the pentose phosphate cycle and the deoxypentose is not formed until a later stage

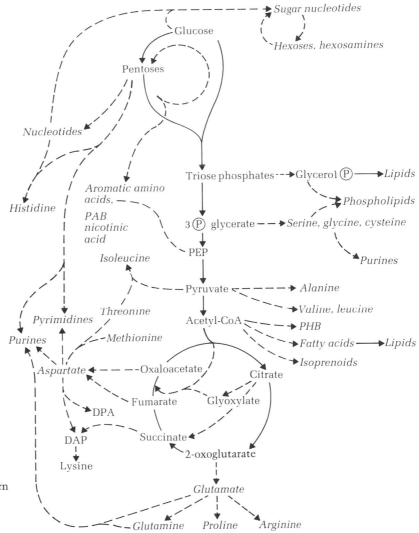

Fig. 5.5 General pattern of monomer synthesis from central metabolites.

in nucleotide synthesis. A common step in the synthesis of both purines and pyrimidines is the activation of ribose-5-phosphate by phosphorylation to the phosphoribosyl pyrophosphate (PRPP):

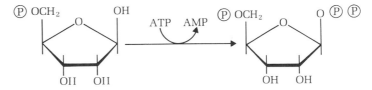

Pyrimidines

PRPP condenses with a base precursor, orotic acid, which is formed in a series of reactions commencing with the condensation of carbamoyl phosphate and aspartate. The enzyme catalysing this step, *aspartate transcarbamylase*, has been extensively studied since it forms an important site of feedback control of pyrimidine nucleotide synthesis. Orotic acid is formed by a cyclization reaction; it condenses with PRPP leading to UMP, and thence UDP and UTP which can be enzymically converted to CTP.

Purines

The synthesis of these differs from pyrimidines in that the bases are built up completely on the ribose-5-phosphate moiety by a lengthy series of steps involving the amination of PRPP and subsequent additions of glycine, amino groups, C_1 groups and aspartate to yield inosine monophosphate. From IMP, divergent pathways exist for forming AMP and GMP.

Nucleotide triphosphates

These are all formed by successive phosphorylations from ATP, catalysed by *nucleoside phosphotransferase*. The deoxyribose of deoxyribonucleotides is formed at the nucleoside diphosphate stage, by a NADPH-linked reduction:

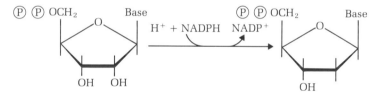

Deoxythymidine phosphates are formed from deoxyCMP via deoxyUMP as an intermediate:

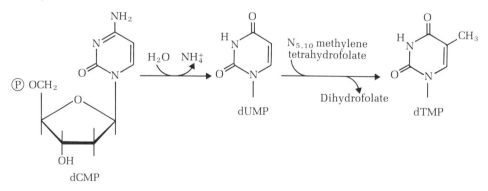

The above reactions are of interest in that free bases do not participate in the normal synthetic reactions. In some organisms, there are pathways by which added adenine, thymine or uracil can be taken up and incorporated into nucleic acid. This is fortunate, since it enables specific labelling of RNA and DNA in many bacteria. In some eukaryotic microorganisms, including yeasts, one of the enzymes needed for incorporating thymine or thymidine—*thymidine kinase*—is lacking and since dTMP is taken up very poorly, specific labelling of DNA is a problem.

Amino acid synthesis

From Fig. 5.5 it can be seen that most of the amino acids are formed from a few major central metabolites. They are therefore often grouped into families on the basis of their precursors (Table 5.2). Histidine is the sole exception. It is synthesized from PRPP and ATP in a sequence of reactions in which the heterocyclic ring is derived from the adenine of ATP.

Lysine biosynthesis

L-Lysine is an essential amino acid in the human diet and methods have been developed to produce it industrially by fermentation. This amino acid also provides an example of separate evolution of two completely different pathways for the synthesis of the same compound. In fungi, including members of the Phycomycetes, Ascomycetes and Basidiomycetes, and in a few green algae including *Euglena*, L-lysine is formed from L-glutamate via α-aminoadipate. In bacteria, cyanobacteria and most green algae, another important pathway exists, starting from aspartate and proceeding via diaminopimelic acid (DAP). The two reaction sequences are shown in Fig. 5.6.

The aspartate pathway for lysine is essential to prokaryotes

Table 5.2 Families of amino acid synthesis.

Family	Precursors	Amino acids
Aromatic amino acids	Erythrose-4-phosphate and phosphoenolpyruvate	→ tryptophan → tyrosine → phenylalanine
Pyruvate	Pyruvate	→ alanine → valine → leucine
Glutamate	α-Oxoglutarate	→ glutamine → glutamate → proline → arginine → lysine (fungi)
Aspartate	Oxaloacetate	Aspartate → lysine (bacteria) → threonine isoleucine → methionine
Serine	3-Phosphoglycerate	→ serine → cysteine → glycine

Histidine is the sole amino acid member of its pathway, but its precursors, PRPP and ATP, are involved in nucleotide synthesis.

(a)

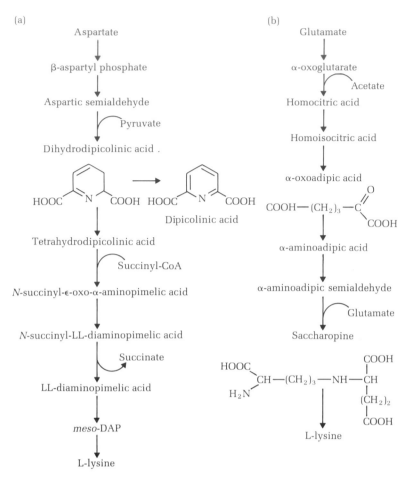

(b)

Aspartate
↓
β-aspartyl phosphate
↓
Aspartic semialdehyde
↓ Pyruvate
Dihydrodipicolinic acid .

Tetrahydrodipicolinic acid
↓ Succinyl-CoA
N-succinyl-ε-oxo-α-aminopimelic acid
↓
N-succinyl-LL-diaminopimelic acid
↓ Succinate
LL-diaminopimelic acid
↓
meso-DAP
↓
L-lysine

Dipicolinic acid

Glutamate
↓
α-oxoglutarate
↓ Acetate
Homocitric acid
↓
Homoisocitric acid
↓
α-oxoadipic acid

$COOH—(CH_2)_3—C\begin{smallmatrix}O\\ \\COOH\end{smallmatrix}$

α-aminoadipic acid
↓
α-aminoadipic semialdehyde
↓ Glutamate
Saccharopine
↓
L-lysine

$HOOC \atop H_2N$ $CH—(CH_2)_3—NH—CH \atop$ $COOH \atop (CH_2)_2 \atop COOH$

Fig. 5.6 Alternative pathways of lysine biosynthesis. (a) Bacteria, blue–green algae and some green algae (aspartate pathway); (b) fungi and most algae (glutamate pathway).

since it provides two compounds unique to their physiology: diaminopimelic acid, occurring in many peptidoglycans, and dipicolinic acid, a major constituent of bacterial spores, formed by the oxidation of dihydropicolinic acid.

Fatty acid synthesis

Various fatty acids are found in microbial cells as components of lipids, but unlike the precursors of proteins and nucleic acids, they do not occur as free acids. Fatty acids may be unsaturated or saturated; relatively large amounts of the former are found in psychrophiles, where their lower melting point is essential in maintaining the fluidity of the cell lipids.

The key compounds in fatty acid synthesis, and hence in lipid formation, are derivatives of coenzyme A and *acyl carrier protein* (ACP). ACP has now been isolated from numerous microorganisms since its initial discovery in *Clostridium kluyveri*, an anaerobe capable of growth on a mixture of acetate and ethanol as carbon sources. The protein contains β-alanine and 2-mercaptoethylamine

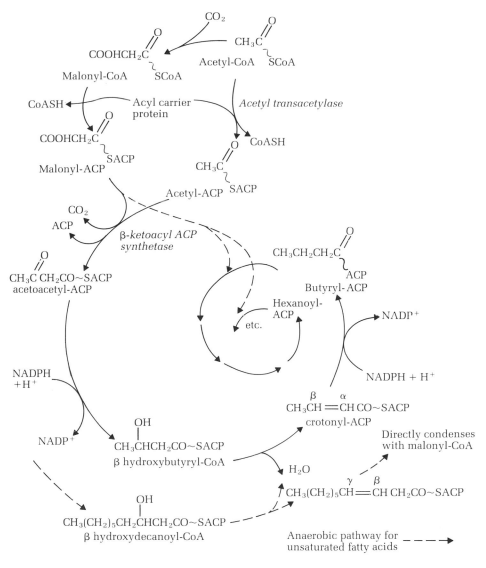

Fig. 5.7 The biosynthesis of fatty acids. The important reaction in the anaerobic pathway of unsaturated fatty acid synthesis is indicated.

and is bound to the fatty acyl moiety at all stages of the biosynthesis, as indicated in Fig. 5.7. In prokaryotes, the ACP and associated enzymes are present in soluble form, whereas in eukaryotes they form tightly particulate fatty acid synthetase complexes. In all microorganisms, the mode of saturated fatty acid synthesis is the same, involving the addition of 2-carbon fragments in the form of acetyl groups, and their subsequent reduction. The initiating acetyl group is carboxylated to malonyl CoA in a biotin-dependent reaction; thereafter, two enzymes convert acetyl CoA and malonyl CoA to their respective ACP derivatives. The higher fatty acids are then built up by the cyclic action of four enzymes as indicated in Fig. 5.7.

As well as saturated fatty acids, most microbial lipids contain a range of unsaturated fatty acids, including such mono-unsaturated acids as oleic acid

$$[CH_3—(CH_2)_7—CH\!=\!CH—(CH_2)_7COOH]$$

as well as those containing two or three double bonds. Two methods are known for the biosynthesis of unsaturated fatty acids. The *aerobic pathway* involves molecular oxygen, NADPH and the acyl CoA derivative of the appropriate acid. The double bond is always inserted between the C9 and C10 regardless of the length of the fatty acid chain:

$$CH_3—(CH_2)_{14}—CO—SCoA \xrightarrow{\qquad} CH_3—(CH_2)_5—\overset{10}{C}H\!=\!\overset{9}{C}H—(CH_2)_7—CO—SCoA$$

$$\tfrac{1}{2}O_2 \qquad H_2O$$

Palmitoyl-CoA   Palmitoleyl-CoA

This process occurs in eukaryotes and in a number of aerobic bacteria, including *Bacillus megaterium* and *Micrococcus lysodeikticus*.

The other pathway, in which there is no requirement for oxygen, is found in anaerobic bacteria and in a number of aerobes such as *Pseudomonas*, *Lactobacillus* and cyanobacteria. This *anaerobic pathway* is a branch of normal fatty acid synthesis introduced at the β-hydroxydecanoyl level (at the 10-carbon fatty acid stage). Instead of the normal α,β dehydration, a β,γ dehydration occurs. Longer chain unsaturated fatty acids are then produced by further addition of 2-carbon fragments. This means that the products of the anaerobic pathway differ from those of the aerobic pathway in the position of the double bond: e.g. the C_{18} products are *cis*-vaccenic acid (Δ_{11}) and oleic acid (Δ_9) respectively.

Branched-chain fatty acids occur in many organisms. Their synthesis can be initiated from corresponding branched-chain amino acids such as leucine or isoleucine:

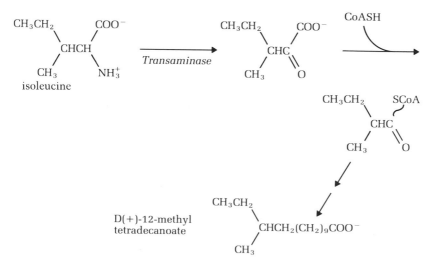

Alternatively, a methyl group can be added to unsaturated fatty acids:

$CH_3(CH_2)_7CH{=}CH(CH_2)_7COOH$ oleic acid

$CH_3(CH_2)_7CCH_2(CH_2)_7COOH$ 10-methylene stearic acid
$$\underset{CH_2}{\overset{||}{|}}$$

$CH_3(CH_2)_7CHCH_2(CH_2)_7COOH$ 10-methyl stearic acid
$$\underset{CH_3}{|}$$

Isoprenoids

A number of terpene derivatives are also found in microbial cells. These are composed of isoprenoid units having the general structure:

$$-(CH_2{-}C{=}CH{-}CH_2)-$$
$$\underset{CH_3}{|}$$

Among the polyisoprenoid compounds are the carrier lipids (bactoprenols) involved in bacterial peptidoglycan, lipopolysaccharide and exopolysaccharide synthesis (Chapter 6). The longer chain dolichols are involved in glycosylation of yeast glycoproteins. Other isoprenoid derivatives include coenzyme Q, vitamin K and different carotenoids present in several groups of microorganisms. Those found in photosynthetic bacteria and in many bacteria isolated from soil resemble hydrocarbons found in plant tissues:

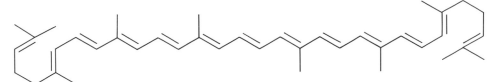

They appear to be absent from anaerobic, non-photosynthetic bacteria. Synthesis of the isoprenoid compound proceeds from acetyl CoA by way of acetoacetyl CoA to *mevalonic acid*, which is phosphorylated by ADP and decarboxylated to yield *isopentenyl pyrophosphate* (Gram-positive but not Gram-negative bacteria can utilize mevalonic acid). In a further series of reactions, the C_{15} compound *farnesyl pyrophosphate* is formed from three isopentenyl pyrophosphate residues. From farnesyl pyrophosphate, sequential addition of isopentenyl groups yields the C_{55} isoprenoid alcohol pyrophosphate. After dephosphorylation to the alcohol phosphate, this is involved in the synthesis of carbohydrate-containing polymers found outside the bacterial cell membrane (Chapter 6). In eukaryotes, the C_{90} isoprenologues (dolichols) perform similar functions. Farnesyl pyrophosphate also undergoes

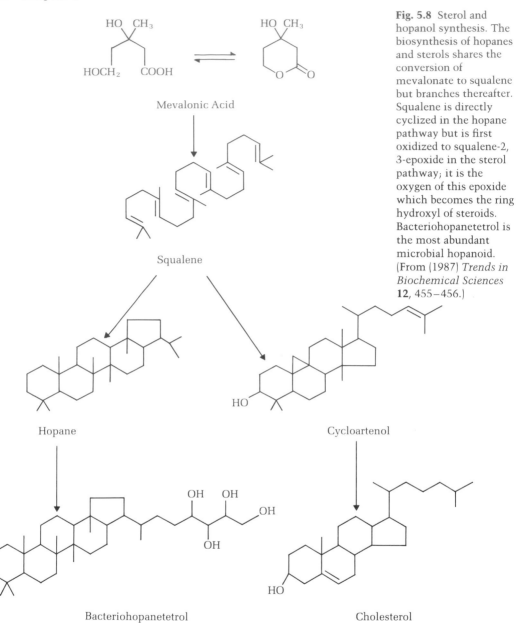

Fig. 5.8 Sterol and hopanol synthesis. The biosynthesis of hopanes and sterols shares the conversion of mevalonate to squalene but branches thereafter. Squalene is directly cyclized in the hopane pathway but is first oxidized to squalene-2, 3-epoxide in the sterol pathway; it is the oxygen of this epoxide which becomes the ring hydroxyl of steroids. Bacteriohopanetetrol is the most abundant microbial hopanoid. (From (1987) *Trends in Biochemical Sciences* **12**, 455–456.)

Mevalonic Acid

Squalene

Hopane

Cycloartenol

Bacteriohopanetetrol

Cholesterol

condensation in eukaryotic cells to form squalene and, subsequently, sterols. This reaction is absent from most prokaryotes, but may be found in some squalene-containing methane-utilizing bacteria. Farnesyl pyrophosphate is also the precursor for parts of the chlorophyll and quinone molecules.

Mevalonic acid is also the precursor for *hopanoids*, pentacyclic compounds resembling sterols which are present in bacterial membranes and in some plants. After conversion to squalene, mevalonic acid is cyclized to form the hopanoid nucleus. Sterol synthesis requires the aerobic formation of the 2,3-epoxide before the cyclic molecule is produced (Fig. 5.8). *Methylococcus capsulatus* contains both hopanoids and sterols and it may use *methane monooxygenase* to convert squalene to the 2,3-epoxide.

Lipid and phospholipid synthesis

Lipids are essentially derivatives of glycerol.

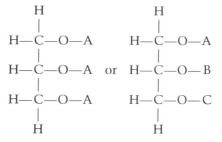

In both prokaryotic and eukaryotic cells, phospholipid synthesis requires cytidine triphosphate (CTP). The reaction between CTP and an L-α-phosphatidic acid produces a cytidine diphosphate diglyceride:

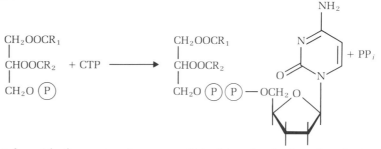

Triglyceride formation is accomplished by the dephosphorylation of L-α-phosphatidic acid by a diphosphatase. The D-α,β-diglyceride then reacts with the CoA derivative of the appropriate fatty acid to form a triglyceride.

In bacteria, phosphatidylethanolamine is synthesized via the intermediate phosphatidylserine:

CDP-diglyceride + L-serine → phosphatidylserine + CMP
Phosphatidylserine → phosphatidylethanolamine + CO_2

This mechanism differs from that in eukaryotic cells, where there is direct interaction between the CDP-ethanolamine and a diglyceride:

CDP-ethanolamine + D-α,β-diglyceride →
phosphatidylethanolamine + CMP

Monosaccharides

In microorganisms, monosaccharides are seldom if ever found as free sugars. Usually, they are present either as components of polysaccharides or other carbohydrate-containing polymers, or in smaller amounts in the cytoplasm as sugar phosphates and 'sugar nucleotides' (nucleoside diphosphate monosaccharides). Monosaccharides and their derivatives can be synthesized from the common sugar substrates, D-glucose, D-fructose or D-mannose, or from other carbon substrates. Microorganisms can vary widely in their ability to utilize external sugars; some such as *Escherichia coli* can take up such sugars as D-arabinose and even the methyl pentose L-rhamnose, while others show a much more restricted range. Some bacteria can even assimilate sugar phosphates or sugar nucleotides without degradation. For those microorganisms growing on lipids, amino acids or citric acid cycle intermediates as carbon sources, monosaccharides are synthesized by some of the Embden–Meyerhof enzymes acting in reverse, with a shunt around the energetically unfavourable pyruvate → phosphoenolpyruvate step via one of the enzymes converting malate or oxaloacetate to phosphoenolpyruvate.

After uptake into the cell, monosaccharides can be phosphorylated by the non-specific enzyme hexokinase at the expense of ATP. Thus D-glucose-6-phosphate is formed from D-glucose and converted to D-glucose-1-phosphate by *phosphoglucomutase*. In enterobacteria, the sugar is usually phosphorylated during entry to the cells via the PEP-dependent reaction sequence described on p. 83.

Sugar nucleotides

Before they can participate in many biosynthetic or interconversion reactions, sugar phosphates are activated by reaction with nucleoside triphosphates to form sugar nucleotides. These are primarily synthesized from hexose phosphates such as α-D-glucose-, α-D-galactose- or α-D-mannose-1-phosphate in the presence of the appropriate nucleoside diphosphate sugar pyrophosphorylase and nucleoside triphosphate as in:

$$\text{D-glucose-1-phosphate} + \text{UTP} \rightarrow \text{UDP-D-glucose} + \text{PP}_i$$
UDP-glucose pyrophosphorylase

The reaction is irreversible and the pyrophosphorylases are specific both for the hexose phosphate and for the nucleoside triphosphate. A wide variety of 'sugar nucleotides' are found in microbial cells, but the function of some of them remains obscure; most cells contain UDP-glucose, UDP-*N*-acetyl-D-glucosamine and GDP-mannose. The role of sugar nucleotides in polymer synthesis is understandable when one considers that hydrolysis of one mole of the glucose phosphate bond of UDP-D-glucose yields 7.6 kcal. By contrast, hydrolysis of the phosphate bond of α-D-glucose-1-phosphate yields only 4.8 kcal.

The nucleoside diphosphate monosaccharides serve two purposes in the microbial cell; they provide a mechanism for the

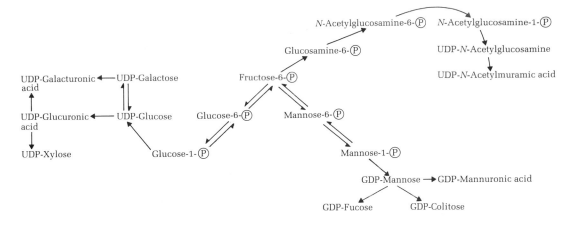

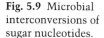

Fig. 5.9 Microbial interconversions of sugar nucleotides.

interconversion of certain monosaccharides and they are the glycosyl donors needed for the formation of polysaccharides and other carbohydrate-containing macromolecules. The glycosyl moiety of the sugar nucleotides can be transformed by a variety of mechanisms, some of which are confined to prokaryotes (Fig. 5.9).

1 *Epimerization* of carbon atom 4 (C4) converts UDP-D-glucose to UDP-D-galactose in the presence of *UDP-galactose-4-epimerase*. Correspondingly, UDP-D-glucuronic acid, UDP-N-acetyl-D-glucosamine and UDP-D-arabinose are epimerized by specific enzymes to UDP-D-galacturonic acid, UDP-N-acetyl-D-galactosamine and UDP-D-xylose respectively. These reactions are all reversible. The cofactor in these reactions is NAD^+; it is probable that the sugar is first oxidized then reduced at the C4 position.

2 *Oxidation*: Uronic acids are formed from the corresponding neutral hexose by oxidation at the C6 position of the sugar nucleotide:

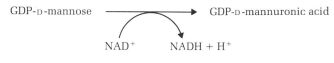

GDP-mannose dehydrogenase

3 *Decarboxylation*: The pentose xylose, in the form of UDP-xylose, is normally formed by the decarboxylation of UDP-D-glucuronic acid. Although this reaction is found in a number of bacterial species, it is more common in yeasts and other eukaryotic microorganisms. This is as yet the only known mechanism for the formation of 'activated' pentoses other than pentose phosphates.

4 One of the reactions which is confined to prokaryotes, and moreover absent from the archaebacteria, is that by which UDP-N-acetyl-D-glucosamine combines with phosphoenolpyruvate to yield UDP-N-acetyl-D-muramic acid, the precursor of the muramic acid pentapeptide involved in eubacterial peptidoglycan biosynthesis (Chapter 6):

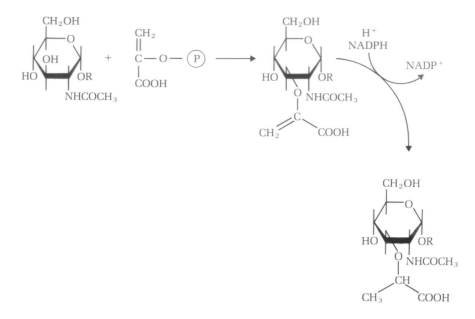

5 The common deoxysugars L-fucose and L-rhamnose are formed from GDP-D-mannose and TDP-D-glucose respectively. The hexose portion of the sugar nucleotide loses a molecule of water to form an intermediate which is oxidized in the presence of NAD^+ to give a nucleoside diphosphate 5-keto-6-deoxyhexose. Further rearrangement leads to the formation of the L-6-deoxyhexoses. Similar mechanisms are involved in the formation of the 3,6-dideoxyhexoses—tyvelose, abequose, paratose and colitose—which are found exclusively in the lipopolysaccharides of certain Gram-negative bacteria, predominantly members of the Enterobacteriaceae.

While most sugar nucleotides are nucleoside diphosphate sugars, the precursor for *ketodeoxyoctonic acid* (KDO) in lipopolysaccharides (and in a small number of exopolysaccharides) is CMP-KDO, and that for sialic acids (found in extracellular polysaccharides of some *E. coli* strains and of *Neisseria meningitidis*) is CMP-sialic acid.

The nutritional requirements of microorganisms vary greatly. Some microorganisms are very exacting, while others can synthesize all their metabolic needs from a minimal medium containing a single carbon source and essential salts.

Pathways for monomer synthesis are very similar from one group of organisms to another, one exception being lysine biosynthesis. Differences have, however, evolved in the way various groups of organisms regulate these pathways, particularly the branched pathways, and these are discussed in Chapter 7. The wide diversity of biosyntheses carried out by microorganisms makes generalization difficult, but the following observations can be made:

1 Most of the pathways require activation of intermediates and therefore expenditure of energy.

2 In lipid synthesis and monosaccharide formation in particular, the intermediates are activated not only for synthetic reactions, but also for interconversions such as desaturation, isomerization, epimerization or oxidation.

3 The presence of a monomeric constituent of a microbial macromolecule does not imply that the microorganism can utilize the monomer. More probably, it is formed from other substrates through a metabolic pathway.

6 Polymer synthesis and metabolism

In Chapter 1, we have seen that more than half of the dry mass of the cell is composed of proteins and carbohydrate-containing polymers. In microbial cells polymers are required for a wide variety of functions. DNA acts as the information storage molecule; peptidoglycan in eubacteria, and cellulose, mannans, glucans and chitin in algae and fungi, have structural roles in providing mechanical strength and resistance to osmotic lysis. Glycogen, poly-β-hydroxybutyrate and polyphosphate act as storage polymers which maintain substrates in a form less accessible to degradative enzymes, as well as exerting reduced osmotic pressure. Other polymers have been adapted in the course of evolution to a variety of functions.

Certain proteins, such as some in ribosomes, may be structural in function, as are several in the outer membrane of the Gram-negative cell, although most are enzymes with specific catalytic activity. Other proteins function in the transport of molecules across cell membranes, while some provide the cell with a means of locomotion or of internal movement of its structures. Diversity of function is best illustrated by RNA, which plays intermediary (mRNA), adaptor (tRNA) and scaffolding (rRNA) roles in protein synthesis.

There are too many polymers in the cell to consider each one in detail; the following discussion is mainly concerned with those polymers involved in the storage and expression of genetic information, since they are of fundamental importance to the cell, and their synthesis is currently of considerable interest in genetic manipulation for commercial purposes. Also included are polysaccharides since some of these (the cell envelope polymers and cell surface antigens) are of importance in medicine or are of commercial value (e.g. *Haemophilus influenzae* capsular polysaccharide, dextrans and xanthans).

Structure of polymers

In chemical terms, microbial polymers can be classified as *homopolymers*, composed of a single repeated subunit, and *heteropolymers*, composed of a number of different subunits. Few homopolymers are found in microorganisms; they include bacterial or yeast glycogen, levans, dextrans and sialic acids, poly-β-hydroxybutyrate and poly-D-glutamate, polyphosphate and the glucans and mannans of fungal cell walls. Heteropolymers are more common; they include many polysaccharides, peptidoglycan and all proteins and nucleic acids. The sequence of monomers in heteropolymers can be of two types. There may be a repeating group of subunits, as in most polysaccharides and in peptidoglycan. For extracellular polysaccharides, these vary from disaccharides to hexasaccharides, while the backbone chain of peptidoglycan is a repeating unit of *N*-acetylmuramyl-1,4-β-*N*-acetylglucosamine. Repeating units of relatively small size may be essential in polymers formed external to the cell membrane. The alternative type of polymer, found in proteins and nucleic acids, has an ordered structure without repeating units. In these, the monomer order is determined by a genetic template.

For many polymers, the three-dimensional arrangement of the subunit monomers is important. Thus peptidoglycan consists of a relatively rigid polysaccharide backbone crosslinked by short peptide chains effectively forming an extended network of high strength, which maintains the shape of the bacterial cell. In bacterial spores, this crosslinking is much reduced, leaving free many ionized groups on the peptide. These may play an important role in maintaining the resistance and dormancy of the endospore.

The molecular architecture of proteins is fundamental to their activity. The primary sequence of amino acids adopts a secondary structure of helical and non-helical regions. These are then organized into a tertiary structure in which ionic, hydrophobic and covalent bonds all play some part. For some enzymes the tertiary structure is sufficient to provide the correct environment for catalysis; in others, a quaternary structure is necessary. In most cases, the tertiary structure of a polypeptide is that most favoured thermodynamically and is adopted spontaneously; in others there are proteins called *chaperonins* which assist the folding process. For other polymers, synthesis of the three-dimensional form depends on a pre-existing framework. A good example is peptidoglycan, which is synthesized by additions of disaccharide-pentapeptide units to the terminal groups of available peptidoglycan; complete removal of the cell wall peptidoglycan of a Gram-positive cell using lysozyme prevents the regeneration of new wall material by the protoplast so formed.

General characteristics of polymer metabolism

While the diversity of polymers implies variety in mechanisms for their synthesis, there are a number of general characteristics common to most:

1 Macromolecular synthesis is a highly endergonic (energy-requiring) process. In most cases, energy is derived from the hydrolysis of high-energy bonds; the substrates either contain these (as in ATP for RNA synthesis) or are activated prior to the polymerization step.

2 A requirement for a mechanism initiating polymerization. This may involve a primer molecule.

3 Once initiated, the polymer needs to be elongated by the addition of subunits.

4 A requirement for termination processes.
5 A template is needed for those heteropolymers with ordered, non-repeating subunits, to specify the correct monomer arrangement.

Another common characteristic of many microbial polymers is their susceptibility to rapid breakdown as well as synthesis. For example, growth requires controlled lysis of wall components to enable insertion of new growing points. When cells face starvation, they can selectively degrade some of their proteins and RNA to provide energy of maintenance of the cell. A molecule in a dynamic state, due to synthesis and degradation acting simultaneously, is undergoing turnover. In general, synthesis and degradation are distinct processes with different sets of enzymes responsible. Furthermore, associated with this ease of breakdown of polymers, there must be either 'compartmentation' to separate the polymers from degradative enzymes, or the enzymes must be inhibited or regulated in such a way that they only act under certain conditions. For proteolytic enzymes, this is achieved in part by the presence of specific inhibitors—proteins which bind to the proteases and maintain them in an inactive state.

DNA

The metabolic fates of DNA must mainly be considered in terms of its function as the repository of the total genetic potential of the cell. When a cell divides, its complete set of genetic information must also be duplicated and must segregate in synchrony with the cell division process. The process of duplicating the genetic information is DNA replication. Its coordination with cell division is discussed in Chapter 8.

Another process of considerable importance is DNA repair, since errors and chemical damage can occur either spontaneously or, more particularly, under extreme environmental conditions (e.g. single-strand breaks occur at high temperatures; dimer formation between adjacent bases is induced by ultraviolet radiation). These defects could lead to loss of cell viability unless efficiently repaired. Genetic recombination is a third process which involves considerable enzymic modification of DNA. In eukaryotes, recombination is an essential feature of sexual reproduction, occurring just prior to meiotic division; in prokaryotes, sexual processes are not common, but recombination mechanisms are involved in at least one type of repair system.

The above processes are all concerned with maintaining the integrity of the cell's DNA. There are also enzyme systems which function to degrade DNA—these are concerned with such processes as the defence of the cell against incoming foreign DNA as, for example, when a bacteriophage injects its nucleic acid into the bacterial cell. This latter process is part of the host cell 'restriction' system and some of the so-called *restriction enzymes* are important tools in the *in vitro* genetic manipulation of DNA. This leads to yet another DNA alteration process used by both the host bacterium and sometimes by the bacteriophage. This is the modification of DNA to prevent its degradation by restriction enzymes.

DNA structure

DNA species are linear heteropolymers composed of the four main deoxyribonucleotide subunits dATP, dGTP, dCTP and dTTP linked by phosphodiester bonds between the 3'- and 5'-positions of the deoxyribose moieties. In most natural systems, it is present as a double-stranded duplex with the two chains arranged in an antiparallel way in a double helix. This arrangement is made possible by the specific base pairing properties of adenine with thymine and guanine with cytosine as illustrated in Fig. 6.1. DNA molecules are very long; the intact *Escherichia coli* chromosome has a relative molecular mass of about 2.5×10^9 and is about $1100\,\mu m$ long. With the advent of restriction enzymes capable of cutting DNA into fragments of specific length, it has become customary to measure the length of DNA fragments in terms of base pairs (bp). One thousand base pairs (1 kbp) is equivalent to a relative molecular mass of about 2.4×10^5; it has a length of about $0.34\,\mu m$, and can encode 333 amino acids.

Supercoiling

Double-stranded DNA molecules often exist in bacterial cells in a circular form, or in eukaryotes in a form in which they are constrained within a complex structure. Under these circumstances, in which rotation of the free ends is not possible, they can adopt a tertiary structure in which a greater, or lesser, number of turns are introduced into the helix than would normally be the case. This often leads to a supercoiling of the molecule, as illustrated in Fig. 6.2. Nicking either strand in a supercoiled struc-

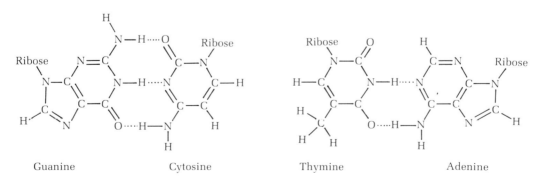

Fig. 6.1 Pairing of bases in nucleic acids.

(a)   nick   (b)   (c)

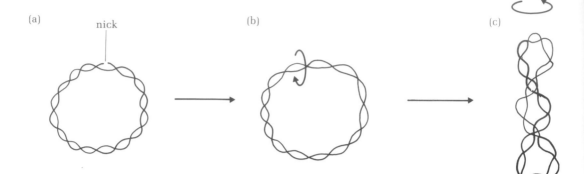

Fig. 6.2 Supercoiling of
DNA. (a) Open circle:
'nicked DNA' (cut in
one strand) is in a
relaxed state; (b)
introduction of twists
reducing turns, and
resealing leads to
torsion in the molecule
(note two less turns); (c)
molecule twists on
itself to relieve tension,
supercoiled form of
closed circle.

ture will lead to free rotation of the strands and a return to the
relaxed state.

Major differences exist between prokaryotes and eukaryotes in
the arrangement, replication and segregation of their DNA, and
these aspects are best considered separately for the two groups of
microorganisms.

Prokaryotic DNA structure and replication

In most bacterial species that have been examined in sufficient
detail by genetic or physical mapping methods, there is normally
one type of circular chromosome of circumference about 1–2 mm,
although several smaller circular DNA plasmids may also be present (see p. 32). However, in the photosynthetic bacterium
Rhodobacter sphaeroides there are two distinct chromosomes.

This bacterial chromosome is not contained within a nuclear
membrane and the DNA is not complexed with basic histone proteins as is found in eukaryotes (p. 145). There are, however, some
basic proteins complexed with the DNA and careful extraction
techniques using buffers containing Mg^{2+} can give a 'nucleoid' of
condensed DNA with its associated proteins.

Since the bacterial genome is a double-stranded completely
closed molecule, its replication is rather more complicated than
might at first be expected. In *E. coli*, the products of at least 14
genes participate. Replication begins from a single region of the
chromosome, the *origin*, and proceeds bidirectionally from the
origin to a *terminus* region. The resultant replication intermediate, a three-armed closed loop structure with two loops of
equal length, has been visualized by autoradiography (Fig. 6.3). The
bacterial chromosome is attached to the cell membrane at several
points: this plays an important role in the segregation of the
replicated chromosomes into the daughter cells formed by cell
division (see Chapter 8), and it seems that both the origin and
the points at which DNA replication occurs are attached to the
membrane.

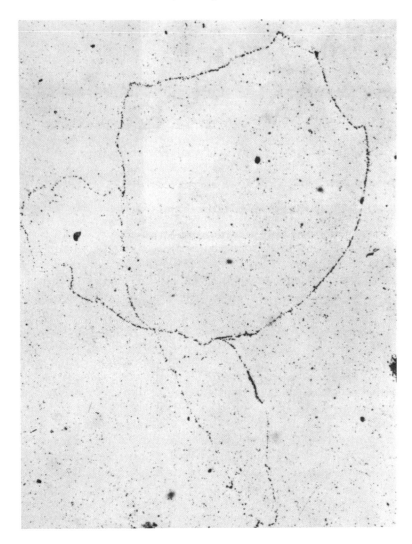

Fig. 6.3 Autoradiograph of the replicating *Escherichia coli* chromosome from a cell labelled with [³H]-thymidine for two generations. (Courtesy of Dr Cairns and the Cold Spring Harbor Laboratory.)

Replication initiation

The rate at which bacterial DNA is synthesized is relatively constant despite wide variations in the growth rate of cells, and hence much of the control of replication is exerted at initiation (see Chapter 8 for the coordination of DNA replication with cell division). The process is complex and not fully understood. It requires a defined sequence of bases (the origin in *E. coli* is defined by the *oriC* locus) and the involvement of several proteins (possibly the products of the *dnaA, dnaB, dnaC, dnaI* and *dnaP* loci) which may form a complex located on the membrane. At least one of these needs to be synthesized shortly before initiation can occur, since the process is sensitive to inhibitors of protein synthesis such as chloramphenicol. Since none of the DNA polymerases that have been isolated are able to initiate semiconservative replication without some form of primer on the template strand to be copied, there is an apparent requirement for a small amount of RNA synthesis to produce this primer. This is accomplished not by the RNA polymerase responsible for transcription, but by a *primase* (product of the *dnaG* gene) which can polymerize deoxyribonucleotides as well as ribonucleotides. The primer is then used by the DNA polymerase to extend replication against the complementary strand. This leaves some RNA which must be removed by an *endonuclease*. There is therefore a requirement for another DNA polymerase to fill the gap that is left, and a DNA ligase enzyme to seal the nick in the newly replicated strand.

DNA synthesis at the replication fork

In those few bacteria examined in sufficient detail there are at least three DNA polymerases (I to III in *E. coli*), all of which can only polymerize nucleotide triphosphates in the 5′ → 3′ direction. DNA is, however, antiparallel, having one strand with 5′ → 3′ polarity and the other with 3′ → 5′. Thus at the replication fork, only one of the two complementary strands can be read in the same direction as that in which replication is proceeding. On the other hand, it is known from autoradiography that recently replicated DNA does not have long single-stranded regions. This problem is overcome by DNA polymerase III (the replication polymerase; in *E. coli* coded by the *dnaE* or *polC* gene) on the antiparallel strand polymerizing in fairly short steps away from the replication fork as shown in Fig. 6.4. This generates short pieces of newly synthesized DNA, known as 'Okazaki fragments'. Again the primase and several 'prepriming proteins' are involved in primer synthesis.

Since replication takes place on a double helical template, there is a requirement to unwind the DNA strands, to relieve the superhelical turns introduced, and to separate and stabilize the single-stranded regions behind the growing replication fork. Unwinding of DNA at the replication fork involves the action of enzymes known as *helicases*, which catalyse the process at the expense of ATP hydrolysis. Several ATPases of this type have been isolated from *E. coli*; that involved in replication is the helicase II (product of the *rep* gene). One helicase molecule will progressively unwind DNA, one base pair at a time, utilizing ATP hydrolysis to provide energy. Stabilization of the single-stranded DNA behind the replication fork also apparently requires the binding of a number of 'single-stranded DNA binding protein' (SSB) molecules.

To relieve the additional turns in the DNA introduced by this unwinding requires the addition of negative superhelical turns in double-stranded DNA ahead of the replication fork. This is catalysed by the enzyme DNA gyrase, which has two subunits encoded by *gyrB* (coumermycin resistance) and *gyrA* genes in *E. coli*. This enzyme works by transiently cutting both strands of the

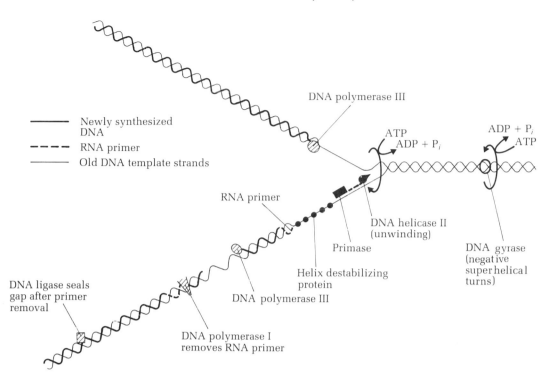

Fig. 6.4 Bacterial DNA replication.

DNA duplex and reforming them, and requires ATP hydrolysis when counteracting the positive supercoiling of DNA induced by helicase. Gyrase is inhibited by the antimicrobial agents nalidixic acid and coumermycin.

DNA polymerases

There are three DNA polymerases in *E. coli* (DNA polymerases I to III) of which enzyme III is responsible for the replication from the RNA primer. All three enzymes are alike in their ability to synthesize DNA in the $5' \rightarrow 3'$ direction only, from an RNA primer against a $3' \rightarrow 5'$ template strand. They also possess a $3' \rightarrow 5'$ exonuclease activity which has an important function in proof-reading to remove mistakes. This enzyme works by transiently cutting both strands of the DNA duplex and reforming them. This requires ATP hydrolysis when counteracting positive supercoiling of DNA is induced by helicase. If an incorrect base is inserted, the enzyme cannot polymerize further, but moves backwards and the nuclease removes the error. This reduces the error in replication from an estimated 1 mismatch per 10^5 nucleotides to 1 per 10^{10}.

DNA polymerase I has an additional $5' \rightarrow 3'$ exonuclease activity, and this enzyme functions to remove the RNA primer and fill the gap by its polymerase activity. The 'nick' left after this is sealed by DNA ligase (*lig* gene) which in bacteria uses NAD^+ to provide the energy needed for the reaction.

Overall, the rate of replication is very rapid—of the order of $1.5\,kb\,s^{-1}$—so that the *E. coli* genome is replicated in about 40 min. At present, little is known about what happens when replication reaches the termination site.

Eukaryotic replication

Structure of eukaryotic chromosomes

The eukaryotic chromosome is a linear structure with a number of important structural elements concerned with its stability, its organization in space, its replication and its segregation during mitosis. The important functional elements are: centromeres, which are the sites of spindle attachment during segregation of chromosomes at mitosis or meiosis; telomeres, which are the terminal regions conferring stability on the linear form; and replication origins from which DNA replication commences. All three of these elements have now been cloned—centromeres (*CEN* regions) from *Saccharomyces*; autonomously replicating sequences (*ARS*) from a number of microorganisms, including *Saccharomyces* and *Schizosaccharomyces*; and telomere regions (*TEL*) from *Tetrahymena* and *Saccharomyces*. Figure 6.5 illustrates the main features of these structural elements from *Saccharomyces cerevisiae*. Yeast artificial chromosomes (YACs) which can func-

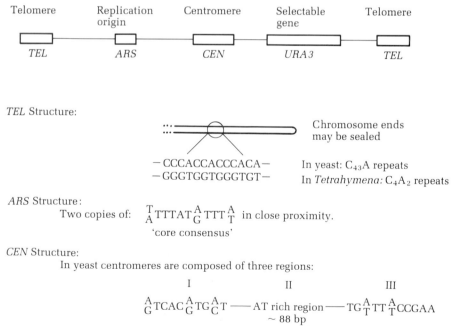

Fig. 6.5 Essential features of a eukaryotic chromosome. The diagram is based on genetic elements used to construct artificial chromosomes which segregate normally during mitosis and meiosis in the yeast host.

tion in yeast mitosis and meiosis in almost the same way as natural chromosomes, have been made *in vitro* by combining these three elements with sufficient DNA inserted to give a reasonable length. These are very useful cloning vectors for very large fragments of DNA (e.g. from human genome).

Eukaryotic DNA is also organized into the chromosome in a very different way from that in bacteria. The eukaryotic chromosome can undergo different degrees of condensation depending on the stage of the cell in its division cycle. Even in its least condensed form, during prophase, the DNA is still highly condensed relative to its linear sequence of bases. Much of this arrangement is brought about by its association with the strongly basic histone proteins. In higher eukaryotes, there are five main types

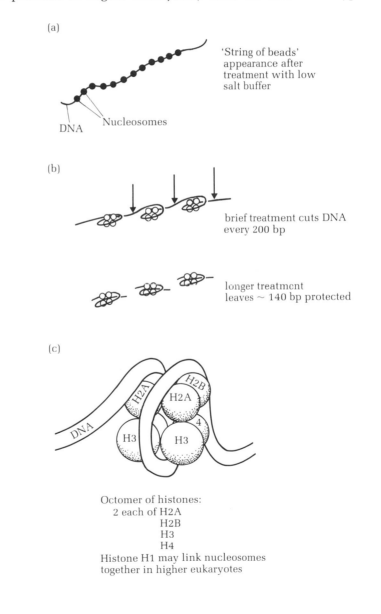

(a)

'String of beads' appearance after treatment with low salt buffer

DNA   Nucleosomes

(b)

brief treatment cuts DNA every 200 bp

longer treatment leaves ~ 140 bp protected

(c)

DNA   H2A   H2B   H2A   4   H3   H3

Octomer of histones:
2 each of H2A
H2B
H3
H4
Histone H1 may link nucleosomes together in higher eukaryotes

Fig. 6.6 Chromatin structure. (a) Chromatin under electron microscope: nucleosomes; (b) after treatment with DNase; (c) model of nucleosome.

of histone—histones 1, 2A, 2B, 3 and 4; in the only microbial eukaryotes examined in detail, these are all present except histone 1. When isolated in buffers of low ionic strength, eukaryotic chromosomes have a characteristic 'string of beads' appearance in the electron microscope. Each 'bead' is termed a nucleosome. This structure is composed of the DNA strand wound around the outside of a complex of eight proteins, two of each of the histones 2A, 2B, 3 and 4 (Fig. 6.6). Nucleosomes are spaced about every 140 bp along the DNA, and this arrangement has many implications with regard to the replication of the DNA and the control of gene expression. Experimentally, the arrangement can be demonstrated by studying the sensitivity of isolated chromatin (DNA carefully extracted to maintain histone binding) to endonuclease activity; the regions between nucleosomes are particularly sensitive to cleavage by the nuclease. Even this extensive coiling cannot account for the condensation of DNA in the typical eukaryotic cell, and there are even higher levels of coiling of the nucleosomes.

Eukaryotic replication mechanism

In bacteria, replication proceeds at a rate of about 1000 monomers/sed^{-1}. Eukaryotic microorganisms, on the other hand, replicate at about one tenth of this rate, and even the simplest contain at least five to ten times as much DNA as *E. coli*. Despite this, some can, under optimal conditions, duplicate their DNA in roughly the same time as *E. coli*. They accomplish this by having multiple replication origins on each chromosome, such that during DNA synthesis there are many replication forks active at any one time. This has been visualized by autoradiography in higher eukaryotes, and by direct electron microscopy in yeast (Fig. 6.7). Replication from each origin is bidirectional, with adjacent origins located between 15 and 70 μm apart. In yeasts, this corresponds to about 5–20 origins on an average-sized chromosome. The *ARS* elements discussed above were identified by their ability to increase the frequency with which circular plasmids containing a selectable marker could be transformed successfully and maintained with some degree of stability in yeast. They probably represent origins or potential origins of replication. While there is as yet no definite proof of this, the number of *ARS* sequences obtained in random screening of the yeast genome was consistent with the expected number of origins (about 400) from direct electron microscopic measurement of replicon size.

The rate of replication is controlled by the frequency of initiation rather than by the rate of propagation of a replication fork or termination of synthesis. Unlike bacteria, the eukaryotic cell always completes a round of replication of its chromosomes before starting another round, and DNA synthesis occurs in a discrete phase (the S phase) of the cell division cycle.

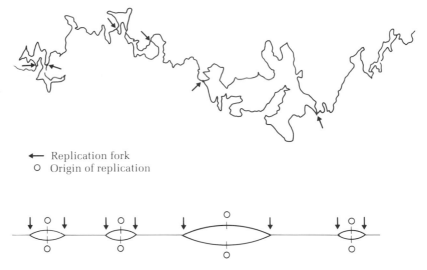

Fig. 6.7 Yeast DNA in the process of replication. Direct tracing of an electron micrograph and a diagrammatic representation are shown. (From Peters, Newton, Byres & Fangman (1973) *Cold Spring Harbor Symp. Quantitative Biology* **38**, 9.)

← Replication fork
○ Origin of replication

Once initiated, the molecular mechanism of DNA replication resembles that found in prokaryotes, although there are some differences associated with the requirement for dissociation of the histones as the replication fork moves.

Other replication processes

It should be emphasized that we have only dealt with two of the possible modes of DNA replication. Other mechanisms have been found to occur in bacteriophage development and in DNA-containing eukaryotic organelles such as the mitochondrion. One example of a different mechanism is seen with bacteriophage T4 of *E. coli*. This is the 'rolling circle' model, in which a nick is introduced in the circular replicative form of the phage DNA, with replication proceeding around the circle as outlined in Fig. 6.8. This leads to a long concatamer containing many copies of the phage genome. T4 codes for an enzyme which cuts this concatamer into pieces which are larger than one complete phage genome. The pieces are then included within the developing phage

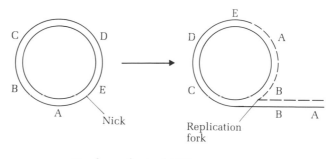

Fig. 6.8 Rolling circle model for replication of bacteriophage T4 DNA.

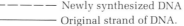

– – – – – Newly synthesized DNA
——— Original strand of DNA.

particles. This means that the virus particles differ from each other in the order of genes on their DNA, but all have a complete set of genes. Other viruses adopt yet other replication strategies. Rolling circle replication also occurs during the transfer of DNA from an Hfr strain of *E. coli* to an F⁻ strain during conjugation.

Modification of DNA in prokaryotes and eukaryotes

DNA repair

There are a number of ways in which DNA is modified after replication has occurred. Most of these processes are concerned with the cell's defence against agents which can damage DNA and therefore prevent the cell from producing viable progeny. For example, when DNA is exposed to ultraviolet light of a wavelength around 260 nm, adjacent pyrimidine bases can form dimers (thymine–thymine being the most common) as indicated in Fig. 6.9. These dimers cannot base pair correctly and hence, unless they are removed from the DNA in some way, they will seriously affect the cell at the next round of replication. Several mechanisms for removal of these dimers are discussed below.

Most microorganisms also possess repair mechanisms to deal with other damage which may arise from: mistakes in base pairing during replication; strand breakage after exposure to ionizing radiations (X- and γ-rays); crosslinkage of DNA strands due to chemical mutagens such as psoralens or mitomycin C; or base mismatches formed by the action of mutagens which modify nucleotides (e.g. by methylation) or which act as abnormal bases and are inserted during replication (2-aminopurine, 5-bromodeoxyuridine).

There are clearly a number of different processes needed to repair such a wide variety of types of damage. In both prokaryotes and eukaryotes, there are multiple repair pathways which have been dissected in some detail by isolating and characterizing mutants defective in repair. For example, in *E. coli* and yeast, there are at least five such pathways. All of these pathways depend on enzymes capable of modifying DNA. In some cases, these are also involved in replication, as is true for DNA ligase activity. In *E. coli* there are two DNA polymerases in addition to the replication enzyme specified by *polC*. One of these (DNA polymerase I) is specially adapted to a repair function since it not only polymerizes

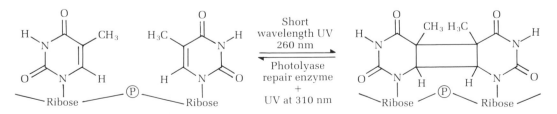

Fig. 6.9 Thymine–thymine dimers formed by exposure of DNA to short-wavelength UV.

DNA in the $5' \rightarrow 3'$ direction against a single-strand template, but it also possesses a $5' \rightarrow 3'$ exonuclease activity which can begin excising nucleotides from one strand of DNA (at a nick in the DNA introduced at the damage site by a specific endonuclease). This enzyme may therefore degrade one strand of the DNA and resynthesize it against the other strand as template.

The main mechanisms for repair found in *E. coli* include those which directly reverse the damage without the need to synthesize any new phosphodiester bonds. Others involve cutting, degradation, resynthesis and ligation. Pathways for repair differ in the extent to which mistakes are made in restoring the original base sequence. They are therefore of interest to the microbial geneticist concerned with mutation and are frequently classified in terms of whether they are 'error-prone' or 'error-free'. The main repair pathways of *E. coli* are outlined in Fig. 6.10, and considered below.

Photoreactivation. Some microorganisms have a photoreactivation enzyme which can recognize pyrimidine dimers formed by ultraviolet (UV) light and use the energy of a photon of wavelength around 300 nm to split the dimer. This direct repair pathway is error-free, hence the need to incubate UV-treated strains in the dark when attempting to induce mutants.

Demethylation. This pathway is specific to the removal of the methyl group from O^6-methylguanine by transfer to the enzyme O^6-alkylguanine transferase. This is a direct and an accurate process removing lesions which are potentially very mutagenic, and it appears to be induced by treatment of cells with alkylating agents.

Excision repair. This pathway (Fig. 6.10) is defective in certain UV-sensitive strains (*uvrA, uvrB* and *uvrC*), and it depends on an endonuclease complex which can recognize base mismatches. This nicks one strand of the DNA and DNA polymerase I then excises a run of bases from the free 5' end and also resynthesizes DNA against the other strand. This leaves a gap which is sealed by DNA ligase activity. The endonuclease is a multi-subunit complex determined by the three *uvr* genes, and it is induced by exposure to UV light.

This excision pathway is relatively free from errors. Excision can also be initiated by the action of DNA glycosylases, which can remove incorrect bases from the sugar phosphate backbone of DNA by hydrolysis of the *N*-glycoside bond.

Postreplication repair. This class of repair process (Fig. 6.10) involves recombination between intact duplex DNA and damaged DNA. This process appears to be a mechanism whereby cells can repair damage when DNA replication forks have advanced beyond a lesion. When the replication polymerase meets a base mismatch

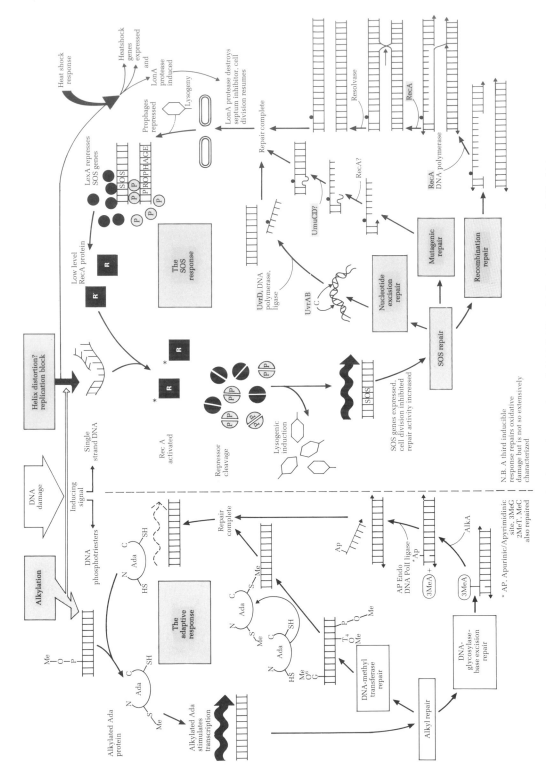

Fig. 6.10 DNA repair mechanisms in *Escherichia coli*. (Redrawn from Sedgwick (1986) *Microbiological Sciences* **3**, 76–83.)

or a thymine–thymine dimer, it pauses then eventually leaves a gap opposite the damaged strand.

Without a recombinational repair process, there is no way of restoring the original sequence. This process is defective in *rec* mutants of *E. coli*. It can, in principle, be error-free, but since *recA* mutants are UV-sensitive but not UV-mutable, whereas the wild-type cells are mutable by UV, the operation of this pathway can be error-prone. Mutation can occur when the postreplication system tries to repair two sites of damage located close to each other on opposite strands; overlapping gaps are formed and there is no way by which the cell can reconstruct one of the lesions with accuracy. An inducible enzyme inserts a random base opposite the lesion with only a one in four chance of being correct.

The SOS system. Most of these repair mechanisms are inducible by damage to DNA. For repair mediated by the *uvr* and *rec* genes, this is referred to as SOS regulation. The SOS system is very interesting since the control acts on a number of functions in the cell, including cell division. It appears to be a major response on the part of the cell to any treatment or injury that leads to the generation of single-stranded regions of DNA. The SOS control process is illustrated in Fig. 6.10, from which it can be seen that the products of two main genes—*recA* and *lexA*—control the expression of a large number of other genes, mostly concerned with repair of DNA.

The *recA* gene product has a proteolytic activity which is activated by damaged DNA, possibly single-stranded regions. This leads to degradation of the *lexA* gene product, which is a repressor preventing transcription of its own gene and about 17 others, including that for the *recA* protein. Thus as damage is repaired by the various *lexA*-controlled mechanisms, the system tends to return to the normal state in which most of the SOS system is repressed since the level of *lexA* repressor increases.

This is one example of a general response to conditions damaging the cell. A similar situation is seen in the *heat-shock* response of cells to heat and other forms of stress. These systems are found in a broad spectrum of organisms other than *E. coli*, including Gram-negative genera such as *Salmonella*, *Proteus*, *Haemophilus*, *Bacteroides* and *Rhizobium*, the Gram-positive *Bacillus*, and eukaryotes from *Saccharomyces* up to mammals.

Recombination

Genetic recombination is a process of considerable importance in genetic analysis, since it forms the basis of all *in vivo* genetic exchange. It involves the replacement of one sequence of a double-stranded DNA molecule by another, which is usually homologous. It is much more common in eukaryotes, occurring at high frequency during the sexual process of meiosis, but also to a small

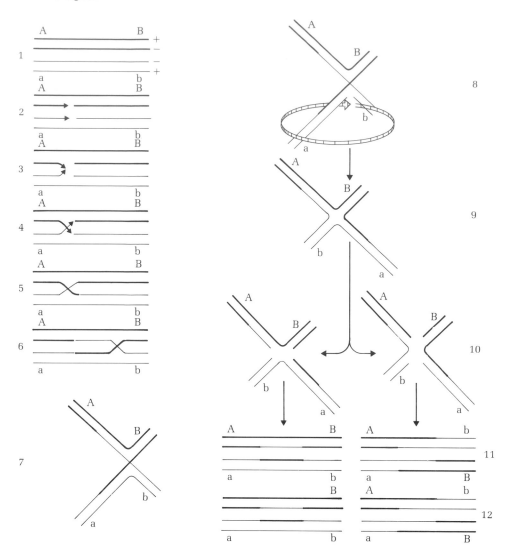

extent during normal cell division by mitosis. In bacteria, it does occur during such processes as conjugation and transformation, and also in the integration of temperate phage genomes into the host chromosome. During meiosis in higher eukaryotes, it is usually reciprocal, involving exchanges between intact chromosomes.

The precise mechanism of recombination is not known. Many models have been proposed; one of the most recent is outlined in Fig. 6.11. This takes into account most of the features of the process. For example, it is clear that it involves breakage and reunion of DNA strands. The currently favoured view is that recombination is initiated by a single-strand break formed by an endonuclease. This strand invades the homologous region of the other DNA double helix and anneals to form a heteroduplex. Some

Fig. 6.11 Model for the mechanism of reciprocal DNA recombination. (Redrawn from Mandelstam *et al.* (1982) *Biochemistry of Bacterial Growth.*)

DNA degradation and resynthesis occurs in the region of this heteroduplex and eventually an isomerization of the structure is formed and ligation leads to crossover. This branch can migrate for some distance and be resolved eventually in one of several ways. Note that a crossover can isomerize to give a chi structure and this can be cut by an endonuclease to yield either reciprocal or non-reciprocal recombination in the region of the exchange. Such chi structures have been visualized by electron microscopy; there is genetic evidence that around the site of the crossover during reciprocal recombination, there is often a region in which gene conversion (a non-reciprocal exchange) occurs. Some of the enzymes needed for DNA repair pathways are involved in recombination, so that in yeast, some *rad* mutations causing defective repair lead to defective meiotic recombination, and in *E. coli* *recA* mutations affect many recombination processes.

Restriction and modification

Bacteria are capable of modifying their DNA as part of a defence system designed to repel invasion by foreign DNA injected by a bacteriophage. This involves a two part system in which the bacterial cell produces a *restriction endonuclease* that can degrade intact double-stranded DNA by recognizing a particular sequence of bases and cutting both strands of the duplex. The host protects its own genome by specific methylation of bases within the recognition sequence; this is the process of modification. Clearly, this is an efficient form of protection and explains the high degree of specificity of both restriction and modification enzymes.

Type I restriction enzymes recognize a specific sequence of bases, but they cut randomly in the vicinity of this site, whereas type II enzymes recognize a specific target, usually a 4-, 5- or 6-base palindromic sequence and cut very specifically in that sequence. In many cases, the cuts are symmetrically staggered and generate *cohesive ends*, as illustrated in Fig. 6.12. Most type II

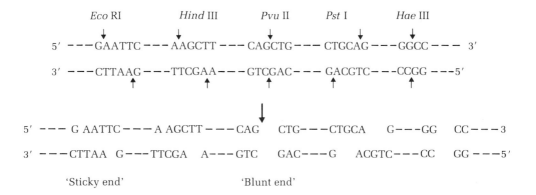

Fig. 6.12 Sequence specificity and cutting pattern of some restriction endonucleases.

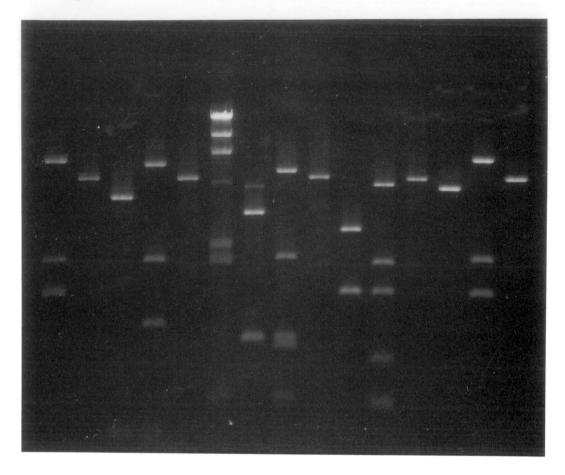

restriction endonucleases produce 5'-protruding ends, some produce 'blunt' ends, and a few, 3'-protruding ends.

The type II restriction enzymes are of fundamental importance for *in vitro* genetic manipulation, since they can be used to cut DNA from any source, e.g. from a mammalian cell, into fragments of defined length with specific sticky ends. These ends can anneal with those from any other DNA molecules cut by the same restriction endonucleases (e.g. bacterial plasmid vector DNA) or by another generating the same sticky ends, and following treatment with DNA ligase, a recombinant DNA molecule is obtained. In the example given, this can be used to infect the bacterial host with a vector carrying a piece of mammalian DNA.

Restriction enzymes can also be used to physically map regions of DNA. The recognition sites for these enzymes occur randomly in any particular DNA sequence. For those enzymes recognizing six bases, these sites may be an average of about 4 kb apart. Treatment of a particular sequence of DNA, for example a plasmid vector carrying an inserted 'foreign' gene, will generate specific fragments which can be sized accurately by agarose gel electrophoresis (see Fig. 6.13). By treating this DNA with several

Fig. 6.13 Restriction digestion pattern of plasmids treated with *Eco IR*. The fragments were separated by electrophoresis on a 0.7% agarose gel containing ethidium bromide and visualized under UV by the fluorescence of DNA associated with the dye.

enzymes, and combinations of them, a restriction map can be obtained giving the location of the restriction sites relative to each other and the physical distance between adjacent sites. Such maps are useful in investigating the fine structure and the sequencing of genes.

TRANSCRIPTION

RNA synthesis

The three major classes of RNA found in microorganisms differ in their size, but all participate in protein synthesis and all are synthesized in a similar way from a DNA template. The process is called *transcription* and is catalysed by the enzyme *DNA-dependent RNA polymerase*. This is an important process, since much of the control over the rate of protein synthesis is exerted at the level of mRNA transcription.

In prokaryotes, only one DNA-dependent RNA polymerase can be isolated, while in eukaryotic microorganisms three or more different enzymes can be found. This difference between eukaryotes and prokaryotes reflects a difference in the way the two groups of organisms regulate the synthesis of the various classes of RNA. In eukaryotes, one enzyme (RNA polymerase I) is specific to rRNA synthesis, another (RNA polymerase II) to mRNA synthesis and a third (RNA polymerase III) to tRNA. Yet another enzyme may be involved in the transcription of mito-chondrial genes. This obviously leads to separate control systems. In bacteria, there is also differential control, so that the rates of synthesis of rRNA, mRNA and of tRNA can vary independently, but this is achieved by a variety of control mechanisms that operate on the one enzyme (see p. 219).

These polymerases are all multimeric enzymes. In *E. coli* and other bacteria which have been examined, except the archaebacteria, gel electrophoresis under denaturing conditions shows that the enzyme is composed of at least four subunits: two alpha, one beta and one beta', which together comprise the 'core enzyme'. When the enzyme is purified gently, one or more other polypeptides are found, of which the best characterized is the sigma factor (Table 6.1).

The eukaryotic RNA polymerases have even more complicated structures with up to 13 subunits. Some of the subunits are common to all three polymerases, as is indicated in Table 6.2.

Enzyme I is concerned with rRNA synthesis, enzyme II with mRNA synthesis (which is highly sensitive *in vitro* to the mycotoxin α-amanitin) and enzyme III with the formation of tRNA and other low-molecular mass RNA species. The need for so many subunits in each of these enzymes is not yet understood and must await the successful dissociation and reconstitution of each enzyme.

156 *Chapter 6*

Table 6.1 Polypeptides of *E. coli* RNA polymerase.

Subunits	Relative molecular mass
Alpha	37 000
Beta	155 000
Beta'	145 000
Sigma	85 000

All of the above polymerases require the four ribonucleotide triphosphates ATP, CTP, GTP and UTP, double-stranded or denatured DNA to act as template, and Mg^{2+} (or Mn^{2+} for the eukaryotic enzyme II). The reaction can be represented as:

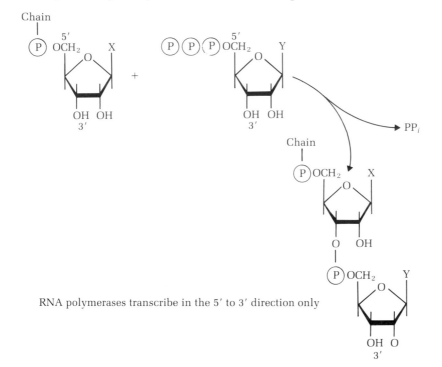

RNA polymerases transcribe in the 5' to 3' direction only

In the bacterial cell, the rate of RNA chain growth at 37°C has been estimated to be between 1000 and 2000 nucleotides min^{-1} $chain^{-1}$; there may be 5000 to 10 000 polymerase molecules per cell, which is about twice the concentration involved in RNA synthesis at any one time. For the eukaryotic enzyme II of yeast, the rate of RNA chain elongation *in vitro* approaches 1800 nucleotides min^{-1} at 30°C, which is similar to the *in vivo* rate.

In vivo RNA synthesis is a highly directed process. The transcripts, whether mRNA, rRNA or tRNA, must begin at a given point on one strand only, and finish after the correct sequence has been read. This specific transcription requires initiation and termination of polymerization at defined sites on the DNA. These

Table 6.2 Polypeptides (relative molecular mass) of RNA polymerases I, II and III of yeast.

Polymerase I	Polymerase II	Polymerase III
	220 000	
190 000		
	185 000	
		160 000
135 000		
		128 000
		82 000
		53 000
49 000		
	44 500	
43 000		
40 000		40 000
		37 000
34 500		
		34 000
	32 000	
27 000	27 000	27 000
23 000	23 000	23 000
19 000		19 000
	16 000	
14 500	14 500	14 500
14 000		
	12 600	
12 200		
		11 000
10 000	10 000	

sites delineate genes or (in bacteria) groups of genes that are co-transcribed. The mechanism of initiation is presently much better understood for bacterial systems in which purified preparations of the enzyme RNA polymerase, in the holoenzyme form, are unable to initiate or terminate transcription correctly and synthesize RNA randomly from both strands of the DNA template.

Initiation

The specificity of initiation is conferred by a protein that, under some circumstances of gentle purification, co-purifies with the core enzyme. This sigma factor interacts with the RNA polymerase, and probably also the DNA at the appropriate sites—called promoters—on the DNA template. From these sites, transcription occurs in one direction only from one (the coding) strand of the DNA template; this is termed asymmetric transcription.

Promoters have a definite structure; comparative studies of a large number of bacterial or bacteriophage promoters have indicated that within the 40 base pairs preceding the start of transcription, there are 'consensus' sequences (Fig. 6.14) which are almost, but not completely, identical from one promoter to

(a)
Consensus promoter for ordinary genes:

                    −35   −10

5′ − − − −TGTTGACAATTT− − − − − − − − − − −TATAAT− − − − − − 3′
    − − − −ACAACTGTTAAA− − − − − − − − − −ATATTA− − − − − −

compare the coding strand for several genes:

trp operon   TGTTGACAATTA − − − − − − − − − −TAACTA

lac operon   GCTTTACACTTT − − − − − − − − − − TATGTT

gal operon   TGTCACACTTTT − − − − − − − − − −TATGGT

(b)
(*i*) ρ-dependent (*cro* gene of phage λ)

                                                                                    U   A
                                                                                    U   U
5′ − − −CTATGG**TGATGCA**TTTATTTT**TGCATCA**TTCAATCAA− − 3′ DNA   U   U
   − − −GATACC**ACTACGT**AAATAAAA**ACGTAGT**AAGTTAGTT − − −   A   U
                                                                                    C   G
         |←───── dyad symmetry ─────→| G   C
                                                                                    U   A
                                                                                    A   U
RNA transcript can form a hairpin loop: G   C   note lack of run of
                                                                                    U   A   U's at terminus
                                                          − − −CUAUGG   UUCAAUCAA

(*ii*) ρ-dependent (6S RNA terminator)

RNA transcript has a run of U's at the terminus

                                                    A   G   U
                                             U   U
                                                                    U   A
                                          A   A
                                          A   U   G   A   G
                                             G   C
                                             G   C
                                             A   U
                                             C   C
                                             G   C
                                             C   U
                                             U   A   A
                                          A   G
                                             C   G
                                             A   U
                                             A   U
                                             A   U
                                             G   C
                                             C   G
                                             C   G
                                             C   G
                                             U   A
                                             A   U
                                             A   U
                                    − − − − − −U G C   U U U U A U

Fig. 6.14 Promoters and terminators in *Escherichia coli*. (a) Promoters. The numbers refer to the start of transcription at +1. The −35 region is involved in strong interactions with the sigma factor, the −10 region with the core RNA polymerase. Note that none of the three real promoters conforms exactly to the consensus sequence, the *lac* is better in the −10 region but not the −35 region, while the *trp* promoter shows the opposite effect. For biotechnological purposes a *tac* fusion promoter has been constructed to have the better features of both. (b) Terminators.

another. These include a run of six bases termed the 'recognition box', located 16 to 18 base pairs upstream of another short sequence known as the Pribnow box, which has the sequence TATPuATG in the 5′ to 3′ direction in the direction of reading. Mutations that alter these bases alter the efficiency with which transcription is initiated. The RNA polymerase holoenzyme (core plus sigma factor) forms stable complexes with promoters. When a molecule of RNA polymerase holoenzyme recognizes a promoter, a complex is formed which rapidly changes conformation to an activated state. This activation probably involves the localized melting of the double-stranded DNA and each promoter has a characteristic transition temperature at which activation occurs. Presumably weak promoters require more energy for their activation and each promoter sequence has evolved to give the appropriate rate of reading of the gene(s) that it controls.

For eukaryotic organisms, the precise mechanism of initiation is less well characterized. Studies with mutants generated by *in vitro* mutation techniques, especially those in which the level of expression of a gene has been altered by introducing defined deletions in the region preceding the start of mRNA transcription, have indicated that an extensive region prior to the start of transcription is important in determining the rate of transcription initiation. There are consensus sequences, including a run of T and A bases (in yeast, TATAAA is common), analogous to the Pribnow box in *E. coli*. These may be located as many as 100 bp before the 5' end of the mRNA and form only part of the process by which initiation is controlled (Fig. 6.15). There are indications, from work on the control of homothallism in yeast, that chromosome structure in the chromatin complex plays a part.

Initiation from tRNA genes by polymerase III is completely different, and is under the control of intragenic promoters, sequences downstream from the start of transcription.

Termination

In bacterial systems, there are two types of termination system. One of these depends on a protein (rho factor), which acts in the opposite way to the sigma factor, in that it assists the core enzyme to release from the DNA. The other type of termination does not depend on any factor. Like initiation, the termination signal is a specific sequence of bases which in a typical case is such that the RNA transcript could form a GC-rich hairpin near the 3' terminus, followed by a tail rich in U (Fig. 6.14). For rho-dependent termination, the U-rich tail is not present. Apparently the ability of the RNA to adopt the hairpin structure causes the RNA polymerase molecule to pause and this helps its release from the DNA. Termination can also play an important part in the regulation of gene expression and this is discussed later (p. 202).

In yeast, both 5S rRNA and tRNA genes possess similar structural features to those concerned with rho-dependent termination in *E. coli*; extensive twofold symmetries within the gene and a cluster of T bases on the coding strand opposite the 3' terminus of the RNA. For termination of mRNA species, there appears to be a different mechanism which may also relate to the addition of a poly(A) tail found on most mRNA species. Many yeast genes have an AT-rich sequence about 20 to 30 nucleotides before the site of poly(A) addition (Fig. 6.15).

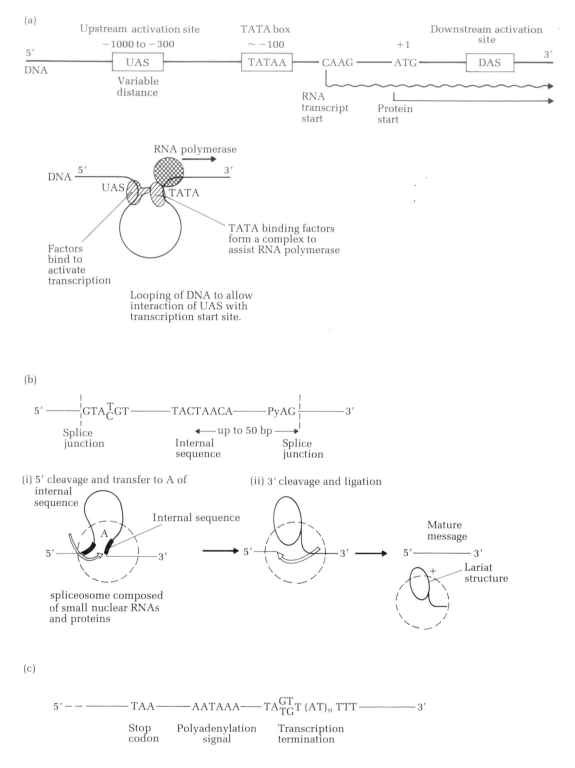

Fig. 6.15 Important aspects of gene structure for transcription in yeast. (a) Promoter; (b) intron splicing; (c) termination.

Post-transcriptional modification

Many RNA species are altered after they have been transcribed from the DNA template. Sometimes, these modifications occur before the gene has been completely transcribed. There are a number of types of modification and each class of RNA has its own set of alterations.

One important modification involves cleavage of a larger precursor RNA by site-specific nucleases; this is most clearly seen in formation of rRNAs. In bacteria, the three species of RNA found in the 70S ribosome, designated 23S, 16S and 5S from their sedimentation behaviour, are encoded in a linear sequence of 16S, 23S and 5S, with one or two tRNAs between the 16S and 23S genes. All of these form a single, long transcriptional unit which is specifically cleaved by the sequential action of endonucleases as indicated in Fig. 6.16. During this processing, some nucleotides are methylated enzymically in either the base or ribose moiety; this may play some part in the accurate assembly of the ribosome. In eukaryotes, rRNA precursors are cleaved in a similar way to give the 28S, 18S and 5.8S species. This processing is so rapid that, under normal circumstances, it is not possible to detect very much of the 45S precursor; this is only found when processing is inhibited.

To provide an adequate supply of rRNA in the growing cells,

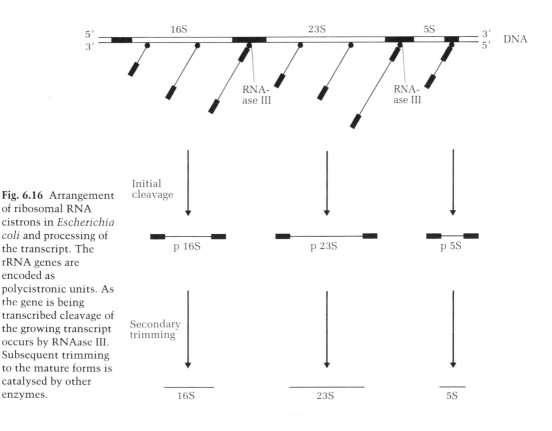

Fig. 6.16 Arrangement of ribosomal RNA cistrons in *Escherichia coli* and processing of the transcript. The rRNA genes are encoded as polycistronic units. As the gene is being transcribed cleavage of the growing transcript occurs by RNAase III. Subsequent trimming to the mature forms is catalysed by other enzymes.

bacteria have at least six sets of these long rRNA cistrons, while in eukaryotic organisms there is a much greater extent of gene amplification—yeast has 150 copies. In all organisms, the transcriptional units are adjacent sequences with short spacers between. This arrangement may be the result of the linear amplification of a single gene, and since closely linked genes are less frequently involved in recombination, there is less likelihood of an adverse mutation in one cistron affecting the others in this type of arrangement. In eukaryotes, the rDNA is organized into a specific structure—the nucleolus—and this is made possible by the close linkage of these genes.

Processing of bacterial mRNAs is not a common occurrence, but in eukaryotes four types of post-transcriptional modification of mRNAs usually, but not always, occur. *Capping* involves the addition of a methylated guanosine residue by a 5' to 5' triphosphate linkage to the first coded nucleotide of the RNA; this and the subsequent nucleotide in the sequence may also be methylated, for example:

$$m7G(5')ppp(5')mXpmYp\ldots$$

Capped mRNAs bind to ribosomes more rapidly and to a greater extent than their uncapped counterparts and hence capping may have some role in initiation of translation. Unlike bacterial mRNAs, those from eukaryotes generally cannot form extensively base-paired complexes with the 18S rRNA in the ribosome; in bacteria, these play a role in mRNA selection by the ribosome. Cap-dependent initiation may be one reason why eukaryotes do not seem to have polycistronic messages which are common to bacteria.

At the 3' end of the eukaryotic primary transcript, there is frequently cleavage by a nuclease followed by the enzymatic addition of a *polyadenylate poly(A) tail*. This occurs in the nucleus before the mRNA is transported to the cytoplasm and the poly(A) tail may therefore be important in transport of mRNA, or in its protection during transport to the site of its translation—the cytoplasmic ribosome. Some methylation of mRNAs can also occur.

Probably the most interesting modification of eukaryotic primary transcripts is the *splicing out of non-coding segments (introns)* which can fall between coding regions *(exons)*. It is not immediately obvious why eukaryotes should have evolved with complicated 'split' genes. One possibility is that accidental recombination events within the introns of different genes would have led to the more rapid generation of new protein combinations made up of functional domains of proteins coded in their exons. The evolution of proteins would thus have been much more rapid in those organisms with a splicing mechanism and some split genes. In lower eukaryotes, such as fungi, apart from rRNA cistrons, and some removal of short introns from tRNA precursors, fewer examples of split nuclear genes have been found; these include inositol dehydrogenase and actin genes in *S. cerevisiae* and the NADP$^+$-dependent glutamate dehydrogenase gene of *Neurospora crassa*. Split genes are, however, more common in the fission yeast *Schizosaccharomyces pombe*.

The splicing mechanism depends on the presence of 'consensus' sequences located in the introns immediately adjacent to the exons (Fig. 6.15). The particle that catalyses the splicing event (the spliceosome) is composed of small RNA molecules as well as protein. From a comparison of the sequences of one of the small RNAs and the consensus sequences at either end of the intron, it is clear that the small nuclear RNA (snRNA) acts as a complementary template to ensure that the splicing is accurate and preserves the correct reading frame for translation. One of the most interesting examples of introns in lower eukaryotes is found in the cytochrome *c* oxidase/cytochrome *b* oxidase region of the yeast mitochondrial genome. One of the surprises of this system was the finding that some of the introns could code for proteins, and mutations within the intron region affected the process of splicing. In this case, the intron codes for a splicing enzyme which, once formed shuts off its own synthesis, since it can only be translated from the unprocessed precursor RNA.

For tRNA species, apart from the enzymes for post-translational modification of bases by methylation, and splicing, others are needed since the terminal nucleotides (. . . pCpCpA) at the amino acyl-accepting end are added sequentially by specific enzymes, not RNA polymerase.

Degradation

Apart from the specific nucleases involved in processing, other enzymes degrading RNA have been found. Some are intracellular and have quite specific functions. One of the more important of these enzymes is the endonuclease responsible for rapid breakdown of mRNA. This enables the cell to adapt rapidly to changes in the environment (see Chapters 2 and 7). Other RNases break down large amounts of cellular RNA in cells facing starvation, providing substrates for endogenous metabolism necessary to keep the cell viable.

Other degradative enzymes are extracellular, either periplasmic or excreted into the medium; these presumably act as scavenger enzymes that degrade RNA into units small enough to cross the cell membrane. In many organisms, these enzymes are excreted when the cells face starvation.

PROTEINS

Synthesis (translation)

Proteins are linear heteropolymers formed from up to 20 precursors, the amino acids. For a particular protein, the order of amino acids is encoded on the organism's genome in a particular sequence of DNA, termed the structural gene for that protein. For a bacterium such as *E. coli*, the genome can encode about 5000 proteins. For simple microbial eukaryotes, the genome may contain about five times more DNA than *E. coli*, although not all of this may encode additional proteins due to the difference in chromosome structure and regulation of gene expression in these organisms.

Each amino acid is coded by a linear triplet of bases on one strand (the coding strand) of the DNA, and these triplets are read sequentially; for example:

DNA coding strand 5'...–A–A–A–T–G–A–G–C–A–...
mRNA transcript   ...–U–U–U–A–C–U–C–U–G–...
Protein   –Phe———Thr——Arg–...

Three bases are the minimum needed to code for 20 amino acids. The code is in fact degenerate, since there are 64 possible triplet combinations so that more than one triplet may represent any particular amino acid. The genetic code, which applies in almost all situations, is given in Table 6.3. Of the 64 possible codons (i.e. three-base sequences), 61 specify amino acids, while three (UGA, UAG and UAA) are responsible for terminating the protein chain at the correct length. This code is not completely universal, since it has been found that UGA is not a termination codon for the yeast mitochondrial genome, but encodes tryptophan instead. In the micronucleus of the ciliated protozoa, such as *Paramecium* and *Tetrahymena*, the codons UAA and UAG specify glutamine or glutamate, and in *Mycoplasma* UGA codes for tryptophan, while UAA is used as a terminator.

The DNA sequence is not translated directly into the protein sequence, but indirectly via messenger RNA (mRNA) which is transcribed on DNA and acts as the template for protein synthesis. There are many reasons why the existence of such an intermediate is vital to the cell, for example:

1 Each gene can be transcribed many times and hence amplification is achieved.
2 Control of the rate of synthesis of a particular protein can be more readily exerted (see Chapter 8).
3 mRNA degradation can also play a part in control.
4 In eukaryotes, an intermediate is necessary since DNA is contained within the nucleus while translation machinery is located in the cytoplasm.

As for the synthesis of most polymers, activated precursors are needed. Each amino acid is activated in a two-step enzymic process requiring ATP and a transfer RNA (tRNA) molecule specific to that amino acid. The result is a tRNA that is 'charged' with the amino acyl group on the 3'-OH of the terminal A residue of the CCA sequence common to all tRNA species. tRNAs, however, serve a multifunctional role during translation and are not just

Table 6.3 The genetic code. Standard abbreviations for the amino acids are given, together with the single letter code used for convenience in describing a protein sequence. The AUG start codon codes for *N*-formylmethionine in bacteria and for methionine within the open reading frame. Amber, ochre and opal are genetic terms given to the different termination codons to distinguish the potential suppression characteristics of mutations to these codons.

5'-base to the left							
UUU	Phe(F)	UCU	Ser(S)	UAU	Tyr(Y)	UGU	Cys(C)
UUC	Phe	UCC	Ser	UAC	Tyr	UGC	Cys
UUA	Leu(L)	UCA	Ser	UAA	Ochre	UGA	Opal
UUG	Leu	UCG	Ser	UAG	Amber	UGG	Trp(W)
CUU	Leu	CCU	Pro(P)	CAU	His(H)	CGU	Arg(R)
CUC	Leu	CCC	Pro	CAC	His	CGC	Arg
CUA	Leu	CCA	Pro	CAA	Gln(Q)	CGA	Arg
CUG	Leu	CCG	Pro	CAG	Gln	CGG	Arg
AUU	Ile(I)	ACU	Thr(T)	AAU	Asn(N)	AGU	Ser
AUC	Ile	ACC	Thr	AAC	Asn	AGC	Ser
AUA	Ile	ACA	Thr	AAA	Lys(K)	AGA	Arg
AUG	Met(M) (Start)	ACG	Thr	AAG	Lys	AGG	Arg
GUU	Val(V)	GCU	Ala(A)	GAU	Asp(D)	GGU	Gly(G)
GUC	Val	GCC	Ala	GAC	Asp	GGC	Gly
GUA	Val	GCA	Ala	GAA	Glu(E)	GGA	Gly
GUG	Val	GCG	Ala	GAG	Glu	GGG	Gly

vehicles for accepting amino acids in a reactive state. Amino acids have no affinity for nucleic acids and cannot recognize a codon. The tRNA serves this function, each having on one loop (the anticodon loop) of its clover-leaf structure, a three-base sequence complementary to the coding triplet in the mRNA. The secondary structure of a tRNA species is shown in Fig. 6.17.

While 61 codons specify the 20 amino acids, fewer than 61 tRNA species are required, since it has been found that some tRNA species can recognize more than one codon. This has been explained in terms of the 'wobble hypothesis', which suggests that some of the bases at the 5' position of the tRNA anticodon can base-pair by hydrogen bonding to more than one other base. For example, G in this position can pair with either C or U; U with A or G, and inosine (which is a modified base often found in the 5' position) can pair with A, U or C. This freedom of pairing of the 5' base presumably arises due to its position in the tertiary structure of the molecule.

For each amino acid, there is a separate *charging enzyme*, catalysing its activation by ATP and transfer to the appropriate tRNA species. The charging enzyme is highly specific and recognizes regions of the tRNAs other than the anticodon.

Aminoacyl-tRNAs do not condense to form peptides in free solution; this takes place on the very complex particles called ribosomes. Ribosomes are composed of two subunits, each containing rRNA species and 20 to 30 proteins. The bacterial ribo-

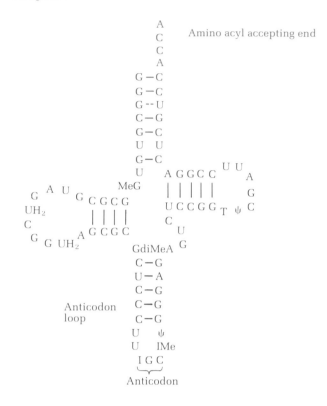

Fig. 6.17 Yeast alanine transfer RNA showing intrachain base pairing and secondary structure. Unusual bases: T = ribothymidylic acid; UH_2 = 5, 6-dihydrouridylic acid; Ψ = pseudouridylic acid; I = inosinic acid.

somes have a sedimentation coefficient of 70S and they can be dissociated into 50S and 30S subunits. In *E. coli*, the 50S subunit contains two rRNA species of size 23S and 5S complexed with 34 proteins; the 30S subunit contains one 16S rRNA molecule and 21 proteins. So far, the three-dimensional arrangement of such complicated structures is not fully understood, although a considerable amount of work has enabled informed suggestions of their shapes and of the interactions of many of the components during ribosome assembly. In eukaryotes, the ribosome differs in size; for instance, in *S. cerevisiae* the 80S particle dissociates to a 60S subunit composed of a 28S rRNA, a 5.8S rRNA, a 5S RNA and 49 proteins, and to a 40S subunit containing an 18S rRNA and 33 proteins. The eukaryotic ribosome is also inhibited by different antibiotics to those affecting bacterial ribosomes (see Table 2.5, p. 67).

At the ribosome, charged tRNAs are successively brought in conjunction with each other and the mRNA template. Each mRNA is usually read by many ribosomes at once and polyribosomes containing ten or more ribosomes can be isolated from cells broken by very gentle means. In bacteria, mRNA is translated as it is synthesized on the DNA template. This has been visualized directly by electron microscopy (Fig. 6.18); thus translation proceeds on the mRNA in the 5' to 3' direction corresponding to protein synthesis from the amino to the carboxy terminal end.

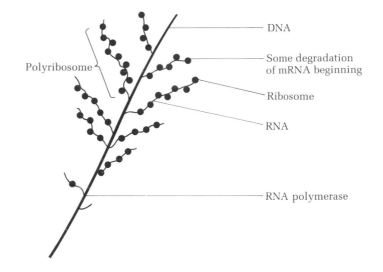

Fig. 6.18 Bacterial gene transcription and simultaneous translation on the DNA template seen by electron microscopy of gently lysed bacteria.

In eukaryotes, transcription occurs in the nucleus and the post-transcriptionally modified mRNA is transported to the cytoplasm. Translation takes place on ribosomes which are either free or attached to the endoplasmic reticulum, depending on the ultimate destination of the protein concerned (see p. 30).

Initiation of protein synthesis

As with transcription, translation requires a mechanism for correct initiation and termination, and there may also be mechanisms to regulate the frequency with which translation is initiated. In bacteria, initiation occurs at the specific codon AUG (or, less frequently, GUG) as long as this codon is preceded on the mRNA by a ribosome binding sequence of about 20 nucleotides located just prior to the initiation codon. This is known as the Shine–Dalgarno sequence; a four to nine base sequence in this region is complementary to the 5′ end of the 16S rRNA (in the 30S subunit) as indicated in Fig. 6.19. This recognition presumably plays some part in the extent of mRNA selection by the ribosome. Cloning vectors designed to express recombinant genes in *E. coli* as efficiently as possible, carry not only strong bacterial promoters, but a Shine–Dalgarno sequence prior to the initiation codon of the recombinant gene.

The initiation codons are recognized by a specific tRNA. In bacteria, there are two methionyl tRNAs; one of these, $tRNA^{Met}$, is charged with methionine and the methionyl moiety is *N*-formylated and is incorporated into the NH_2-terminal position during initiation. The other methionyl tRNA, $tRNA_m^{Met}$, acts at codons internal to the structural gene.

Initiation in eukaryotes differs in important respects. First, there appear to be no regular features of the 5′ sequence of the mRNA

16S rRNA sequences at 3' terminus

B. stearothermophilus	AUCUUUCCUCCAC
Caulobacter crescentus	UCUUUCCU . . . .
Ps. aeruginosa	AUUCCUCUC . . . .
E. coli	AUUCCUCCACUAG

lacZ 5' . . . . AAUUUC ACACAGGAAACAGCU**AUG**

lacI 5' . . . . AGUC AAUUCAGGGUGGU GAAU**GUG**

araB 5' . . . . UUUUUUGGAUGGAGUGAA ACG**AUG**

trpA 5' . . . . GA AAGCACG AG GGGAAAUCUG**AUG**

galT 5' . . . . UAUC CCGAUUAAGGAACGACC**AUG**

galE 5' . . . . AUAAGCCUAAUGGAGC GAAUU**AUG**

Fig. 6.19 The 3' termini of 16S rRNA species from *Escherichia coli* and other bacteria and the Shine–Dalgarno sequences of several *E. coli* genes with the bases complementary to the *E. coli* 16S RNA terminus indicated in bold type. Initiation codons are shown in normal type.

which might direct ribosomes and the ribosomes always seem to start at the first AUG sequence in the mRNA. So no equivalent of a Shine–Dalgarno sequence exists. It is currently held that the eukaryotic ribosomes bind at or near the 5' end of the RNA, using the 'cap' as a guide, and work their way towards the first AUG codon. Note that a few mRNA species are not capped, but that removal of a cap from an mRNA species does lead to lowered rates of translation *in vitro*. Secondly, there is no requirement for *N*-formylation of the initiation methionyl tRNA^{Met}.

In both prokaryotes and eukaryotes, the process of initiation of translation involves a complicated sequence of interactions between the mRNA, *N*-formylmethionyl tRNA, GTP, several protein initiation factors and the smaller ribosomal subunit. This is outlined for *E. coli* in Fig. 6.20. It should be noted that the complete 70S or 80S ribosomal particle is not assembled until the above complex has been made, and that binding of the initiating tRNA^{Met} to the smaller subunit is not codon directed.

For prokaryotes, there is some, but not a great deal, of control over protein synthesis at the level of translation. For eukaryotes, however, the physical separation of transcription from translation allows for more control at the initiation of translation. There are indications that such control does occur via the initiation factors, of which there are more than in bacteria.

Elongation of the polypeptide chain

The ribosome has two binding sites for aminoacyl tRNAs: one is called the peptide or donor site (P), the other the acceptor (A) site. At the end of the initiation step, the *N*-formylmethionyl tRNA occupies the P site and there follows three reactions in a sequence which is repeated for the addition of each successive amino acid in the growing polypeptide chain. This sequence of three steps is shown in Fig. 6.20 and includes:

1 Binding of the incoming aminoacyl tRNA specified by the next codon at the A site. This involves protein elongation factors and

Protein synthesis in *E. coli*

Initiation

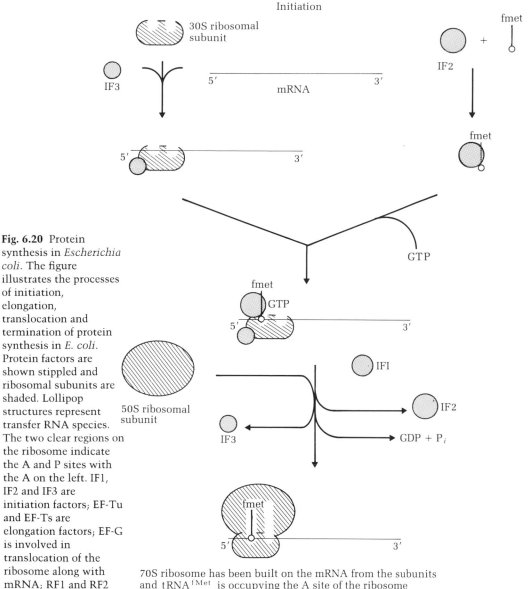

Fig. 6.20 Protein synthesis in *Escherichia coli*. The figure illustrates the processes of initiation, elongation, translocation and termination of protein synthesis in *E. coli*. Protein factors are shown stippled and ribosomal subunits are shaded. Lollipop structures represent transfer RNA species. The two clear regions on the ribosome indicate the A and P sites with the A on the left. IF1, IF2 and IF3 are initiation factors; EF-Tu and EF-Ts are elongation factors; EF-G is involved in translocation of the ribosome along with mRNA; RF1 and RF2 are release factors.

70S ribosome has been built on the mRNA from the subunits and tRNA^{fMet} is occupying the A site of the ribosome

the hydrolysis of GTP.

2 Transfer of the peptidyl group from the tRNA at the P site to form a peptide bond with the aminoacyl tRNA at the A site, catalysed by a protein of the larger subunit. The tRNA is then released from the P site.

3 Translocation of the elongated peptidyl tRNA from the A site to the P site enabling another sequence to follow. This step involves another protein factor (the GTP-requiring elongation factor, EF-G) and the hydrolysis of another molecule of GTP.

Elongation & translocation

EF-Tu and EF-Ts are elongation factors

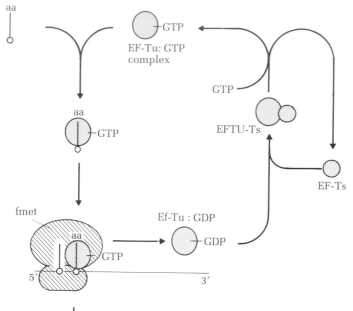

aa

aa
–GTP

EF-Tu: GTP
complex

GTP

EFTU-Ts

EF-Ts

Ef-Tu : GDP
–GDP

fmet

aa
+GTP

5′   3′

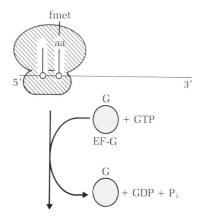

fmet

aa

5′   3′

G
+ GTP

EF-G

G
+ GDP + P$_i$

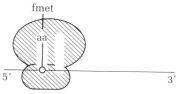

fmet

aa

5′   3′

Fig. 6.20 Cont.

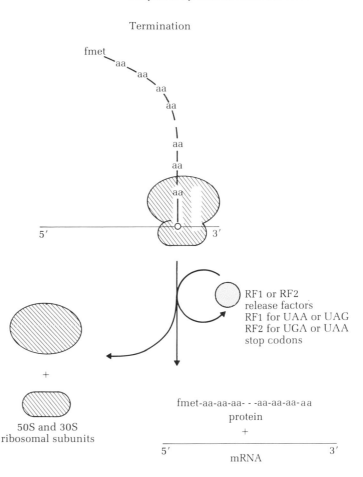

Fig. 6.20 Cont.

Termination

The above sequence continues with extension of the polypeptide chain until a termination codon (UAA, UAG or UGA) is reached. Termination is achieved via the binding of a protein release factor (RF) to the A site of the ribosome. This catalyses the release of the complete protein from the ribosome by hydrolysis of its bond to the final tRNA. In bacteria, the ribosome can continue on the mRNA and re-initiate synthesis of another protein if the message is polycistronic. In eukaryotes, this is not known to occur. Eventually, however, the last termination step is reached. Yet another protein factor may be involved in the dissociation of the mRNA from the ribosome, which can dissociate in the presence of the initiation factors to allow the whole process to recommence on another mRNA.

Protein modification

During synthesis, or just after, the nascent polypeptide folds into its functional configuration. In many cases, this occurs spontaneously with the polypeptide adopting the thermodynamically most favoured state. Exceptions do occur, particularly when the protein is assembled into a complicated multicomponent structure (e.g. during assembly of the phage T4 head structure, see p. 261). The GroEL protein (a major heat shock protein) is involved in protein folding and phage assembly. It is a member of a very highly conserved family of proteins found in all organisms.

There are, however, a number of modifications which can occur before the polypeptide reaches its final location and becomes fully functional.

At the simplest level, the *N*-formylmethionyl moiety is often removed, S–S bonds are formed, prosthetic groups, lipid or carbohydrate moieties are attached. Other important post-translational modifications that can occur are concerned with transport of proteins either to, or across, the cytoplasmic membrane, or for eukaryotes, into the various organelles. These aspects, which involve removal of signal peptides by specific proteolytic cleavage and (in eukaryotes) glycosylation of proteins, are discussed in Chapter 1.

Reversible covalent modification can also play an important part in regulation of the activity of a protein. This can be seen in the phosphorylation of proteins by transfer of a phosphate group from ATP or GTP to tyrosine, threonine or serine residues via the action of a protein kinase. This type of modification is important in the amplification of the signal received when a hormone interacts with a receptor at the target cell surface (p. 222) and also seems to play an important role in the control of cell division processes (p. 229). Some ribosomal proteins are phosphorylated, as are a number of subunits of the eukaryotic RNA polymerases. Other, less frequently encountered, modifications of this type include: methylation (important in bacterial chemotaxis, see p. 72) usually via methyl transfer from *S*-adenosylmethionine; acetylation; and adenylylation in which tyrosine residues in the protein accept the adenylyl groups from ATP (for example, glutamate synthetase involved in NH_4^+ assimilation in bacteria, p. 218). These modifications can be reversed in most cases and they provide the cell with a rapid way of modulating the activity of an enzyme. Such changes are more frequently seen in eukaryotic cells in which enzyme induction may be less obvious than in bacteria.

PROTEIN EXPORT IN PROKARYOTES

Gram-negative bacteria

Proteins present in the outer membrane of the Gram-negative bacterial cell or secreted into the extracellular environment (extracellular enzymes, see p. 77) must pass from the cytosol across two membranes and the periplasm. Their passage may be facilitated by zones of adhesion between the inner and outer membranes. As well as these proteins, a number of different enzymes and transport proteins are secreted into the periplasm. Synthesis of these groups of proteins occurs in the cytoplasm; after leaving the ribosome, the proteins are translocated to their final destination by a common mechanism. Each protein is synthesized as a precursor with a signal sequence or leader peptide of 15–30 amino acids on the amino terminus. Energy is needed in the form of ATP and electrochemical potential. The signal sequence is removed by either of two signal peptidases—one for proteins and one for lipoproteins. An export system is also necessary and soluble cytoplasmic factors may couple the precursor protein to the export apparatus.

The signal sequences of periplasmic proteins, such as β-lactamase, and extracellular proteins show sufficient homology to function normally in heterologous systems. The leader peptides therefore do not designate the final location of the protein but may instead direct the protein to the export apparatus and across the cytoplasmic membrane. Indeed, not all exported proteins carry leader peptide sequences; they appear to be lacking in *E. coli* haemolysin and from colicins. The N-terminal amino acid sequence in the former may itself act as a signal. In the case of the periplasmic maltose-binding protein, the leader sequence appears to be involved in at least two aspects of the process. It is needed to mediate the initial binding of the precursor to the membrane, a process also seen in mutants with altered leader sequences which prevent export. Secondly, the correct leader sequence is clearly needed for translocation. Translocation is found at discrete sites on the cytoplasmic membrane. These sites possess higher density than the bulk of the membrane and are distributed non-uniformly.

Translocation requires an unfolded conformation and cytoplasmic components maintain the precursor proteins in the required conformation. Using cell fractions it is also possible to achieve some translocation of proteins which have been unfolded by chemical treatments such as 8 M urea. For translocation across inverted membrane vesicles to occur, ATP is required together with 'trigger factor', a polypeptide of molecular mass *c.* 63 kDa. The trigger factor and precursor protein combine in a stoichiometric ratio, perhaps formed co-translationally, and are targeted to the cytoplasmic membrane. The trigger factor may be recycled back to the ribosome to form further complexes. The membrane-bound precursor protein interacts with the product of the *secA* gene, which functions as an ATPase. The trigger factor may only function for certain of the exported proteins; the product of the *secB* gene may serve in a similar capacity for other proteins, including the maltose-binding protein found in the periplasm.

In bacterial systems, it is not clear whether the trigger factor is also involved in targeting. In mammalian cells, a signal recognition particle with affinity for a docking protein targets the polysome to the membrane.

Does the protein to be exported to the outer membrane or extracellular environment enter the periplasm? A number of proteins which possess amino terminal signal sequences apparently do. They include cellulase and polygalacturonase from *Erwinia chrysanthemumi*, cholera toxin, and others. Mutants unable to secrete these enzymes accumulate them in the periplasm. Other proteins apparently fail to pass through the periplasm and possibly pass through intramembrane adhesion zones or trans-envelope channels. No intermediate forms of this group of proteins are detectable in the periplasm of mutants defective in secretion.

There may be a number of different factors required for the secretion of each group of extracellular proteins. The factors may also be species-specific or at least functionally limited to a group of closely related bacterial species. *E. coli* will not secrete cloned cholera toxin or pullulanase from *Klebsiella aerogenes* (a lipoprotein), although it will secrete an alginase from a *Klebsiella* species. Cloning of larger DNA fragments from *K. pneumoniae* leads to the identification of two loci facilitating secretion of pullulanase by transferring the enzyme across from the outer membrane and (possibly) releasing it from the outer surface of the outer membrane. Some of the factors required for protein secretion may be ATP-binding proteins involved in supplying the energy needed for the secretory process.

The signal peptidase needed to cleave the leader sequence from the bacterial protein has a similar processing specificity to leader peptidases from eukaryotes. Several eukaryotic secreted proteins, when expressed in *E. coli*, can be processed by *E. coli* signal peptidase. The enzyme is an integral protein of the bacterial cytoplasmic membrane, which it spans, the amino terminal domain being exposed to the cytoplasm while the carboxy terminal is within the periplasm. Like most proteins of the cytoplasmic membrane, the signal peptidase is not itself synthesized with a leader peptide.

Lipoprotein export

The lipoprotein of *E. coli*, shown by Braun to be associated with peptidoglycan in the cell envelope, has provided information on the mechanisms of modification and processing of lipoproteins. This lipoprotein is found (i) associated with peptidoglycan in the periplasm; and (ii) as a peptidoglycan-free lipoprotein in the outer membrane. At the amino terminus of the peptidoglycan-linked form is a lipoamino acid. The precursor prolipoprotein differs from the mature molecule in several respects. It is free from fatty acids and peptidoglycan and carries a signal sequence. Export of lipoprotein is affected in two types of *E. coli* mutant, *secA* and *secY*, which are defective in the secretion of several outer membrane and periplasmic proteins. In both types of mutant, the prolipoprotein (free of glyceride) accumulates in the cytoplasmic membrane. The early stages of protein export are therefore the

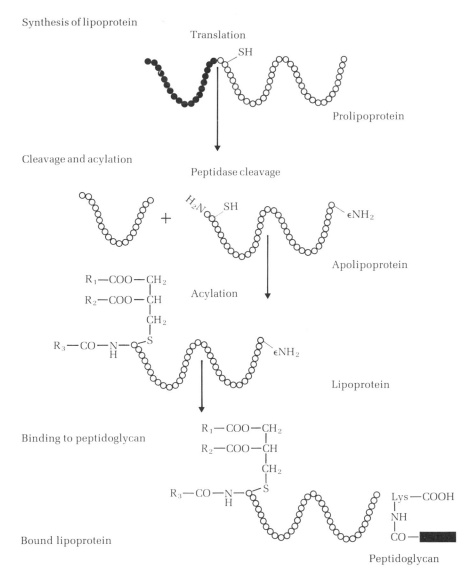

Fig. 6.21 The post-translational modification of bacterial lipoprotein. Prolipoprotein is first cleaved to yield apolipoprotein; this product is then acylated by the addition of fatty acids. Finally, the molecule is covalently attached to the carboxyl terminus of peptidoglycan.

same for a group of structurally diverse proteins and lipoproteins and clearly do not distinguish the different signal peptides. Thereafter the processing mechanisms diverge.

Prolipoprotein signal peptides differ from the precursors of exported proteins in the amino acid sequence in the vicinity of the cleavage site. Leu-Ala-Gly-Cys is recognized by the glyceryl transferase and the cysteine is modified by the presence of the glyceride. The modified amino acid is in turn recognized by signal peptidase II (the lipoprotein signal peptidase). Thus the prolipoprotein is modified by the addition of lipid *then* processed by signal peptidase II. This signal peptidase is also distinguishable by its binding to and inhibition by the cyclic peptide antibiotic, globomycin. No charged residue is present in the hydrophilic core of the lipoprotein signal peptide.

The lipoprotein signal sequence can be divided into three regions—basic, hydrophilic and cleavage (Fig. 6.21). Alteration of the amino acids through mutagenesis has permitted some indication of the functions of the different regions. The basic residues at the amino terminus may aid in protein secretion, perhaps in releasing nascent protein from a translational block. Some mutations in the hydrophilic region lead to elevated synthesis of lipoprotein, but alteration to the cleavage region does not affect synthesis because of the involvement of cleavage late in protein secretion. Studies on protein secretion using the *malB* (maltose-binding protein) system indicate that the overall hydrophobicity and absolute length of the signal peptide are important for functionality.

Gram-positive bacteria

In Gram-positive bacteria, all exported proteins must be extracellular as there is no periplasm. The secreted proteins can, however, be maintained at relatively high concentrations near the surface. The penicillinase from *Bacillus licheniformis* is an example of this. About 50% of this enzyme is located in a highly hydrophobic form on the outer surface of the bacterial cell membrane. The rest is truly extracellular and water soluble but is in two distinct forms differing in length by eight amino acids due to post-translational modification. The protein may either be cleaved of a signal sequence of 26 residues or linked to diglyceride at residue 27. The extracellular forms represent further processing events at residues 34 and 42.

Extracellular proteins from Gram-positive bacteria are initially synthesized as precursors with amino-terminal extensions. These extensions are removed during export, thus yielding the mature extracellular proteins. In the case of proteases, the molecules are synthesized with *propeptides*, additional polypeptide segments, inserted between the signal peptide and the mature, active protein. Propeptides are a feature almost unique to extracellular proteases. Their probable role is to maintain the proteins in inactive conformation; however, they may also be necessary for ensuring that the proteins are correctly folded or are anchored onto the cell envelope.

PROTEIN DEGRADATION

Microorganisms have to adapt rapidly to changes in culture condi-

Table 6.4 Proteinases of the yeast *Saccharomyces cerevisiae*.

Enzymes	Structural gene	Localization	Cellular role
Proteinase yscA	*PRA*1	Vacuole (soluble)	Protein degradation, nitrogen metabolism
Proteinase yscB	*PRB*1	Vacuole (soluble)	Protein degradation, nitrogen metabolism
Proteinases yscD, E		Non-vacuolar (soluble)	Unknown
Proteinase yscF	*KEX*2	Membrane	Precursor processing (alpha factor)
Proteinases yscG, H		Membrane fraction	Unknown
Proteinase K		Unknown (soluble)	Unknown
Proteinase yscmMpI nuclear-encoded		Mitochondrial matrix	Processing of mitochondrial proteins
3 mitochondrial proteinases		Inner mitochondrial membrane	Unknown
Propheromone convertase Y		Unknown	Unknown
Proteinases yscM, P etc.		Unknown	Unknown
Aminopeptidase yscI	*LAP*4	Vacuole (soluble)	Nitrogen supply
Aminopeptidase yscII	*APE*2	Periplasm (soluble)	Nitrogen supply
Aminopeptidases yscIV–XV		Unknown	Unknown
Carboxypeptidase yscY	*PRC*1	Vacuole (soluble)	Protein degradation, nitrogen metabolism
Carboxypeptidase yscS	*CPS*1	Vacuole (soluble)	Protein degradation, nitrogen metabolism
Carboxypeptidases ysc		Unknown	Unknown

In addition there are at least five dipeptidyl aminopeptidases (yscI–V) and a dipeptidase yscI which have been reported.

tions, especially to starvation, and cells facing starvation begin to break down some of their protein complement to provide amino acids for synthesis of new enzymes capable of dealing with any alternative substrate which may exist, or for providing the necessary energy to maintain the cell via further metabolism of the amino acids. This process is known as protein turnover.

In most bacteria, this protein degradation does not occur significantly during exponential growth; two-dimensional gel electrophoretic studies of doubly-labelled proteins of *E. coli* have shown that only three major proteins undergo breakdown during growth. However, *E. coli* cells can rapidly degrade proteins with an abnormal configuration via an ATP-dependent protease (the *lon* or *capR* gene product). This proteolysis can be a problem when trying to express foreign proteins (recombinant gene products) in *E. coli*.

In eukaryotes, there is in general more turnover of proteins during vegetative growth, and proteases play an important role in cell physiology, since mutations affecting protease activities can impair such functions as sporulation. As an indication of the variety and number of enzymes found in yeast, Table 6.4 lists some of the activities that have been identified to date and, where known, functions that can be ascribed to them from studies of the effects of mutations. Some of these enzymes have broad specificity and are presumably involved in more general degradation, while others have a much higher specificity and may cleave only a few proteins at one particular sequence to achieve very selective control of a metabolic process (e.g. polypeptide secretion).

POLYSACCHARIDE SYNTHESIS

The polymers discussed so far are synthesized on templates, an essential requirement for gene expression. Many cellular polymers are, however, composed totally or in part of repeating units for which no direct template is required. The ordering of subunits within the polymer molecules is due to the specificity of the transferase enzymes adding the subunits in strict sequence.

There are many polymers which fall within this category; some such as poly-β-hydroxyalkanoic acids (e.g. PHB) have already been discussed (Chapter 5) and most of the essential principles have emerged from studying polysaccharides.

Homopolysaccharides

Microbial cells form several types of homopolysaccharide, some being linear molecules while others are branched. The most common is glycogen, found intracellularly in bacteria, yeasts and slime moulds. Its synthesis in prokaryotes follows a similar pattern to that in eukaryotes, with one major difference in the nature of the glycosyl donor. In eukaryotes, the polymer is formed by the sequential addition of D-glucopyranose units from UDP-D-glucose; in prokaryotes, the enzyme catalysing this reaction shows a primary specificity for ADP-D-glucose. *In vitro* activity of this enzyme with ADP-glucose is 100-fold that with UDP-glucose, while other glucose-containing sugar nucleotides are inactive.

Thus the first specific stage in the synthesis of bacterial glycogen is an activation, forming ADP-glucose (see p. 88). Subsequently, a linear polymer is formed by *glycogen synthetase* (ADP-glucose: 1,4-glucan-4-α-glucosyl transferase). A third enzyme, the *branching enzyme*, transfers a segment of 6–8 glucose residues from the main chain to form a 1,6 α-linkage at a branch point. Mutants lacking either of the first two enzymes fail to form glycogen, while lack of the branching enzyme leads to the accumulation of an unbranched 1,4 α-linked glucan staining blue with iodine. *Glycogen phosphorylase*, an enzyme long thought to be involved in the synthesis of glycogen, functions solely in the breakdown of the polymer. In *E. coli*, the three enzymes responsible for glycogen synthesis are controlled by genes mapping at a chromosomal locus adjacent to that for glycerol-3-phosphate dehydrogenase.

The requirement for ADP-glucose is interesting since it may provide the prokaryotic cell with a way of controlling glycogen synthesis independently from the processes requiring UDP-sugars as substrates. *ADP-glucose pyrophosphorylase* is an allosteric enzyme which can be activated by various glycolytic intermediates (Table 6.5). The activation leads to an increased affinity and an increased V_{max} for ADP-glucose synthesis. The observed differences in activators are probably due to the utilization of the Embden–Meyerhof pathway by some of the species listed in Table 6.5, and the Entner–Doudoroff pathway by others, except the cyanobacteria. This latter group grows poorly on organic substrates and depends on CO_2 fixation for carbon assimilation. D-Glycerate-3-phosphate is the primary product. No other ADP-linked sugars are known to be of metabolic importance in bacteria.

Much less is known about the synthesis of other homopolysaccharides such as the poly-*N*-acetylneuraminic acid 'Vi' antigen of *Salmonella* strains or the extracellular cellulose fibres secreted by *Acetobacter* species. These polysaccharides also require sugar nucleotides for their synthesis, but levans and dextrans (poly-D-fructose and poly-D-glucose respectively) are formed by a different mechanism. A specific substrate, sucrose, is required and, in the presence of *levansucrase* or *dextransucrase*, both extracellular lipoprotein complexes, the polymers are formed:

$$x \text{ sucrose} + (\text{fructose})_n \rightarrow (\text{fructose})_{n+x} + x \text{ glucose}$$
$$\text{levan} \qquad\qquad \text{levan}$$
$$x \text{ sucrose} + (\text{glucose})_n \rightarrow (\text{glucose})_{n+x} + x \text{ fructose}$$
$$\text{dextran} \qquad\qquad \text{dextran}$$

Although 'mutan', the 1,3 α-D-glucan formed by *Streptococcus mutans*, is essentially unbranched, most dextrans are substituted at the C2 or C3 positions, perhaps due to the activity of a *transglucosylase* causing internal rearrangement of the molecule.

Table 6.5 Activators of ADP-glucose pyrophosphorylase.

Activator	Species
Pyruvate	*Rhodospirillum* spp.
3-Phosphoglycerate	Cyanobacterial species
Pyruvate, fructose-6-phosphate	*Agrobacterium tumefaciens, Arthrobacter viscosus, Rhodopseudomonas* spp.
Fructose-6-phosphate, fructose-1,6-diphosphate	*Aeromonas hydrophila, Rhodopseudomonas viridis*
Pyruvate, fructose-6-phosphate, · fructose-1,6-diphosphate	*Rhodopseudomonas* spp.
Fructose-1,6-diphosphate, NADH, pyridoxal phosphate	*Enterobacter aerogenes, E. cloacae, E. coli, Salmonella* spp.
None	*Clostridium pasteurianum, Serratia* spp.

Heteropolysaccharides

Microorganisms synthesize a large number of different hetero-polysaccharides. Several of these are composed, at least in part, of regular repeating units. Rather than enumerate many different types it is better to concentrate on one or two well-characterized systems. The biosynthesis of the lipopolysaccharide found in the outer membrane of *Salmonella typhimurium* has been intensively studied and illustrates many features common to heteropolysac-charide synthesis. In particular, it provides a clear example of how extracellular polysaccharides are formed at the cytoplasmic membrane from intracellular components, then transported to their final location in the outer membrane. It also typifies the two types of synthetic process in which a 'core' portion of the molecule is formed which then acts as an acceptor for the addition of side-chains (the O-antigenic determinants in this case).

The acceptor for the pentasaccharide 'core' of the lipopolysac-charide is formed by the sequential addition of ketodeoxyoctonate (KDO) from CMP.KDO (Fig. 6.22), one of a small number of nucleoside *mono*phosphate sugars known to function in biological systems. Subsequently, heptose is added and phosphorylated. In the laboratory, KDO addition to the lipopolysaccharide is essential for cell viability, whereas transfer of subsequent monosaccharides may be lost with viability of the bacteria maintained. Glucose is transferred from UDP-glucose to the acceptor, then two molecules of galactose from UDP-galactose. Finally, addition of a further molecule of glucose and one of *N*-acetyl-D-glucosamine complete the formation of the core (Fig. 1.9). An incomplete polymer may be formed either through mutations in the sugar nucleotide synthetic enzymes or in the specific sugar transferases. Sugars distal to the block are not attached, nor are the side-chains, although the latter may still be synthesized. As a result, phage receptors and serological determinants of the cell surface are altered.

Although the 'side-chains' are also synthesized at the cyto-plasmic face of the inner membrane using sugar nucleotides from the cytoplasm, the initiation of synthesis and transposition to the periplasmic face are independent of 'core' synthesis. A different receptor molecule is initially used, one which has an important function in all syntheses of extracellular and wall polysaccharides. This is a polyisoprenoid lipid phosphate which has been termed *bactoprenol* or *antigen carrier lipid (ACL)*:

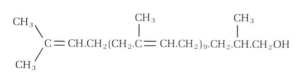

$$CH_3\!\!\diagdown$$
$$C = CH.CH_2(CH_2.C = CH.CH_2)_9.CH_2.CH.CH_2OH$$

The primary reaction involving this receptor requires the addi-tion of a *sugar phosphate* from the appropriate sugar nucleotide. Other sugars are added successively by specific transferase en-

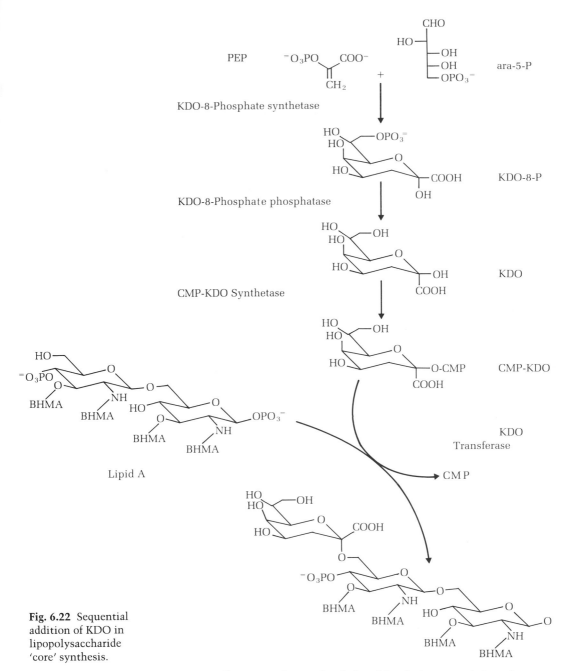

Fig. 6.22 Sequential addition of KDO in lipopolysaccharide 'core' synthesis.

zymes until a repeating unit of the side-chain, containing three to four sugar residues, is formed. Transfer of repeating units leads to the formation of a polymer of increased chain length, polymerization taking place in such a way that the monosaccharide adjacent to the lipid phosphate is added to the terminal sugar on another oligosaccharide–ACL complex. Thus in bacteria, in which the side-chain repeating units are trisaccharides of galactose, rhamnose and mannose, the sequence of reactions is:

$$\text{UDP—Gal} + \text{ACL—P} \rightarrow \text{ACL—P—P—Gal} + \text{UMP}$$

$$\text{ACL—P—P—Gal} + \text{TDP—Rha} \rightarrow$$
$$\text{ACL—P—P—Gal—Rha} + \text{TDP}$$

$$\text{ACL—P—P—Gal—Rha} + \text{GDP—Man} \rightarrow$$
$$\text{ACL—P—P—Gal—Rha—Man} + \text{GDP}$$

$$\text{ACL—P—P—Gal—Rha—Man} + \text{ACL—P—P—Gal—Rha—Man}$$
$$\rightarrow \text{ACL—P—P—(Gal—Rha—Man)}_2 + \text{ACL—P—P}$$

Buildup of the repeating units continues until the normal 'side-chain' of about eight units is formed. Then, as in the case illustrated of *Salmonella* lipopolysaccharide, the entire side-chain is transferred to the lipopolysaccharide 'core' along with the release of the lipid pyrophosphate:

$$\begin{array}{ccc} & \text{Glc.NAc} & \text{Gal} \\ & | & | \\ \text{ACL—P—P—(Gal—Rha—Man)}_n + & \text{Glc—Gal—Glc—Hept} \ldots \end{array}$$

$$\begin{array}{ccc} & \text{Glc.NAc} & \text{Gal} \\ & | & | \\ \text{ACL—P—P—(Man—Rha—Gal)}_n - & \text{Glc—Gal—Glc—Hept} \ldots \end{array}$$

The ACL molecules are located in the cell membrane and have the important role of transferring repeating units formed on the cytoplasmic side of the cell membrane across the membrane to the periplasmic side. After attachment of the 'side-chains' to the 'core', the polymer is transferred to its location in the outer membrane. This transfer occurs at sites of close apposition between inner and outer membranes and is dependent on membrane potential and intracellular ATP pools.

Although the side-chains are composed of several repeating units, not all the core acceptor molecules in wild-type cells are substituted; some may carry a single repeat unit only, others chains of varying length. Modification of the lipopolysaccharide structures may occur through the process of phage (lysogenic) conversion. The modified polymer may have different linkages or may carry an additional monosaccharide such as D-glucose.

Other microbial polysaccharides are also synthesized by processes involving assembly of their repeating unit structures on a similar lipid intermediate. This mechanism appears to be used in the synthesis of all such polymers found external to the bacterial cell membrane. Thus the extracellular capsules of the genus *Klebsiella* and the polysaccharide of *Xanthomonas campestris* are formed using a lipid diphosphate (Fig. 6.23); others such as the mannan of *Micrococcus lysodeikticus* and the teichoic acids of *Bacillus licheniformis* are assembled on the lipid monophosphate. Isoprenoid lipid-linked intermediates have also been identified in the synthesis of polysaccharides and glycoproteins in yeast and other fungi.

Many polysaccharides, particularly those excreted extracellularly by bacteria, are acylated—they contain *O*-acetyl groups or ketal-linked pyruvate. Addition of acetate or pyruvate to the polymer from acetyl CoA and phosphoenolpyruvate, respectively, occurs during the sequential addition of the sugars to the lipid intermediates (Fig. 6.23).

The regulation of polysaccharide synthesis has been studied recently in several systems, revealing both common features and some intriguing differences. Thus all the genes controlling enzymes involved in xanthan biosynthesis are found in a 17 kb region on the chromosome of *Xanthomonas campestris* (Fig. 6.24). This group of genes is responsible for enzymes synthesizing the repeating pentasaccharide subunit as well as those necessary for acylation and polymerisation and for export. In some *E. coli* strains there are distinct groups of genes controlling synthesis, export and postpolymerization modification.

Peptidoglycan

This characteristic structural polymer of prokaryotic cell walls is much more complicated than other polysaccharides and indeed

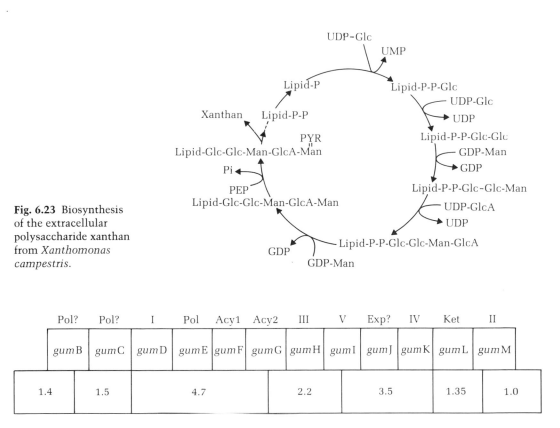

Fig. 6.23 Biosynthesis of the extracellular polysaccharide xanthan from *Xanthomonas campestris.*

Pol?	Pol?	I	Pol	Acyl	Acy2	III	V	Exp?	IV	Ket	II
*gum*B	*gum*C	*gum*D	*gum*E	*gum*F	*gum*G	*gum*H	*gum*I	*gum*J	*gum*K	*gum*L	*gum*M
1.4	1.5	4.7			2.2		3.5			1.35	1.0

Fig. 6.24 The genetic control of xanthan synthesis.

has some of the features of a polysaccharide and others of a peptide. Part of the molecule is a repeating carbohydrate unit structure to which are attached peptide subunits of regular sequence (Fig. 1.9). These linear strands are usually crosslinked by a second type of peptide, creating a giant network of considerable strength. As might be expected from both its structure and its extracellular location, formation of the peptidoglycan is a complex process. In intact cells the synthesis proceeds in four stages as illustrated in Fig. 6.25.

1 Formation of UDP-aminosugars. These are UDP-*N*-acetyl-D-glucosamine and UDP-*N*-acetylmuramic acid (see Chapter 5).

2 Amino acids to form the peptides are added sequentially by specific ligases requiring Mg^{2+}, Mn^{2+} and the hydrolysis of ATP. The amino acid sequence is determined by the enzyme specificity. The fourth enzyme involved, D-*alanyl-D-alanine ligase*, transfers a dipeptide, which is itself formed by two enzymes specifically required for peptidoglycan formation—D-*alanine racemase* and D-*alanyl-D-alanine synthetase*. The genes controlling synthesis of the UDP-muramyl pentapeptide are situated close to one another on the *E. coli* chromosome, that for D-alanyl-D-alanine synthetase being adjacent to the one controlling septation; synthesis of UDP-*N*-acetylmuramic acid is under the control of a different locus (*murB*). The concentration of the different UDP-*N*-acetylmuramic acid derivatives (Park nucleotides) in the cell is regulated by feedback inhibition, probably via the concentration of the UDP-*N*-acetylmuramyl pentapeptide. It should also be noted that the precursor is a pentapeptide attached to the sugar nucleotide, whereas the final macromolecule generally carries tetrapeptides. This is essential for the crosslinking stage described in 4 below.

3 Phosphoryl-*N*-acetylmuramyl pentapeptide from the UDP derivative is transferred to the isoprenoid lipid phosphate carrier by an enzyme requiring Mg^{2+} and K^+; *N*-acetylglucosamine is then added from UDP-*N*-acetylglucosamine. This forms the repeating unit of the polymer, which is transported across the cytoplasmic membrane while attached to isoprenoid lipid and transferred to an acceptor of partially degraded polymer (see p. 187). Chains containing from 10 to 30 or more repeating units are formed (Fig. 6.25).

4 The linear chains are crosslinked. In some Gram-positive bacteria crosslinks are formed directly as an amide bond between the DAP or lysine residue and the penultimate D-alanine of the peptidoglycan precursor. Formation of the crosslink is simultaneous with the release of the terminal D-alanine through the action of a carboxypeptidase, an enzyme which is one of the major penicillin-binding proteins (PBPs) of the bacterial cell. Formation of the peptide bond involves a tRNA which is probably specific to peptidoglycan synthesis. None of the peptide linkages is formed on a template, their order being determined by the specificity of the enzymes needed at each successive step. Since crosslinking

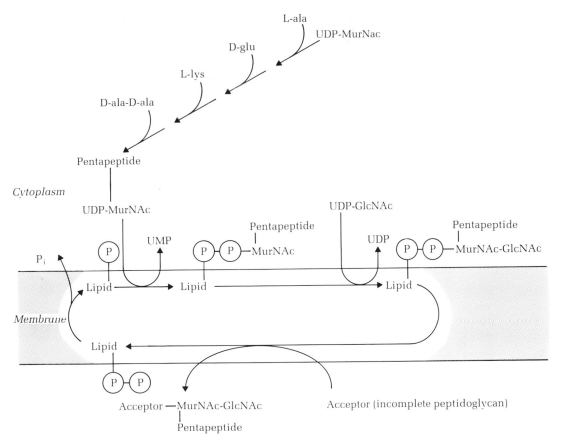

Fig. 6.25 Peptidoglycan biosynthesis.

Table 6.6 Penicillin-binding proteins of *E. coli*.

PBP	M_r	No. of molecules/cell	Function	Effect of inhibition
1a	92 000	100	Elongation (transglycosylase–transpeptidase)	
1b	90 000	120	Cell integrity; elongation (transglycosylase–transpeptidase)	Lysis
2	66 000	20	Cell shape–rod growth (transpeptidase)	Ovoid forms
3	60 000	50	Septation–division (transglycosylase–transpeptidase)	Filaments
4	49 000	110	Crosslink in elongation (DD-endopeptidase/DD-carboxypeptidase)	None
5	42 000	1800	Murein maturation (DD-carboxypeptidase)	None
6	40 000	60	Destroy unused pentapeptide (DD-carboxypeptidase)	None

occurs outside the membrane, ATP is not available to supply the energy needed for formation of the cross-bridge; it comes instead from cleavage of the D-alanyl-D-alanine moiety. Not all peptides carry crosslinks. The terminal D-alanine from unlinked peptides is normally also removed by a carboxypeptidase. The whole process of peptidoglycan synthesis and degradation is complex. In *E. coli*, where there are at least eight PBPs, two or three of these proteins are probably bifunctional enzymes (Table 6.6). Some function as repair enzymes to the peptidoglycan structure.

An interesting feature of both peptidoglycan and lipopolysaccharide synthesis is that the isoprenoid lipid pyrophosphate is inactive, as is the free lipid, although both forms are found in cells. Both a pyrophosphatase and a kinase have been found in *Staphylococcus aureus*, and these may function in controlling the availability of the carrier lipid, and possibly the location of cell wall synthesis.

Degradation of peptidoglycan

Most, if not all, bacteria produce one or more enzymes capable of depolymerizing peptidoglycan (Fig. 6.26); their function in growth of the cell wall and cell division is discussed on p. 233. These *murolytic enzymes* or autolysins are essential for bacterial growth. They can be *amidases*, cleaving the polypeptide chains from the polysaccharide backbone, or *endoglycosidases*, acting at one or other of the glycosidic linkages between the amino sugars. The best known of the latter type is lysozyme; although this occurs in human tears and egg white, similar enzymes are found in bacteria and some bacteriophages. These enzymes cleave between *N*-acetylmuramic acid and *N*-acetylglucosamine, and lysozyme is widely used in the preparation of protoplasts and spheroplasts of sensitive bacterial species.

Cleavage of the peptide cross-bridges in peptidoglycan by peptidases allows the intercalation of new peptidoglycan during the growth of the cell, permitting the expansion of the cell envelope prior to cell division. At the same time peptides derived

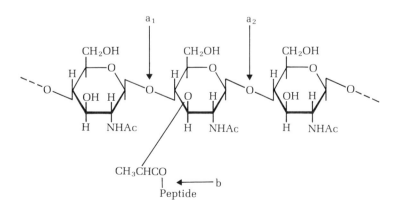

Fig. 6.26 Enzymic degradation of peptidoglycan. $a_{1,2}$ = glycanases acting at sites as indicated; a_1 = endo-*N*-acetyl-glucosaminidase; a_2 = muramidase (e.g. *lysozyme*); b = peptidoglycan amidase.

from peptidoglycan are released during growth and re-used for the synthesis of new polymer. In the case of Gram-negative bacteria, release is into the periplasm, and recovery and re-utilization are relatively efficient. The peptides are taken up intact into the cytoplasm by a specific *oligopeptide permease*; as much as 50% of the peptides are recycled per generation.

7 Regulation

The growth, or even just the survival, of a cell requires a phenomenal degree of coordination of its activities. Almost all physiological processes are subject to some form of regulation, and in previous chapters some specific instances have been discussed. This chapter is concerned with a general review of the various methods by which cells control their activities, especially those concerned with metabolism and growth. The requirement for control can be readily appreciated by a glimpse at a biochemical pathway chart showing how many compounds can be synthesized in a complex of interwoven chemical reactions. For a cell to grow normally it is essential that the flow of metabolites through the various pathways be under a high degree of control, ensuring that no products are deficient or manufactured to excess. This is particularly so for microorganisms since they must respond to much wider fluctuations in environmental conditions than the cells of higher organisms. The reactions essential to cell growth are in a state of dynamic balance with a continuous, and tightly controlled, flux of metabolites through each pathway.

Microorganisms can use a wide range of organic and inorganic substrates, such as hydrocarbons, catechols and phenols by *Pseudomonas* spp., N_2 by *Azotobacter*, *Rhizobium* and cyanobacteria, long-chain alkanes by yeast, sugar alcohols by fungi, and starch and other polymers by a wide variety of bacteria, especially *Bacillus* spp. and myxobacteria. However, in the presence of more readily assimilated substrates these organisms do not waste energy synthesizing enzymes needed to handle these substrates. Cells have the genetic potential to carry out a large number of reactions, but control the expression of this potential according to demand. A very dramatic example of the ability of cells to respond to changes in nutritional conditions is illustrated in Fig. 7.1. This illustrates the amazing difference in the appearance of cells of the yeast *Hansenula polymorpha* when grown on glucose or on methanol as C substrates. The methanol-grown yeasts contain huge peroxisomes loaded with so much methanol oxidase that this enzyme appears in crystalline arrays. In glucose-grown cells a more familiar yeast organization is seen.

In addition to controlling the entry of substrates and metabolic pathways in the cell, there is a need for coordination of the various rates of macromolecular synthesis leading to balanced cell growth. This is a more general level at which control is exerted to ensure, for example, that the cell envelope grows at a rate adequate to match the increase in cell mass due to growth of the internal components. At an even more complex level, the cell must coordinate the changes in its structures so that division or

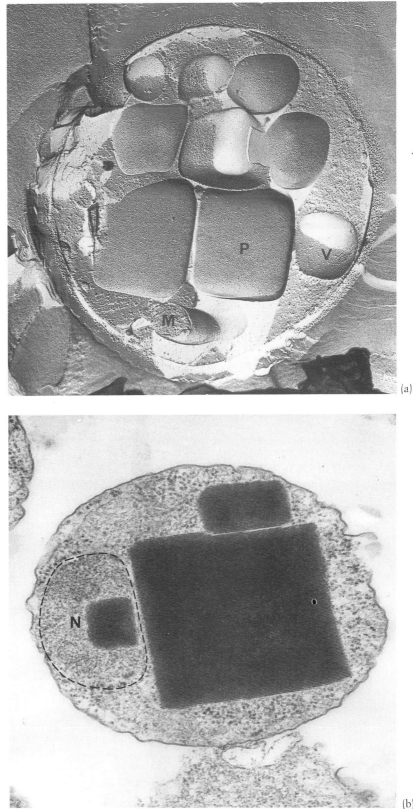

Fig. 7.1 *Hansenula polymorpha* grown under different conditions. (a) Freeze-etch replica of cells grown in methanol-limited chemostat. Note the extensive peroxisomes, the mitochondrion and vacuole; (b) cytosolic and nuclear crystalloids of alcohol oxidase in a mutant deficient in protoplast peroxisome (grown in chemostat on glucose/methanol); (c) *Hansenula polymorpha* grown on glucose and shifted to methanol. These cells display a more normal morphology for a microbial eukaryote but reveal induction of a peroxisome. N = nucleus; V = vacuole; M = mitochondrion; P = peroxisomes.

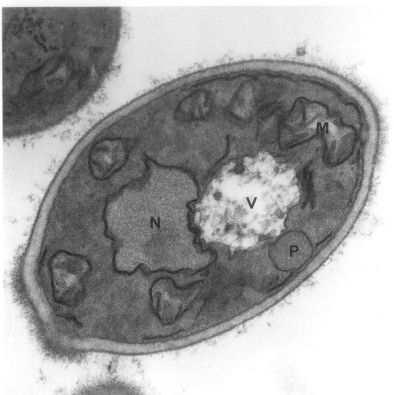

(c)   **Fig. 7.1** Cont.

developmental changes occur at the right time and in the right
place to produce the correct pattern. Discussion of this type
of control is left to Chapter 8; this section concentrates on the
regulation affecting cell metabolism.

In addition to an academic interest in what makes cells tick,
there are a number of practical reasons for studying regulation
at this level. Metabolic pathways can be manipulated to suit
the demands of research and industry. For example, the essential
amino acid L-lysine is produced quite cheaply by fermentation
using overproducing strains of *Corynebacterium glutamicum*.
These were selected on the basis of knowledge of the controls
affecting the branched pathways leading from aspartate to
methionine, threonine, isoleucine and lysine (Fig. 7.2). The field is
still rapidly expanding, especially with regard to regulation of gene
expression, due to the current interest in biotechnology. Much
of the present extensive ability to manipulate a gene from one
organism and express it in another host is based on earlier studies
of bacteriophage, plasmid and cellular control. This, coupled with
the ease of growth of microorganisms, means that many valuable
proteins will probably be produced commercially in organisms
such as *Escherichia coli* and to a lesser extent *Bacillus subtilis* and
Saccharomyces cerevisiae.

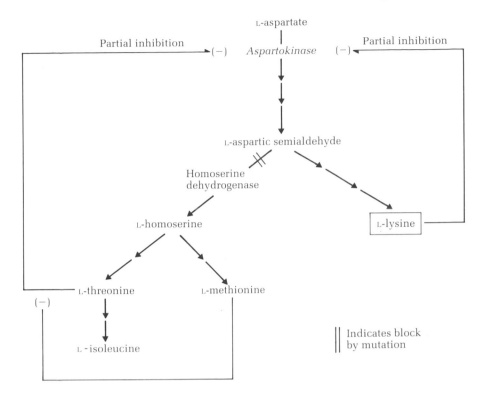

Fig. 7.2 Production of L-lysine by homoserine-requiring mutants of *Corynebacterium glutamicum*. By blocking homoserine dehydrogenase the flow of metabolites is diverted to L-lysine. The mutant requires feeding of limiting amounts of L-methionine and L-threonine. The L-threonine must be kept limiting to avoid feedback inhibition of aspartokinase. In other bacteria, such as *Escherichia coli*, there are multiple forms of aspartokinase each subject to repression by a different amino acid and hence, in these, homoserine autotrophs do not accumulate L-lysine.

CONTROL AS A FUNCTION OF METABOLIC ROLE OF A PATHWAY

The controls that have evolved for metabolic processes in each organism depend a great deal on the nature of the substrates and products concerned, and their role in the overall metabolism of the cell. For example, the enzymes of the Embden–Meyerhof pathway are required under most conditions of growth either for the production of energy, or the supply of compounds needed for biosynthetic purposes. These need to be produced in relatively large amounts and they are usually controlled by modulation of *enzyme activity* rather than at the level of enzyme synthesis. Not all enzymes in the pathway need to be controlled; those occurring just after major branch points in metabolism are the most economical sites for control.

For enzymes that are central to metabolism, regulation is often complicated and one enzyme may respond to many metabolites. A good example is *citrate synthetase*, which in some species of aerobic Gram-negative bacteria is inhibited by 2-oxoglutarate and NADH, and NADH inhibition is reversed by AMP. In other species, ATP acts as an inhibitor, while in yet others the substrates (acetyl CoA and oxaloacetate) stimulate the activity of the enzyme. These controls reflect the importance to the various organisms of the need to generate ATP and reducing equivalents on the one hand, and citric acid cycle intermediates for biosynthesis on the other. They also show that different organisms have evolved different strategies for the same type of control.

For a synthetic pathway with one major end product (e.g. an amino acid) it is advantageous to a cell if control of a pathway responds to the final concentration of the product in the cell. This is *feedback control*, and can be exerted either on enzyme synthesis or enzyme activity, in many cases both. For a degradative pathway it is more likely that control responds to the presence of a substrate and not its final product. This control is usually found to affect the amount of enzyme synthesized and/or entry of the substrate into the cell.

SITES OF MICROBIAL REGULATION

There are many mechanisms whereby cells regulate their metabolism, but in general terms the control is usually exerted at one or more of a specific number of sites. For example, Fig. 7.3 indicates some controls involved in the utilization of an external nutrient.

Entry. The cell membrane acts as a barrier to most hydrophilic molecules, but it has systems for the transport of specific compounds (see Chapter 3). Most of these mechanisms are dependent on energy. Entry can thus be controlled by the availability of ATP or PEP for the permease function, by regulating the synthesis of the permeases, or by inhibiting their activity in some way.

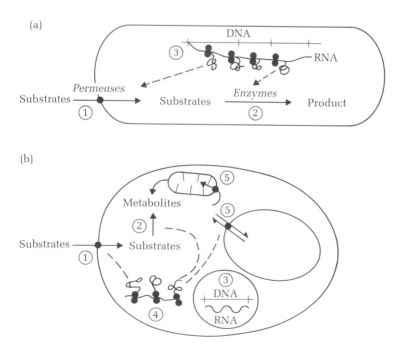

Fig. 7.3 Sites of microbial control. (a) Prokaryotic: 1 = solute uptake, 2 = enzyme activity, 3 = enzyme or permease synthesis; (b) eukaryotic: 1 = solute uptake, 2 = enzyme activity, 3 = transcription in the nucleus, 4 = translation in cytoplasm, 5 = uptake and separation of compounds into organelles.

Flux through the metabolic pathway. There are two major ways in which the flow of the metabolites through a sequence of enzyme-catalysed steps is controlled: by regulation of the *concentration* of enzyme present (i.e. by increasing or decreasing the rate of *synthesis* or *degradation* of crucial enzymes in the pathway, relative to that for other cell proteins); or by modifying the *activity* of enzyme molecules already present. In prokaryotes, by virtue of the coupling between transcription and translation, most but not all of the control over the rate of enzyme synthesis occurs at the level of transcription. In eukaryotes there is more scope for translational control due to the spatial separation of the processes of transcription (nucleus) and translation (cytoplasm).

Limiting physical access of enzymes to their substrates. This is more evident in eukaryotes where substrates can exist in separate *pools* by virtue of their location within different membrane-bound organelles. For example, in *Neurospora*, arginine is found in two kinetically distinct pools, one in the cytoplasm for biosynthetic reactions, the other in the vacuole in which the enzymes involved in arginine degradation are located. This spatial type of control can exist in prokaryotes when the enzymes of a reaction sequence exist as a multi-enzyme complex, or as membrane-bound entities.

CONTROL OF ENZYME SYNTHESIS

Some of the enzymes in a cell are synthesized at about the same rate relative to other proteins under a broad range of conditions. This includes the enzymes of central metabolism such as the Embden–Meyerhof pathway; such enzymes are said to be *constitutive*. However, the concentrations of many other enzymes in microorganisms, especially prokaryotes, are subject to considerable variation depending on the conditions in which the organisms are growing. This is particularly so for pathways which are required only under some but not all conditions of growth. Such enzymes are produced in response to the presence of a compound such as a metabolizable sugar (*induction*), or are prevented from being synthesized by a metabolite such as an amino acid (*repression*).

There are many ways in which control of the rate of enzyme synthesis can be achieved, including:

1 Altering the rate of initiation of transcription (a major method).
2 Preventing termination of transcription giving read-through into subsequent genes (seen in the development of some bacteriophages, and in a few specific cases of metabolism).
3 Altering the rate of initiation of protein synthesis (a minor, but significant method seen in controlling the quantity of subunits of ribosomal components and in affecting the quantity of subunits formed in bacteriophage development).

Since there are major differences in the processes of gene expression between prokaryotes and eukaryotes, the nature of the control systems are rather different, and the following treats each separately.

REGULATION OF PROKARYOTIC GENE EXPRESSION

Most of the regulation of gene expression in prokaryotes occurs at the level of transcription. There are several ways in which this can be achieved.

Promoter strength

Different proteins, even those produced constitutively, are required in the cell at different molar concentrations. Organisms have this static control over quantity via the evolution of differences in the base sequence in the promoter region, such that highly expressed genes have a sequence that is closer to the ideal (see p. 158). This has an obvious consequence for biotechnology, when high levels of expression of a heterologous gene may be desired, and many genes with 'strong promoters' have been identified and cloned. In fact, a combination promoter using the 'better' regions of the *lac* and the *trp* promoters of *E. coli* (the *tac* promoter) has been produced for high-level expression.

Altered transcription factors

The above control is fixed, and does not lead to the cell responding to different conditions by altering the rate of enzyme synthesis. This can be achieved in bacteria by producing a change in the transcription initiation factor(s). This occurs when conditions change and a new set of genes needs to be read. The best examples are seen during morphogenesis in *Bacillus* and *Streptomyces* (see Chapter 9), but the same processes occur during the response of *E. coli* to heat shock (see p. 219). A new σ factor is formed, which directs transcription to a relatively small set of genes until the cell has adjusted to the high temperature.

Induction and repression

This is the most common form of control over synthesis of enzymes in bacteria. Table 7.1 lists some of the many metabolic processes that are controlled by induction and repression. Of these, the most extensively studied control system is that affecting lactose fermentation in *E. coli*. While the lactose operon is a very useful example for general discussion it should be understood that it is only one of a large number of variations on a theme, and

Table 7.1 Some processes controlled by induction and repression in bacteria.

Process	Type of response
Utilization of sugars	Induction by sugar or its metabolite
Synthesis of amino acids, nucleotides and cofactors	Feedback repression of synthesis by excess product
Catabolite repression	Repression of catabolic enzyme synthesis by rich carbon sources
Nitrogen repression	Repression of utilization of alternative nitrogen sources to NH_4^+
Synthesis of transcriptional and translational apparatus	Autoregulation by repression in presence of excess subunits
SOS response to DNA damage	Induction by damage to DNA
Heat shock response	Induction by heat or osmotic shock

there are differences not only from one control system to another, but also between bacterial species in the details of control of a single pathway.

The lactose operon

One of the early findings by Monod in studying the utilization of the disaccharide lactose was that in mixtures of glucose and lactose *E. coli* cultures use the glucose preferentially. There is then a slight lag period of about 15 min after glucose is exhausted before the cells start to grow on lactose. This effect, shown in Fig. 7.4, is termed *diauxic growth*, which results from several control systems operating on the uptake and metabolism of lactose. One system is the more general phenomenon of carbon catabolite repression, discussed above and described in more detail later. Another, however, is specific to lactose. Unless lactose or a related β-galactoside was added to the cells, the enzyme needed for the degradation of lactose was not synthesized. An extensive

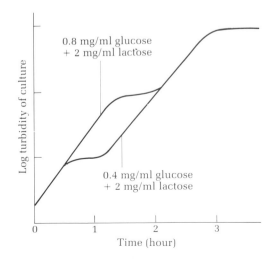

Fig. 7.4 Glucose repression of lactose utilization. The diauxic growth curve.

biochemical and genetic analysis of this system led to the *operon theory of regulation*, which is generally applicable to prokaryotes, but not eukaryotes.

Induction of enzyme synthesis

Entry of lactose into a cell is mediated by a permease system (Chapter 2), which requires only one protein (the *lac permease*, product of the *lacY* gene) specifically for lactose transport. Once inside the cell, the disaccharide is hydrolysed to glucose and galactose by *β-galactosidase* (*lacZ* gene product). Neither the permease nor β-galactosidase is synthesized in large amounts in *E. coli* unless either lactose or certain other β-galactosides are present in the medium. The β-galactosides *induce* synthesis of the two proteins (and also of a third, *thiogalactoside transacetylase; lacA* gene product) from a basal level of about 10 molecules per cell to an induced level which may be about 1000-fold greater.

Induction occurs quite rapidly after the addition of the inducer and is usually studied using an analogue, *isopropyl-thiogalactoside* (IPTG), which acts as an inducer, but not as a substrate, for β-galactosidase. When studying induction in a growing culture, it is important to express the results to show clearly that there has been a change in the rate of synthesis of the enzyme relative to the total rate of protein synthesis. One method, used in Fig. 7.5, is to plot enzyme activity per millilitre of culture against protein per mililitre; one can also follow specific activity (enzyme activity per milligram protein in the culture) as a function of time. On removing the inducer, the rate of enzyme synthesis decays rapidly with a half-life of about 1 min. This rapid response in bacteria means that no energy is wasted on unnecessary enzyme synthesis when lactose is exhausted.

The control system

The operon model for induction of lactose-utilizing enzymes is outlined in Fig. 7.6, which illustrates the arrangement of genes determining the important elements of the *lac* system and their interaction with the inducer molecule (lactose or β-galactoside

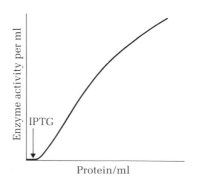

Fig. 7.5 Induction of β-galactosidase in *Escherichia coli* by the lactose analogue IPTG.

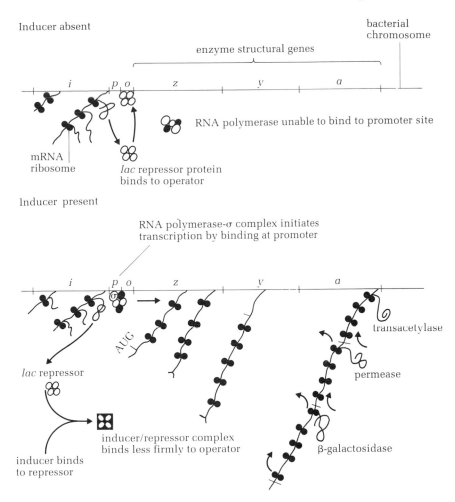

Inducer absent

enzyme structural genes

bacterial chromosome

i   *p o*   *z*   *y*   *a*

RNA polymerase unable to bind to promoter site

mRNA ribosome

lac repressor protein binds to operator

Inducer present

RNA polymerase-σ complex initiates transcription by binding at promoter

i   *p o*   *z*   *y*   *a*

transacetylase

AUG

permease

lac repressor

inducer/repressor complex binds less firmly to operator

β-galactosidase

inducer binds to repressor

Fig. 7.6 The *lac* operon in *Escherichia coli*.

analogue) and each other. This model is the culmination of extensive genetic and biochemical study and is based largely on: mapping of mutations affecting lactose fermentation; analysis of control mutants (e.g. mutations leading to constitutive β-galactosidase production) by diploid genetics to test the interaction of various elements in the system; and eventual biochemical isolation and purification of all components of the system and their use in *in vitro* systems for synthesizing the *lac* proteins from the DNA template and essential substrates.

The essential features of the model are:

1 The structural genes coding for the three proteins, β-galactosidase (*lacZ*), permease (*lacY*) and transacetylase (*lacA*), are adjacent on the *E. coli* chromosome.

2 The expression of these genes (synthesis of the proteins) is regulated at the level of the initiation of transcription by control regions which map outside, but close to, the structural gene *lacZ*. The control gene, *lacI*, codes for a protein (repressor protein) which binds specifically and with very high affinity (dissociation constant: 10^{-13} M) at another control site, the operator (*lacO*), which is a short sequence of about 24 bases that does not code for a protein. These control sequences were initially defined by mutations which affected the inducibility of the system by lactose, and which were not located in the structural genes.

In the absence of inducer molecules the *lacI* gene product binds as a tetramer to the operator site and prevents transcription of the *lacZ*, *lacY* and *lacA* genes by RNA polymerase. *In vitro* this complex decays with the incredible half-life of 30 min, and this has enabled the binding sequence to be determined precisely since the repressor protein protects the operator region from digestion with DNase.

When inducer is present it binds to the repressor protein as a ligand, and the complex so formed has reduced affinity for the operator site (the tetrameric repressor protein is therefore an allosteric protein, see p. 220).

Transcription of *lacZ*, *lacY* and *lacA*, therefore, is initiated from a distinct binding site for the RNA polymerase–σ factor complex, the promoter region *lacP*.

3 The three genes, *lacZ*, *lacY* and *lacA*, are all transcribed as a single mRNA transcript. This polycistronic message contains three initiation sites recognized by *E. coli* ribosomes and acts as a template for the synthesis of all three proteins. These are therefore produced in a coordinately controlled way under normal conditions, that is, regardless of the level of induction all three proteins are synthesized in the same proportions.

4 Rapid degradation of mRNA (its half-life is about 2 min) by a specific endonuclease ensures that the rate of synthesis of the enzymes rapidly decreases on the depletion of lactose.

The essential features of an operon are a clustering of genes for related functions transcribed from a single promoter site under the control of a single operator region.

The *lac* operon is under *negative control* of the *lac* repressor since this protein prevents transcription when bound to the operator. There are other situations, such as the maltose (*mal*) operon in *E. coli* and certain elements in the lytic development of bacteriophage λ (see Chapter 8) in which the presence of a control protein activates transcription: this is *positive control*. In the *lac* operon there is also positive control for the catabolite repression system. The control protein in the arabinose (*ara*) operon is of special interest since in the absence of arabinose it acts negatively to repress transcription, and in the presence of the inducer it is an activator.

The nature of the control region and repressor binding

The whole of the *E. coli lac* region has been sequenced, and the control region between *lacI* and *lacZ* is shown in Fig. 7.7, with an indication of the sites at which various molecules interact. The

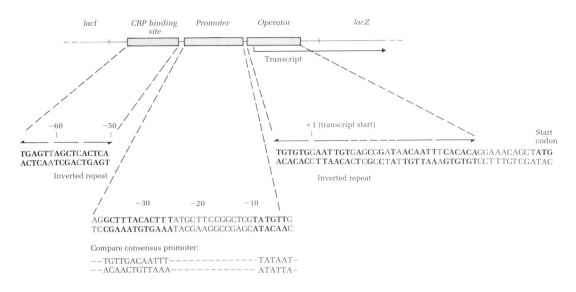

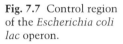

Fig. 7.7 Control region of the *Escherichia coli lac* operon.

promoter (RNA polymerase binding site) has been discussed in the previous chapter. There are two other important regulation sites, the operator at which the *lac* repressor binds, and the cyclic-AMP receptor protein (CRP) binding site involved in the general control process of catabolite repression (p. 215). Both of these have near palindromic sequences (showing twofold rotational symmetry), a feature common to many sites at which a bacterial regulatory protein binds; such symmetry probably contributes significantly to the high affinity displayed by repressor or activator proteins.

The mechanism by which repressor proteins (including those affecting other operons) bind to operator regions has received considerable attention.

Some repressor proteins have a domain which is characterized by a 'helix-turn-helix' motif, that is, they have a group of about 12 or so amino acids which fold to form an α-helix, followed by a short group of hydrophobic amino acids about a glycine residue (this introduces a sharp turn in the structure) and another α-helical region. Such a structure can match the major groove in the DNA helix, and recognize a specific base sequence. The likely secondary structure of the λ repressor and DNA is shown in Fig. 7.8.

Characteristics of operon control

In summary, the important principles of operon control in prokaryotes are:

1 In addition to structural genes there are control genes which code for proteins that bind with high specificity to control sequences to inhibit or activate transcription. Control is therefore largely at the level of transcription and not translation.

2 The DNA-binding activity of control proteins is modified by small molecule ligands (e.g. inducers or repressors), in the same way as the activity of allosteric enzymes (see p. 220).

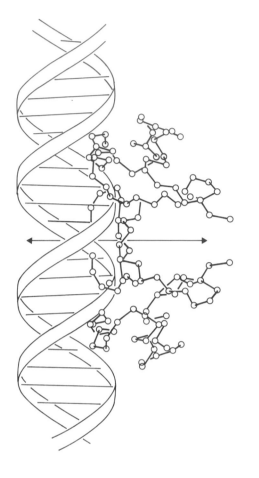

Fig. 7.8 Presumed interaction of the bacteriophage λ cro repressor with its binding site on DNA. Two monomers of cro protein interact with the DNA with a pair of α-helices occupying successive major grooves of the DNA about a two-fold axis of symmetry indicated by arrows. (Redrawn from Anderson *et al.* (1981) *Nature* **290**, 754–758.)

3 Response to a particular molecule in the environment is rapid, due to a rapid alteration in the rate of protein synthesis. However, there is no sudden change in the activity of enzyme already present in the culture. This must be diluted out by growth unless it is unstable and degraded by proteases. In bacteria most enzymes do not undergo turnover (i.e. proteolytic degradation) until the culture is starved.

4 Clustering of related genes so that they are read from a single promoter can provide a simple way of coordinating the response to a particular environmental change. The fully induced levels are a function of the strength of the promoter.

VARIATIONS ON THE OPERON THEME AND OTHER MECHANISMS OF CONTROLLING ENZYME SYNTHESIS IN PROKARYOTES

The above is a brief outline of the *lac* operon to illustrate general principles of prokaryotic control. Other systems differ in details, and these often reflect differences in the role of the pathway in question. The following are far from comprehensive, and are mainly from studies of enterobacteria which have sufficiently well-developed genetic systems (especially partial diploidy) essential to the analysis of control. Other bacteria occupying niches completely different from the human gut may show even more fundamental, as yet undiscovered, differences.

Feedback control

Lactose utilization is a catabolic process; many other controlled enzyme pathways are anabolic, including those forming amino acids, nucleotides, vitamins and cofactors. In these the important variable in overall control is the *end product*, not the substrate of the pathway. Repressor proteins are still formed, but these interact with the end product of the pathway to prevent further enzyme synthesis when end product is in excess. Thus the tryptophan (*trp*) operon in *E. coli* is a negatively controlled operon in which protein binds to prevent transcription in the presence of tryptophan (Fig. 7.9).

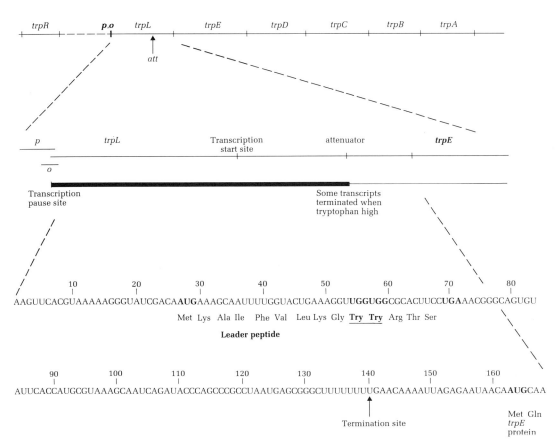

Fig. 7.9 The tryptophan operon of *Escherichia coli*.

Termination and attenuation control

Control of gene expression by modulating the rate of initiation of transcription is an obvious strategy; less obvious is regulation by *termination* of transcription, yet this mechanism does occur in a number of situations. One is the read through from one block of genes to an adjacent one during bacteriophage development (Chapter 8, p. 256). However, transcription termination sites can be located within an operon and act to control the level of gene expression. This mechanism of regulation is termed attenuation.

The most studied examples of attenuation control are those in the operons concerned with biosynthesis of a number of amino acids, including tryptophan, histidine, leucine, threonine and isoleucine/valine (*ilv* operon), but also in the operon coding for the β and β' subunits of RNA polymerase and the ribosomal protein genes *rpoL* and *rpoJ* (see Fig. 7.15); of these the *trp* operon of *E. coli* has been most extensively characterized.

The terminal steps in tryptophan biosynthesis are catalysed by enzymes encoded by five structural genes forming an operon under the control of a regulatory region. The operon is fairly large, about 7 kb, and is under dual control—from both *repression*, mediated at an operator site located within the promoter region by a tryptophan-binding repressor protein (the product of the unlinked regulatory gene *trpR*), and by *attenuation*, from a site located within the 162 bp transcribed region prior to the first major structural gene *trpE*. This is called the *leader* region and is designated *trpL* (Fig. 7.9).

Transcription from the *trp* operon can be regulated over a 600-fold range; repression is the most effective and it can reduce transcription by about 70-fold, while attenuation can only exert about an eight to tenfold effect.

The mechanism of attenuation

The leader region for the *trp* operon is shown in Fig. 7.9. Similar leaders have been sequenced for a number of amino acid

Operon	Leader Sequence
trp	Met Lys Ala Ile Phe Val Leu Lys Gly **Try Try** Arg Thr Ser
pheA	Met Lys His Ile Pro **Phe Phe Phe** Ala **Phe Phe Phe** Thr **Phe** Pro
his	Met Thr Arg Val Gln Phe Lys **His His His His His His His** Pro Asp
leu	Met Ser His Ile Val Arg Phe Thr Gly **Leu Leu Leu Leu** Asn Ala Phe Ile Val Arg Gly Arg Pro Val Gly Gly Ile Gln His
ilv	Met Thr Ala **Leu Leu** Arg **Val Ile** Ser **Leu Val Val Ile** Ser **Val Val Val Ile Ile Ile** Pro Pro Cys Gly Ala Ala **Leu** Gly Arg Gly Lys Ala
thr	Met Lys Arg **Ile** Ser **Thr Thr Ile Thr Thr Thr Ile Thr Ile Thr Thr** Gly Asn Gly Ala Gly

Fig. 7.10 Amino acids in leader peptides of various operons. (From Yanofsky (1981) *Nature* **289**, 751.)

biosynthetic operons, and all have several features in common:

1 They all have a short open reading frame beginning with an AUG codon and capable of encoding a polypeptide of from 14 to 32 aminoacyl residues (14 in the *trp* operon). The open reading is terminated by a stop codon.

2 This short polypeptide contains runs of the amino acid(s) which regulates the operon as shown in Fig. 7.10. Thus the *his* operon contains seven adjacent histidine codons in the leader peptide, while the *trp* operon contains two adjacent tryptophan codons.

3 Further downstream in the leader region is a site at which attenuation of transcription occurs. This is characterized by a termination site with a G+C-rich region followed by an A+T-rich region. When attenuated, the *trp* transcript terminates at base 140 from the start of transcription.

4 Between the start of transcription and the attenuation site there are regions in which the RNA transcript can adopt alternative secondary structures. In the *trp* operon the two likely hairpin loop structures are shown in Fig. 7.11. These have almost equal binding energy.

How is attenuation brought about by this arrangement? The theory proposed by Yanofsky and his colleagues is that transcrip-

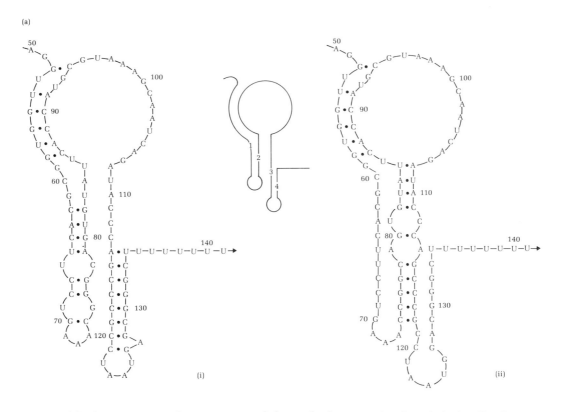

Fig. 7.11 (a) Alternative secondary structures of the *trp* leader transcript. Intrachain bonding between strands 1:2 and 3:4 is shown in (i) and between 2:3 in (ii).

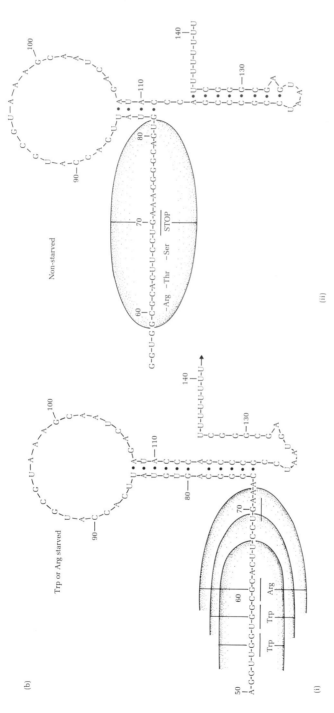
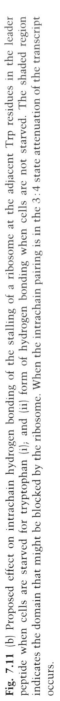

Fig. 7.11 (b) Proposed effect on intrachain hydrogen bonding of the stalling of a ribosome at the adjacent Trp residues in the leader peptide when cells are starved for tryptophan (i); and (ii) form of hydrogen bonding when cells are not starved. The shaded region indicates the domain that might be blocked by the ribosome. When the intrachain pairing is in the 3 : 4 state attenuation of the transcript occurs.

tion is initiated at the promoter and continues through the leader region. Translation of the leader polypeptide is also initiated by a ribosome attaching to the nascent transcript. If there is too low a level of charged tryptophanyl-tRNA^{Trp} then the ribosome will stall at the two adjacent tryptophan codons at nucleotides 54–59. It is proposed that a stalled ribosome sterically blocks about ten nucleotides on the downstream side of the transcript, and thereby determines which secondary structure it will adopt. For the *trp* operon, it is only when the cells are starved for tryptophan (or arginine, the adjacent codon) that the transcript is unable to adopt the secondary structure with the 3:4 arrangement shown in Fig. 7.11. It is assumed that transcription terminates at the attenuator only when this 3:4 structure is formed. It has been found that transcription of the leader region pauses at nucleotide 90: this may allow the ribosome translating the leader peptide time to reach the appropriate position on the transcript and synchronize the movement of the RNA polymerase and ribosome.

Attenuation is thus a curious phenomenon since it is *translational* effects on the secondary structure of an RNA transcript which determine whether or not transcription can continue past a potential termination site. Other aspects of this control are covered in the elegant review by Yanofsky cited under 'Further reading'.

Autogenous control

The *lac* repressor is synthesized constitutively. Autogenous systems differ in that the repressor protein is directly involved in controlling its own synthesis. On theoretical grounds such an arrangement can make negative control systems more stable and

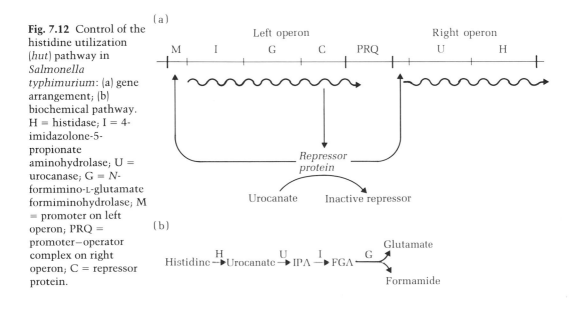

Fig. 7.12 Control of the histidine utilization (*hut*) pathway in *Salmonella typhimurium*: (a) gene arrangement; (b) biochemical pathway. H = histidase; I = 4-imidazolone-5-propionate aminohydrolase; U = urocanase; G = *N*-formimino-L-glutamate formiminohydrolase; M = promoter on left operon; PRQ = promoter–operator complex on right operon; C = repressor protein.

responsive to the environment than those involving constitutive repressor synthesis. This type of control is not common, but has been found in the histidine utilization (*hut*) operon (Fig. 7.12) and in a sense in the control of SOS repair via *recA*.

Mixed and divergent operons

In some pathways not all enzymes are coded on a single polycistronic messenger RNA; several operons, or an operon and several scattered genes are found. In many of these, e.g. the pyrimidine pathway in *E. coli*, regulation is still coordinate for the unclustered genes; one repressor protein can recognize a number of separate operator sites located at different points on the bacterial genome. This is an important point which has considerable relevance to both regulation in eukaryotic microorganisms and the phenomenon of catabolite repression, discussed later.

The arginine pathway in *E. coli* illustrates a case of divergent operon control in which the operator region maps between two structural genes in a cluster. Transcription of these genes occurs in opposite directions (on different strands of the DNA) but is controlled from the same operator region.

Sequential induction and branched-chain pathways

A number of bacteria, particularly *Pseudomonas* species, can use a very wide variety of organic compounds as carbon substrate. These include phenols and other aromatics which are quite toxic to most organisms. The pathways for conversion of many of these compounds to succinate merge (Fig. 7.13 illustrates just two examples), and some substrates are intermediates in the metabolism of others. Such pathways are controlled in sections, rather than as a single operon, so that bacteria can grow on any one of a number of aromatic substrates without inducing unnecessary enzymes. This is accomplished by a process of *sequential induction*, the product of one 'induction block' acting as the inducer for the next group of enzymes in the pathway.

The reverse situation applies when a single intermediate is involved in the synthesis of two or more products by branched pathways in which a common intermediate may feed more than one final product. There are several types of control of enzyme synthesis found for branched systems:

1 Feedback repression control on the first enzymes after the last common intermediate (Fig. 7.14).

2 Partial feedback repression by each product on the first enzyme in the overall pathway.

3 Synthesis of different enzyme species catalysing the same reaction (*isozymes*), with each isozyme species controlled by one particular end product. This is less commonly found, but a good example occurs in *E. coli* for the family of amino acids derived

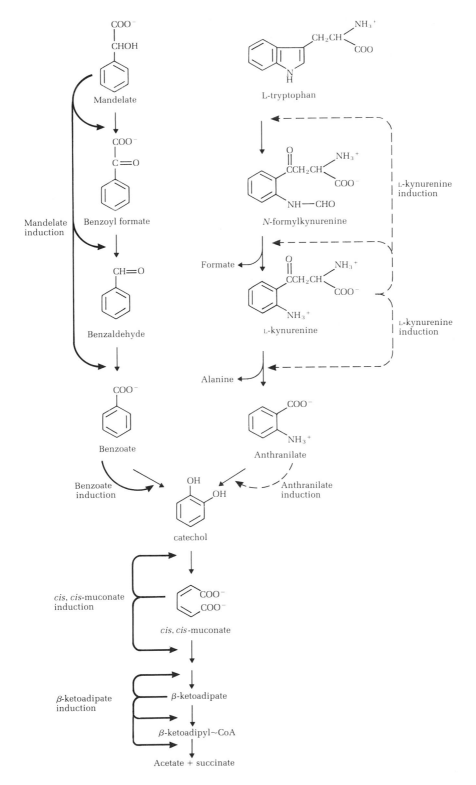

Fig. 7.13 Sequential induction of the aromatic degradation pathways in *Pseudomonas*.

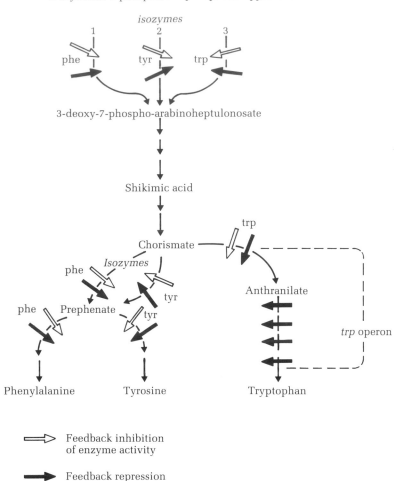

D-erythrose-4-phosphate + phosphoenolpyruvate

isozymes

phe   tyr   trp

3-deoxy-7-phospho-arabinoheptulonosate

Shikimic acid

Chorismate

trp

Isozymes

phe

Anthranilate

phe   Prephenate   tyr

tyr

trp operon

Phenylalanine   Tyrosine   Tryptophan

⟹ Feedback inhibition
    of enzyme activity

➤ Feedback repression
    of enzyme synthesis

Fig. 7.14 Control of aromatic amino acid synthesis in *Escherichia coli*.

from aspartate. There are three isozymes for aspartate kinase: one is repressible by lysine, one by methionine, and the other jointly by threonine and isoleucine.

Translational control

All of the above examples involve reduction of the rate of protein synthesis by a lowering of the rate of initiation of transcription of a gene. This type of control is by far the most common form affecting enzyme synthesis, and is economical since mRNA is not produced when not needed.

There are, however, some important examples of control at the level of translation, probably none more so than those concerned with synthesis of the ribosomal proteins and RNA polymerase. In *E. coli* the rates of synthesis of most of the 55 ribosomal proteins are identical, and respond coordinately to changes in growth rates.

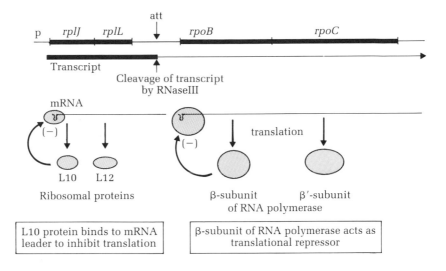

att

p   *rplJ*   *rplL*   *rpoB*   *rpoC*

Transcript

Cleavage of transcript
by RNaseIII

mRNA

(−)

translation

(−)

L10   L12

Ribosomal proteins

β-subunit   β′-subunit
of RNA polymerase

L10 protein binds to mRNA
leader to inhibit translation

β-subunit of RNA polymerase acts as
translational repressor

Fig. 7.15 The β operon of *Escherichia coli*. This operon encodes two genes for proteins of the large ribosomal subunit (L10 and L12) and the two genes for the β and β′ subunits of RNA polymerase. The L10 protein acts as a translational repressor by binding to secondary structure in the leader region of the transcript to block ribosome attachment. A similar process may occur for the β subunit of RNA polymerase on its transcript after processing by the RNase III. The attenuator att leads to a fivefold reduction in transcription into the *rpoB, C* region. The promoter is indicated by p.

The ribosomal proteins are coded in groups of operons, and one reason for the coordinate control is that their synthesis is coupled to the assembly process so that certain free ribosomal proteins (S4, S7, S8, L1, L4 and L10) act as *translational repressors*, each inhibiting the synthesis of some or all of the other ribosomal proteins in the same operon. Figure 7.15 shows one of the more complex of these operons composed of the genes for subunits L7/12 (*rplL*) and L10 (*rplJ*), as well as for the β and β′ subunits of RNA polymerase. This operon is a superb example of several variations on the operon theme. Transcription begins at the promoter before the *rplJ* gene, and proceeds through *rplL*, to an attenuation site, at which all but 20% of the transcripts terminate. Those that read through this site continue to transcribe the *rpoB* and *rpoC* genes. All of the transcripts that read through are cleaved by RNase III at the site shown. Superimposed on this is translational repression of the reading of their mRNA by both free β subunits and the protein L10 (*rplJ* product). The net result is a tight control of the quantity of each protein produced, and inhibition if free subunits accumulate.

TWO-COMPONENT CONTROL SYSTEMS

Many genes in bacteria are regulated in response to a particular set of environmental conditions such as the availability of such nutrients as nitrogen or phosphate, or the osmolarity of the medium. These conditions are sensed and the signal has to be received by a receptor and transmitted to the transcriptional apparatus of the cell.

There are a relatively large number (probably about 50) of such systems which conform to a very similar pattern, with closely related proteins performing the key roles. These are known as two-

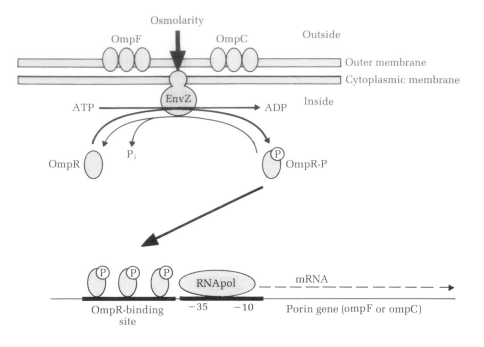

component systems, since each has two active elements. The first is a protein that acts as a signal receptor. When activated, it acts as a protein kinase to phosphorylate the second protein component in the cell. The second protein is, when phosphorylated, a positive activator of transcription of those genes whose expression responds to the particular set of environmental conditions.

Examples of such two-component systems include control mechanisms involved in: nitrogen metabolism in enterobacteria (NtrB/NtrC); chemotaxis in *E. coli* (CheA/CheB); phosphate regulation in *E. coli* (PhoR/PhoB) and plant infection in *Agrobacterium tumefaciens* (VirA/VirB). In each of the above examples, the first component (NtrB, CheA, PhoR and VirA) is the protein which acts as the *sensor* for the environmental signal (they are encoded by the genes *ntrB*, *cheA*, *phoR* and *virA* respectively). The second component (NtrC, etc.) is the protein which functions as a positive effector regulating gene expression or cellular behaviour in response to a particular stimulus.

In some cases, the signal receptor is soluble and is located in the cytoplasm (e.g. NtrB and CheA). For others, however, the signal has to be transduced across the cytoplasmic membrane, and in this case the receptor is located across the cytoplasmic membrane.

The system involved in the osmotic regulation of the porin genes is outlined in Fig. 7.16. In this case the porin genes *ompF* and *ompC* are regulated by the binding of the phosphorylated form of the *ompF* gene product to the binding site (60 bp) just upstream of the RNA polymerase binding site (−10, −35 region). This polymerase binding site does not conform very well to the con-

Fig. 7.16 The two-component system for osmotic regulation of the *ompF* and *ompC* porin genes in *Escherichia coli.* (Redrawn from Mizuno & Mizushima (1990) *Molecular Microbiology* **4**, 1077–1082.)

sensus promoter sequence and the binding of OmpR-P is needed to assist the polymerase to initiate transcription. In this case, the osmolarity of the surrounding medium is detected by the *envZ* gene product located across the cytoplasmic membrane. EnvZ is a protein kinase and can phosphorylate OmpR in response to the external osmotic conditions. Note that EnvZ can also act to dephosphorylate OmpR-P, so that expression of *ompC* and *ompF* is also down-regulated by the same system. This situation is slightly complicated since OmpF is preferentially synthesized under conditions of low osmolarity whereas OmpC is made by the cell under higher osmolarity. The phosphorylated form of OmpR is needed to activate transcription of both genes; when its concentration is low it preferentially binds to the *ompF* gene control region and at high concentration to the *ompC* gene.

CONTROL OF ENZYME SYNTHESIS IN EUKARYOTIC MICROORGANISMS

So far the discussion has been of prokaryotes, and since there are major differences between prokaryotes and eukaryotes in transcription and translation, it is important to know whether the phenomena of induction and repression, and the organization of genes of related function into operons, apply in eukaryotes.

There are many examples in eukaryotic microorganisms of induction and repression in which the rate of synthesis of an enzyme responds to a particular metabolite. The difference between the basal and the fully induced enzyme levels is usually, but not always, less for eukaryotes than for prokaryotes. For example, arginase in *E. coli* can be induced about 100-fold over the basal level, whereas in *Saccharomyces cerevisiae* the maximal change is about tenfold; β-galactosidase can be induced over a 1000-fold range, whereas in the yeast *Kluyveromyces lactis* the range is about 100-fold.

There is, however, no example of a clustering of genes into a true operon in any of the eukaryotic microorganisms examined in detail, including *S. cerevisiae*, *Schizosaccharomyces pombe*, *Neurospora crassa* and *Aspergillus nidulans*. This is a reflection of the mechanism whereby the eukaryotic ribosome recognizes the first AUG codon in a messenger RNA and its inability to reinitiate transcription on a message once translation has been terminated; bacterial operons fused behind yeast promoters are not translated beyond the first open reading frame. Usually in eukaryotes the structural genes for enzymes concerned with a particular biosynthetic pathway are scattered widely and are not linked to each other; for example, the enzymes for histidine biosynthesis in *S. cerevisiae* are coded on six of the 16 chromosomes. There are a few cases in which gene clusters are found, including the *HIS*4 locus in *S. cerevisiae* (which codes for three enzymic activities), the *GAL*1,10 cluster in the same organism, and the genes for proline oxidation in *Aspergillus*. For those systems studied in detail, either the gene cluster encodes a single, multifunctional polypeptide translated as a single entity (e.g. *HIS*4 in *S. cerevisiae*) or there is divergent transcription from a common control region (as in *GAL*1,10). There is, however, no lack of examples in eukaryotic systems of regulated genes or genes coding for regulators, or of sites that may be involved in binding of proteins to activate or repress enzyme synthesis. In fact the control circuits may be even more complex than in prokaryotes.

Considerable progress has been made recently in analysing the control of gene expression in lower eukaryotes, especially yeast. One of the most striking differences between prokaryotes and eukaryotes is seen in the extent to which the 5′ region upstream of the start of transcription is involved in the control. Regulation in some yeast genes, for example that involved in homothallic switching (HO), is exerted from sequences extending 1.4 kb upstream, although 250 to 500 base pairs is more common. Sequence information, together with deletion and other mutational analysis of cloned control regions, has shown that there are *upstream activation sequences* (UAS) at which control is exerted by DNA-binding proteins (see Fig. 7.17); moreover, there is often more than one UAS. The DNA-binding proteins bind in a similar way to bacterial repressor or activator proteins, recognizing specific sequences; examples of these sequences and the control associated with them are given in Table 7.2. These sequences can work in either orientation, they are often palindromic (i.e. inverted repeats) and are sometimes repeated in the upstream region, and their precise location in the upstream region does not seem to matter. That they are the site of binding by specific DNA-binding proteins can be illustrated by 'footprinting' experiments in which DNA-binding proteins protect the DNA from digestion by DNase I (see

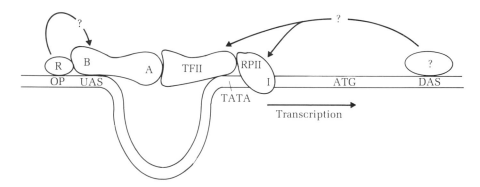

Fig. 7.17 Regulation of transcription in microbial eukaryotes. UAS = upstream activation site; B = DNA-binding domain of activation factor; A = activation domain of activation factor; TFII = complex of TATA-binding factors (these assist RNA polymerase binding); RPII = RNA polymerase II; TATA = sequence near site of initiation of transcription; OP = operator site for binding of repressor protein; I = site of initiation of transcription; DAS = downstream activation site.

Table 7.2 Control motifs in upstream activation sites of yeast genes.

Motif	Binding protein	Function
TGACTCattttt	*GCN*4 product	General control of amino acid synthesis: controls many genes involved in amino acid and nucleotide synthesis
CGGAAGACTCTCCTCCG	*GAL*4 product	Confers inducibility by galactose
T-ATTGGT	*HAP*2/*HAP*3 products	Control of genes involved in respiration
G--GAA--TTC--G	Heat shock regulator	Response of genes induced by heat shock
CACGAAAA	?	Cell division cycle control of homothallism
ACGTGGGTATGGAAG	TUF, GRFI, RAP	Activates transcription of a wide variety of genes involved in growth, including glycolytic genes and genes for ribosomal proteins
TCACGTGA	GFII, CPI	Function unknown, but found upstream of a number of nuclear genes encoding mitochondrial functions as well as some unrelated genes; this is also present in the centromere I element
RTCR-------ACG	GFI, ABF, SUF	Function unknown, found upstream of genes with various functions, including some involved in respiration. Also found near origins of replication (*ARS* elements)

Note that some motifs may vary by several bases from the consensus sequence shown and still retain activity. Moreover, there may be more than one protein in the cell that can recognize the same motif. For example, there are two ABF binding proteins which can bind to the sequence shown.

Fig. 7.18). It remains to be shown how the binding of protein molecules 200 to 500 bp or more away from the site at which transcription is initiated can control that initiation. One theory is that the DNA is looped between the UAS and a site near the TATA box by interactions between proteins binding to the DNA in both regions (as shown in Fig. 7.17).

Genetic dissection of the function of the *GAL*4 and *GCN*4 activator proteins from yeast has shown that they have a domain which confers specific DNA binding to the UAS, and a second region containing acidic residues which may be involved in activating transcription. Interestingly, this acidic domain can be replaced by a randomly chosen 15-residue amphiphilic helix (i.e. one in which acidic residues form a negative charge on one face of the helix, while the other face is hydrophobic) with retention of some activity.

There is also some indication that the extent of transcription from some genes may also be determined in part by *downstream activation sequences* (DAS) located within the open reading frame for the gene. This has important, and to some extent unfortunate, implications for biotechnologists trying to express genes of mammalian origin in yeast or other lower eukaryotes.

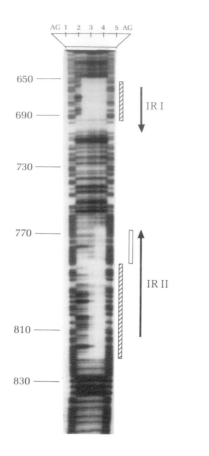

650 ——
690 ——
730 ——
770 ——
810 ——
830 ——

IR I

IR II

Fig. 7.18 Footprinting of the interaction between DNA and a DNA-binding protein. The figure illustrates the protection of a DNA fragment (from the terminus of DNA replication in *Bacillus subtilis*) by a replication terminator protein which binds at two specific sites indicated by the boxes. The DNA fragment was labelled on one strand and subjected to brief DNase I treatment to nick the DNA. Lanes 1–5 represent a sequencing gel analysis of the results of adding increasing concentrations of the protein to the DNA. The outside lanes are derived from a sequencing reaction used to localize the precise sequences to which the protein binds. Photography by courtesy of Professor R.G. Wake. (See Lewis *et al.* (1990) *Journal of Molecular Biology* **214**, 73–84.)

SYSTEMS EXERTING MORE GENERAL CONTROL OVER METABOLISM IN PROKARYOTES AND EUKARYOTES

Induction and feedback repression are *specific* responses to a particular metabolite or closely related group of metabolites, e.g. induction of the lactose utilization system by β-galactosides. In both prokaryotes and eukaryotes there are other important controls which are superimposed on the various induction systems. These are more general in their action and affect many operons, enabling the cell to use a 'preferred' substrate in the presence of a mixture of several others. Thus there is at least one system in which a readily metabolized source of carbon, such as glucose, shuts off the utilization of other, poorer, carbon sources. Another system responds to rich sources of nitrogen such as NH_4^+ or glutamine, and even phosphate represses the formation of about 80 proteins in the cell. Table 7.3 is a summary of some of the better known systems in which this type of phenomenon has been studied. The advantages to microorganisms of these repression systems are obvious. If an easily assimilated growth substrate is

Table 7.3 Systems and enzymes subject to catabolite repression.

Organism	System or enzyme	Repression exerted by:
Escherichia coli	Lactose operon Galactose operon Arabinose operon Glycerol kinase	Carbon sources, particularly glucose, gluconate and 6-phosphogluconate
	Histidine utilization	Carbon and nitrogen sources
	Tryptophan utilization	Carbon and nitrogen sources
Bacillus subtilis	Sucrase	Carbon source
	TCA cycle enzymes	Carbon source
	Sporulation	Carbon and nitrogen sources
Rhizobium species and *Azotobacter*	N$_2$ fixation	Ammonium ions
Klebsiella aerogenes	Nitrate reductase	Nitrogen source, particularly NH$_4{}^+$
Pseudomonas species	Glucose oxidation	Succinate
Saccharomyces	Mitochondrial biogenesis	Carbon source
	Maltase	Carbon source
	Arginase	Carbon and nitrogen sources
Aspergillus nidulans	Proline utilization	Carbon and nitrogen sources
	Arginine utilization	Carbon and nitrogen sources
	Amidase	Nitrogen source

available the cell does not expend considerable amounts of energy synthesizing the enzymes needed for a less efficient pathway, and can direct more of its metabolism to producing proteins (such as those involved in protein synthesis) that are essential for growth. A good example is afforded by N$_2$-fixing bacteria such as *Azotobacter* and *Klebsiella* species, in which the very ATP-expensive fixation of N$_2$ is completely repressed in the presence of NH$_4{}^+$.

Catabolite repression

The best studied example of this type of control is the *glucose effect* in bacteria, which contributes to the phenomenon of diauxic growth illustrated in Fig. 7.4. In the presence of lactose and glucose mixtures, *E. coli* cultures use glucose preferentially, and lactose is not consumed until the glucose is exhausted. Despite the presence of lactose the *lac* operon is not effectively transcribed when a more readily metabolized carbon source than lactose is available. This phenomenon is more usually termed *catabolite repression*, since it is not restricted to glucose, and it acts on many catabolic pathways in the cell. In fact, carbon substrates can be arranged in a hierarchy, in which those higher in the list repress the utilization of those lower down:

gluconate > glucose > fructose > maltose >
lactose > galactose > glycerol > succinate

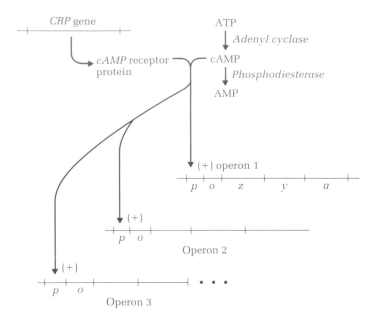

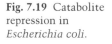

Fig. 7.19 Catabolite repression in *Escherichia coli*.

For this reason, when studying induction systems in *E. coli*, cells are usually grown on glycerol to avoid catabolite repression.

How is catabolite repression mediated at the molecular level? In trying to answer this question it must be stressed that there are a number of different mechanisms operating in these organisms that have been carefully studied. So far the best understood is that for catabolite repression in *E. coli* cells growing aerobically. This system works on many operons including *lac*, *gal* (galactose), *mal* (maltose), *ara* (arabinose), *gly* (glycerol) and *hut* (histidine utilization). The mechanism (Fig. 7.19) resembles in many ways the control circuit for enzyme induction, with the following salient features:

1 The control is mediated directly by the concentration in the cell of cyclic-3′ : 5′AMP (cAMP).

2 This nucleotide binds to the tetrameric cAMP receptor protein (CRP, product of the *crp* gene) and the complex becomes an activator of transcription at *many* operons. Mutants with an inactive CRP are unable to induce the synthesis of any catabolite repressible system, and can only grow on a rich carbon source such as glucose.

3 Binding of the cAMP–CRP complex occurs adjacent to the promoter site. Figure 7.7 illustrates the location for the *lac* operon. It is thought that the CRP assists RNA polymerase to bind to the promoter by making up for some of the deficiencies of the −35 σ-factor binding region of the *lac* promoter. This CRP-binding site is palindromic.

4 cAMP and CRP together act positively, and they must both be added to an *in vitro* transcription system to obtain maximal levels of *lac* expression.

5 The intracellular level of cAMP reflects in some way the energy status of the cell. There are several models of how this may occur. One is based on the observation that cAMP can be excreted from cells and suggests that the internal concentration of cAMP is modulated by the amount of energy available for its excretion. The other is that the activities of the two enzymes involved in cAMP metabolism are regulated according to the energy status of the cell. Under conditions of lowered energy status, ADP levels are increased; ADP is an inhibitor of phosphodiesterase, hence the cAMP is broken down less rapidly. ADP may also affect the activity of adenyl cyclase to promote cAMP formation:

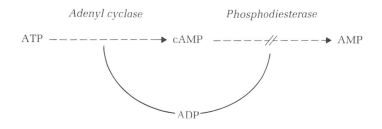

A mutation in the gene encoding adenyl cyclase (*cyr*) prevents cells growing on any of the repressible carbon substrates such as lactose, maltose and arabinose; unlike CRP-deficient mutants they will respond to exogenously added cAMP.

This form of catabolite repression is quite general in its effect in *E. coli*, since mutations affecting CRP or adenyl cyclase affect most of the glucose repression effects studied so far. It should be noted, however, that two-dimensional gel electrophoretic studies of the proteins synthesized in various mutants have shown that there are also operons which are switched off by cAMP-dependent effects, so there may be some operons in which CRP binding inhibits transcription.

A second system in *E. coli*, very closely related to the CRP system, has recently been identified in studies of the control of the citric acid cycle (CAC). Under anaerobic conditions this facultative anaerobe switches off the section of the CAC from 2-oxoglutarate to succinate, and the remaining CAC enzymes (or replacements such as fumarate reductase for succinate dehydrogenase) act as two-branched pathways to succinate and 2-oxoglutarate respectively. This switch is mediated by the product of the *fnr* gene, which has been sequenced and shown to have strong homology to the CRP. The molecule(s) to which the FNR protein responds has not yet been identified.

Note that while cAMP has a central role in catabolite repression in *E. coli*, it has not been detected in some other bacterial genera (including *Bacillus*) which are also subject to catabolite repression, and it does not seem to mediate glucose repression in microbial eukaryotes (where cAMP has a different role). Some other metabolite may be important in these organisms. Another variation is that glucose is not always the preferred substrate since *Pseudomonas* and related genera utilize succinate in preference to glucose. These organisms have the less efficient Entner–Doudoroff pathway for glucose breakdown, and have a metabolism geared to the breakdown of a wide range of aromatic compounds to form succinate.

Nitrogen control systems

In bacteria NH_4^+ is often the preferred N substrate, and the mechanism whereby cells control this N repression system is very interesting. The enzyme *glutamine synthetase* (GS) acts in the high-affinity NH_4^+ uptake system:

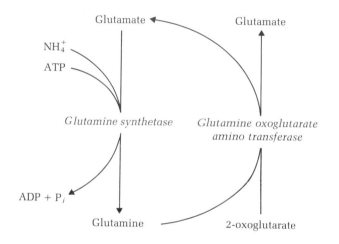

Glutamine synthetase also acts, however, as the repressor molecule for N repression, binding near the promoter region of, for example, the *hut* operon in *E. coli* or the *nif* gene clusters in *Klebsiella* to promote transcription.

The activity of GS is modulated not by the allosteric binding of a small molecule, but rather by covalent modification of the enzyme. This is an *adenylylation*, in which each GS molecule can react with up to 12 ATP molecules with the covalent attachment to GS of AMP residues. This adenylylation (and also deadenylylation) is catalysed by an enzyme (PII) which responds to the concentration of 2-oxoglutarate and glutamine such that in high NH_4^+, when the glutamine : 2-oxoglutarate ratio is high, the GS is adenylylated to its inactive form, and it cannot promote transcription. This is illustrated in Fig. 7.20 for the *hut* operon, which also shows that the enzymes involved in histidine utilization are subject to catabolite repression—this fits with the fact that in *E. coli* histidine can act as a poor source of either carbon or nitrogen.

Stringent response

When cells face starvation of a ready supply of amino acids, they respond by shutting down a large number of functions that are not needed to maintain the cell. These include rRNA and tRNA synthesis (reduced by about 90%) and formation of many mRNA species (by about 60%) as well as other small molecules.

The response was first noticed in amino acid auxotrophs starved for the requirement; in these the rate of RNA synthesis decreased markedly despite the presence of the necessary components for nucleic acid synthesis. This was described as the stringent response, and it has been found to occur in microbial eukaryotes as well as prokaryotes, although the mechanism probably differs between these groups.

In *E. coli*, the response is mediated by a reaction, known as the *idling reaction*, of ribosomes that are not continuing translation due to the presence of an uncharged tRNA in the A site of the ribosome. This reaction leads to the synthesis from GTP and ATP of the highly phosphorylated nucleotides ppGpp and sometimes pppGpp, which are produced in the presence of a *stringent factor* (product of the *relA* gene). Mutations in *relA* lead to 'relaxed' strains which do continue RNA synthesis in the face of starvation for an amino acid. How does ppGpp act? One suggestion is that it

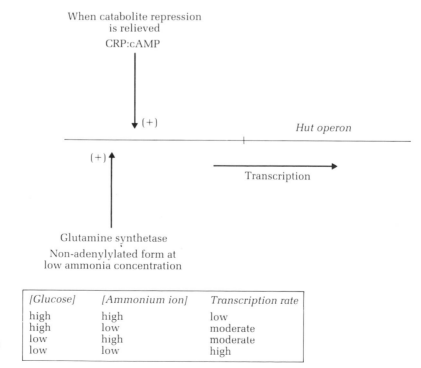

When catabolite repression
is relieved
CRP:cAMP

(+)

Hut operon

(+)

Transcription

Glutamine synthetase
Non-adenylylated form at
low ammonia concentration

[Glucose]	[Ammonium ion]	Transcription rate
high	high	low
high	low	moderate
low	high	moderate
low	low	high

Fig. 7.20 Dual regulation of the *hut* operon by catabolite repression and nitrogen source repression.

acts as an allosteric modifier of RNA polymerase in bacteria, causing RNA polymerase to select some promoters much less frequently, especially those for rRNA.

This mechanism appears to be limited to prokaryotes. In yeast, at least, the effect may be mediated in a rather different way. In the 5′ upstream region of many genes, including those for ribosomal proteins, elongation factors for protein synthesis, and many other enzymes including those of the glycolytic pathway, there is a consensus sequence for binding of the RAP (or TUF) protein, which is therefore a candidate for a general starvation regulator. Its activation may depend on phosphorylation by protein kinases that respond to the nutritional status of the cell (see p. 252).

Other stress response systems

There are, in both prokaryotic and eukaryotic cells, mechanisms for responding to conditions causing injury or stress. One that is found in all organisms is heat shock, which is a slight misnomer, since it also involves a response to other types of stress (e.g. osmotic stress) than heating to above optimal temperatures. In response to these stimuli the cells stop making most of their proteins, but produce a limited number of proteins that are not normally found in the cell. These may have a protective or repair function. The mechanism of this response is currently under study, especially in eukaryotes in which genes that are activated by heat shock have an upstream sequence which is involved in the binding of a heat shock activator protein. This protein is probably present in the cell in an inactive form, but is activated directly by phosphorylation and probably indirectly via the ubiquitinylation system for dealing with damaged proteins (p. 224).

In *S. cerevisiae* and presumably other microbial eukaryotes there is a similar response (*general control of amino acid biosynthesis*) to starvation for amino acids, which leads to a severalfold increase in the rate of transcription of many genes concerned with amino acid synthesis. Such genes have a consensus sequence rrTGACTCatttt located in their 5′ upstream region, and this is the site for binding of a protein which controls the activity.

Another stress response in bacteria is the SOS repair system, which is activated by damage to DNA (p. 151).

CONTROL OF ENZYME ACTIVITY

An alternative to changing the amount of enzyme present in a cell is to affect the flux of compounds through a metabolic pathway by altering the *activity* of one or more key enzymes in the pathway.

Modulation of activity of enzymes usually provides a fine, continuous control of metabolite flux, and is much more responsive to sudden fluctuations in a cell's environment than is either induction or repression. Induction leads to a relatively fast response by the cell to the presence of a compound in the environment, but feedback repression acts more slowly since the cells containing the enzymes for synthesis of an amino acid (for example) only gradually lose the activity of these enzymes by dilution due to growth. In such pathways both repression of synthesis and inhibition of enzyme activity usually operate.

Enzyme activity can be modulated by a number of general mechanisms.

Reversible binding of a low-molecular weight metabolite

This is by far the most common form of control. The metabolite may be a substrate or product of a reaction sequence, or another compound which reflects the need for that sequence (e.g. in some organisms ATP controls certain key glycolytic enzymes). Such metabolites can be either *activators* or *inhibitors*, and they are usually termed *effectors* or *ligands*. There are some enzymes whose activities are modified by more than one effector; for example, phosphofructokinase from *E. coli* has at least three.

Enzymes under the control of effector molecules have a number of important general properties:

1 They are composed of polypeptide subunits assembled into multimeric complexes, often tetramers. The subunits can differ, with one type having catalytic and the other regulatory functions (e.g. aspartate transcarbamylase), or be identical, with both functions on the same polypeptide subunit. An example of the latter (and more common) case is the *lac* repressor protein, which is a tetramer of identical subunits each with a binding site for allolactose and DNA.

2 The effectors are usually of very different chemical structure from the substrates, and they bind to the subunit polypeptides at different sites from the catalytic site on the three-dimensional enzyme structure.

3 Physical studies of these proteins have shown that they undergo conformational changes in the presence of the effectors. This implies that the enzymes can exist in different conformations (hence their name allosteric enzymes). The change from one form to the other is either brought about by the binding of the ligand inducing the change, or by altering the equilibrium between two conformations. In either of these models, in one of the conformations the enzyme is much more active than the other, and the effector therefore modulates the activity.

4 Allosteric enzymes do not show normal Michaelis–Menten kinetics in which the rate of enzyme reaction is a hyperbolic function of the substrate concentration. Instead, as shown in Fig. 7.21, the curve is *sigmoidal* and shows a cooperative effect at low substrate concentration; thus a small increase in substrate concentration leads to a much greater than proportional increase in reaction velocity.

It is thus easy to visualize allosteric enzymes as dynamic entities in which the structure of the enzyme is responsive to relatively small changes in the level of both substrate and allosteric activators or inhibitors. These structural changes affect enzyme activity by altering the affinity of the enzyme for its substrate; this differs markedly from the inactivation of enzyme molecules by covalent binding of inhibitors.

Covalent modification of enzymes

Another way the cell can regulate the activity of an enzyme is to modify it covalently. This is less frequently found than the non-covalent type discussed above, but there are still many cases in which important controls are the result of either binding of a relatively small moiety (e.g. by phosphorylation) or by proteolytic cleavage.

Table 7.4 lists some of the main examples of the binding of small groups to enzymes. Of these the most common is probably phosphorylation, and feeding cells with ^{32}P-phosphate can lead to the labelling of about 50 or so proteins. The phosphorylation of proteins is brought about by protein kinases, which transfer the terminal phosphoryl group from ATP. There are several such enzymes in cells; in yeast at least ten distinct activities have been identified by mutation or gene cloning experiments. The substrates of these protein kinases include enzymes involved in glucose storage and metabolism (glycogen phosphorylase, glycogen synthase, hexokinase, fructose bisphosphatase, phosphofructokinase and trehalase), in protein synthesis (RNA

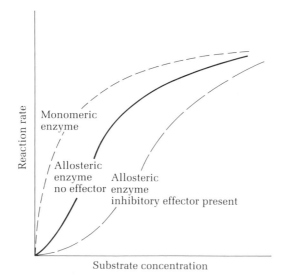

Fig. 7.21 Sigmoidal kinetics of allosteric enzymes.

polymerase and several ribosomal proteins), in glutamate metabolism, and even in the control of the protein kinases themselves. The phosphorylation is reversible. Several phosphatases exist which can remove the phosphoryl group from the proteins.

This type of phosphorylation/diphosphorylation is of considerable current interest since the mechanisms controlling cell division involve protein kinases (see Chapter 8).

Note that these modifications can lead to the amplification of a response. The phosphorylation of one enzyme molecule can lead to the synthesis of many molecules of the product of the enzyme reaction; such events occur in the amplification of hormone reception signals.

Methylation is another form of post-translational protein modification; this has importance in the chemotactic response in bacteria. Methylation is catalysed by specific methylases which often use *S*-adenosylmethionine as the methyl donor. In bacterial chemotaxis the membrane proteins involved in the reception of the chemotactic signal, and in the processes of 'sensory adaptation' and de-adaptation (whereby the cells gradually lose their response to a sudden change in the concentration of an attractant), are methylated and demethylated in this way.

Other types of modification in which a small group is attached to a protein include acetylation, adenylylation (AMP residues) and uridylylation (UMP residues). One of the more curious control systems in *E. coli*, and one which acts in conjunction with regulation of N metabolism at the level of gene transcription (see p. 218), is the adenylylation of glutamine synthetase (which acts in the modified form as a repressor of N metabolic genes). As discussed earlier, glutamine synthetase can have as many as 12 AMP residues added from ATP, and the interchange between these two forms is catalysed by an enzyme (the PII regulatory protein). What is rather bizarre in this arrangement is that the PII activity is itself modified by uridylylation, such that in its UMP-containing form it removes the AMP residues from glutamine synthetase, while in its non-modified form it promotes the transfer of AMP from ATP to the enzyme. Moreover, to show that in this organism control of N metabolism uses all the available control tricks, the PII enzyme is an allosteric one, responding to the concentrations of glutamine and 2-oxoglutarate in the cells.

Table 7.4 Covalent modifications affecting enzyme activity.

Modification	Group	Donor
Phosphorylation	Phosphate	ATP
Methylation	Methyl	*S*-adenosylmethionine
Acetylation	Acetyl	Acetyl CoA
Adenylylation	AMP	ATP
Uridylylation	UMP	UTP
Glycosylation	Sugars, especially mannose	Nucleotide sugars

Probably the best examples of modifications involving the addition of larger groups are the glycosylations by eukaryotes of proteins which are involved in the pathways of protein trans-location to some organelles or for secretion (p. 30). Bacteria cannot carry out such glycosylations, and the glycosyl groups added by fungi are not identical to the mammalian type. This presents a problem in biotechnology when trying by recombinant DNA techniques to produce some human proteins in a microbial host.

Proteolysis

There are a number of general situations in which a pre-enzyme polypeptide is processed to a mature active form. These include the removal of signal sequences from proteins transported across membranes during secretion or as they are transferred into cellular compartments (p. 173). In other cases an enzyme is maintained in the cell in an inactive form until required, at which point it is cleaved by a specific protease. The best example of this is the activation of the proteases themselves, many of which are syn-thesized as an inactive *zymogen*. Another very good example is seen in the SOS repair pathway in *E. coli* in which a protein repressor of many repair-related functions is inactivated by the product of the *recA* gene, which encodes a protease that is activated by damage to DNA (p. 151). This type of activation is irreversible.

In addition to this specific cleavage, there are more general proteases which are responsible for removing unwanted proteins when they are no longer required, or for removing abnormal proteins arising from mistakes during translation events. In eukaryotes unwanted proteins are marked for degradation by the covalent attachment of the protein *ubiquitin* (so called because of its wide distribution in different species). The mechanism of ubiquitinylation is not fully understood, but the system recognizes in some way either denatured proteins, or ones with a N-terminal amino acid that is not normally found at the end of a protein. Experiments with yeast strains in which the N-terminal amino acid of a single protein (the *E. coli* β-galactosidase) was modified genetically by substitution with other amino acids have shown that some amino acids that are not normally found at the N-terminal end (such as leucine, lysine, phenylalanine, aspartate and arginine) are destabilizing, and provoke an initial ubiquitin attachment at the end of the molecule, while the amino acids methionine, serine, alanine, glycine, threonine and valine are stabilizing. This is followed by subsequent ubiquitin attachments elsewhere in the unwanted protein, and proteolytic degradation of the complex. In some cases the half-life of the protein in the cell was reduced from 10 h (with methionine at the terminus) to 2 min (with lysine) by the alteration of just the terminal amino acid. In yeast there are four separate genes for ubiquitin, one of which is a stress-specific gene under heat-shock control: its role is to degrade proteins that have been denatured by heat injury.

When cells of most organisms face starvation, they can survive for relatively long periods by gradually degrading structures which are not required for growth and cell division, and using the amino acids so produced to synthesize new proteins needed for survival or to provide energy. This gradual degradation of proteins is called *protein turnover*. For most organisms during exponential phase cells have very low rates of protein turnover, but as soon as the growth rate decreases protein turnover increases as proteases are activated.

Clearly proteolysis is of importance in biotechnology when trying to express a heterologous gene in a host, and some steps may need to be taken to prevent or minimize it. These have included the use of hosts with mutations in various protease genes, although with the plethora of such proteases present in the cell this may be a difficult task (at the last count *S. cerevisiae* had about 40 proteinase or peptidase activities identified), or deliberately constructing the heterologous gene with signals to target its secretion from the cell.

PATTERNS OF CONTROL

Most reaction pathways are controlled not by just one of the types of control we have discussed, but by a combination of many different systems. Rather than discuss this in great detail, it is better to look at one example and be aware that there are many variations on the control themes. For different organisms there may be varying demands on a particular pathway, and they will often have different patterns of control. Let us consider the biosynthetic pathways leading to aromatic amino acids in several organisms to see how each has evolved a different pattern (Fig. 7.22). These illustrate:

1 In *E. coli* the occurrence of three different isozymes (different proteins with the same catalytic activity) for the first step in the pathway as a way of regulating the demand on this bit of the pathway for the three different branches. Each enzyme is controlled by one of the end products, either by feedback repression or feedback inhibition, or both. A later step, catalysed by *chorismate mutase* and common to the phenylalanine and tyrosine pathways, also has isozymes controlled in the same way. An alternative way of achieving the same objective is to have one enzyme subject to multiple regulation as in *B. subtilis*, and in this case the control is sometimes exerted by intermediates in the pathway. Tryptophan only partly represses the first enzyme, which is an allosteric protein responding to the three different effectors.

2 Feedback repression and inhibition are commonly found just

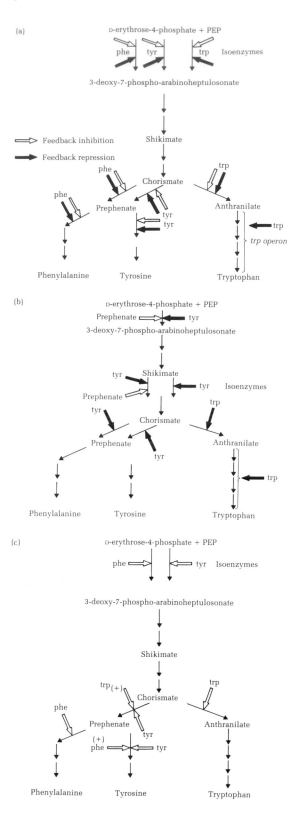

Fig. 7.22 Three different biosynthetic pathways leading to aromatic amino acids (a) *Escherichia coli*; (b) *Bacillus subtilis*; (c) *Saccharomyces cerevisiae.*

after a branching of the pathways. This enables the cell to avoid accumulating intermediates in a pathway when the product of that branch is not required. Sometimes these intermediates are toxic if they accumulate.

3 In bacteria the tryptophan branch forms an operon (and one in which attenuation plays a part), so that none of the enzymes are synthesized when there is no requirement for their activity. There is, however, feedback inhibition imposed on this to modulate the flow of metabolites through this branch when it is functioning.

4 The different control strategies that have evolved in the three organisms should be noted. In particular the *S. cerevisiae* example illustrates that in eukaryotes there is less emphasis on feedback repression, with most of the control at the level of inhibition or activation of the enzymes after the branch points. Moreover, in this case some of the control depends on the kinetic properties of the enzymes after each branch point. From chorismate the flow to tryptophan is favoured, and the tryptophan concentration rises until it activates chorismate mutase, which then feeds the phenylalanine and tyrosine branches. Phenylalanine is then favoured due to the kinetic properties of prephenate dehydratase until the phenylalanine concentration rises and feedback inhibits this enzyme, and some of the activity of the first enzyme in the whole pathway. Finally the tyrosine pool fills until there is sufficient, when the activities of chorismate mutase, and the first enzyme, DHAP synthase, are shut down completely by feedback inhibition.

Finally it should be noted that patterns of control can evolve very rapidly, particularly under conditions of high selection. It is not unusual to find that a strain carrying a mutation affecting part of a reaction pathway undergoes mutation at a second, control site. When branched pathways are involved this can lead to marked changes in cellular metabolism. This has wider implications than its mere nuisance or positive value to the biochemical geneticist or biotechnologist; isolates of microorganisms removed from their natural habitat may rapidly undergo heritable changes in their control patterns on subculture in the laboratory.

8 Growth of individual cells

CELL CYCLE

The term 'cell cycle' has been coined for the process whereby a newborn cell grows by increase in size and ultimately undergoes division to form two cells. In previous chapters, we have been concerned with the processes that lead to the growth of cells. We now consider the way in which this growth is coordinated with the division process to ensure that the progeny resemble their parent cells and contain a correct complement of both genetic information and cell material to ensure continued viability.

There are a number of ways in which microorganisms grow and divide; some are outlined in Fig. 8.1. Most bacteria, algae and protozoa divide by binary fission, each mother cell increasing in volume and eventually dividing to give two identifiable daughters. In some microorganisms, fission is asymmetric and two non-identical cells result. A good example is the bacterial genus *Caulobacter* in which stalk cells divide to form motile cells and stalk cells. Another example is seen with division of some diatoms; these eukaryotes have rigid silica walls (*frustules*) which fit together like overlapping plates. The inner of these decreases in size at each successive division. Ultimately, some of the daughters are so small that they can no longer divide by mitosis, so they undergo meiosis to form an auxospore; this resumes a larger size on germination.

Most yeasts, with the exception of the fission yeast *Schizosaccharomyces*, divide by budding, the mother cell barely changing in volume during the division cycle. A bud emerges at some point on the cell surface and increases in size until it almost matches the mother cell. Mother and daughter cells can be distinguished in this system by the number of bud scars present on the cell surface. Daughters are smaller than the mothers and take longer before the next cell division commences.

Most fungi and the prokaryotic *Streptomyces* species have a hyphal habit in which growth is usually restricted to the apical tip. In aseptate fungi, it is difficult to define a cell cycle, since long multinucleate hyphae are formed. The difference between yeast budding and hyphal growth is not as great as it appears; both involve cell extension at a restricted site and there are fungi which can reversibly switch from a mycelial to a yeast phase. This usually occurs after an increase in temperature or CO_2 concentration. Many of these fungi are potential pathogens.

Another form of growth is shown by the true slime moulds, e.g. *Physarum polycephalum*. These eukaryotes are acellular, increasing in size during growth but without dividing. A large

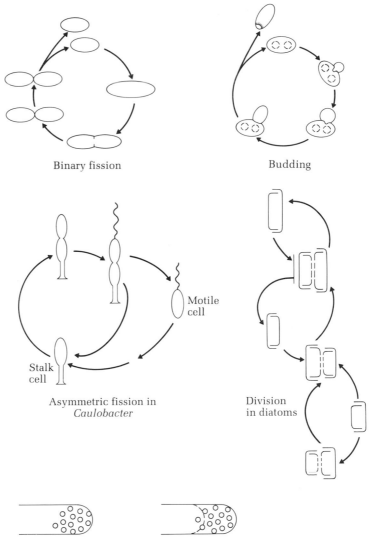

Binary fission

Budding

Motile cell

Stalk cell

Asymmetric fission in *Caulobacter*

Division in diatoms

Hyphal growth

Fig. 8.1 Modes of cell growth and division.

plasmodial mass is formed, which moves by cytoplasmic streaming. These amoeboid masses can divide and fuse randomly; they are multinucleate, but their nuclei divide synchronously.

Kinetics of cell growth

Direct microscopic observation has shown that individual cells of most microorganisms increase in mass linearly with time. Volume changes are also roughly linear. Most growing cultures of microorganisms are *asynchronous*, cells from all stages of the cell cycle being represented in the culture at any one time. Theoretically, there are twice as many young cells of age 0 as there are old cells of age T_d (mean cell age at division). In fact, the observed age distribution of cells in a growing culture deviates from theory since some cells divide at an earlier age than others, as indicated in Fig. 2.1 (p. 40). This means that for synchronized populations, synchrony will decay fairly rapidly on further growth of the cells due to the distribution of individual generation times.

Synchronization procedures

In order to obtain enough material to study biochemical changes taking place during the cell cycle, it is often necessary to synchronize the division of cells within a population. Since microorganisms can adapt very rapidly to changes in their environment, it is important that methods used to obtain synchrony do not introduce artifacts. There are two general ways of obtaining synchrony, either by *induction* (e.g. alternate temperature changes, light pulses to photosynthetic organisms, or the use of metabolic inhibitors affecting essential cell functions in the cell cycle) or by *selection* (e.g. on the basis of cell size, using zonal density gradient centrifugation, or filtration, or by elution of newly divided cells from immobilized parents). Selection methods are less likely to introduce artifacts since the cells are selected on the basis of a physical characteristic (usually size) with the minimum of chemical disturbance; two methods in current use are outlined in Fig. 8.2. One of the best techniques for avoiding perturbations involves the use of an elutriator rotor in a centrifuge. In this technique, cells are separated by centrifugation through a flow of nutrient medium such that they do not move very far, since the flow almost balances movement due to gravity.

Cell cycle events

There are many processes within a cell which are essential to its continued growth and division. Some of these are of a general metabolic nature (e.g. uptake of important substrates, energy production, biosynthesis) which, while important to growth, are not specifically concerned with maintaining the cell cycle. Here we are interested in those functions which are most intimately involved in the cell cycle. How can we determine what functions are relevant? In some cases, including the replication and segregation of DNA, the answer is obvious; in others it can be more difficult to determine. Possibly the most useful criterion available is an inhibition test; if a cell function is specifically affected by either an inhibitor or a mutation, does it cause an accumulation of cells in a particular stage of the cell cycle? If so, then it is probably connected with the cell cycle in a fairly specific way. This is the criterion that has been used in selecting cell division cycle mutants in a number of organisms. For example, mutations affecting cell division in *Escherichia coli* lead to filamentation—long cells without a division septum.

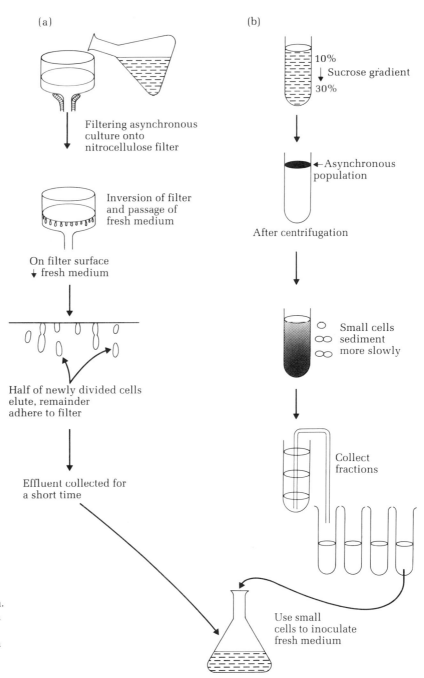

(a)

Filtering asynchronous
culture onto
nitrocellulose filter

Inversion of filter
and passage of
fresh medium

On filter surface
↓ fresh medium

Half of newly divided cells
elute, remainder
adhere to filter

Effluent collected for
a short time

(b)

10%
↓ Sucrose gradient
30%

←Asynchronous
population

After centrifugation

Small cells
sediment
more slowly

Collect
fractions

Use small
cells to inoculate
fresh medium

Fig. 8.2 Selection
methods for obtaining
synchronous cultures:
(a) membrane elution;
(b) zonal centrifugation.
The membrane elution
method only works for
those organisms which
attach to the
membranes used.

BACTERIAL CELL CYCLE

The major cytological changes seen during the bacterial cell cycle
are cell growth, division by septum formation and DNA segregation into daughter cells. These, and the biochemical changes
associated with gene expression, have received most attention.

Growth of surfaces

This involves extension of cell walls and membranes. How does this occur—by random insertion of newly synthesized material or by addition to a few regions of the cell surface? For the cell wall, it is quite clear that synthesis is restricted to particular regions of the pre-existing wall. This has been shown by immunofluorescent staining techniques, using antibodies prepared against cell wall material, to distinguish newly synthesized material from old. In one organism, *Streptococcus faecalis*, electron microscope studies have given a clear picture of the way new cell wall material is organized. This represents a relatively simple situation, the division of a coccus in a single plane (Fig. 8.3). From this study, several points emerge:

1 Wall synthesis begins at an equatorial band formed during the previous division cycle and continues at the leading edge of the nascent cross wall.

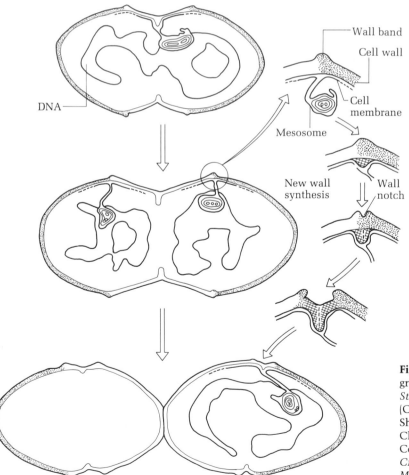

DNA

Wall band
Cell wall
Cell membrane
Mesosome
New wall synthesis
Wall notch

Fig. 8.3 Model for the growth of cell walls in *Streptococcus faecalis*. (Courtesy of Dr Shockman, and the Chemical Rubber Company (1971) *Critical Reviews in Microbiology* **1**, 1.)

2 The mesosome appears to play a role in organizing the site of initiation of new cell wall synthesis, as well as attaching DNA to the membrane.

3 There is some indication in the figure, supported by much data from studies of the surface distribution of wall lytic enzymes, that growth of a new cell wall depends on a limited breakdown of pre-existing cell wall peptidoglycan. This is consistent with the observation that autolysin-deficient mutants of *S. faecalis*, *E. coli* and *Bacillus subtilis* are unable to grow and divide properly unless lysozyme is added.

The mechanisms of wall synthesis and septum formation in bacilli and cocci dividing in more than one plane are less well understood, although similar principles of site-specific initiation and insertion of new cell wall, and of requirement for lytic enzymes, apply. In bacilli, two separate processes can be recognized— lengthwise growth and septum formation—involving different *penicillin-binding proteins* and other enzymes (see pp. 184–187).

Little is known about the synthesis of cell membrane. This is mainly because components of the membrane are semifluid and also undergo degradation and resynthesis (turnover). Site-specific labelling of membrane components is therefore impossible. There is some evidence that membrane synthesis is restricted to an equatorial band around the *B. subtilis* cell. When rod-shaped organisms divide, there is an increase in the rate of incorporation of glycerol and phosphate into lipids, presumably reflecting the synthesis of the division septum.

DNA replication

Cell division is a very closely regulated periodic process. In steady state cultures of *E. coli* and related genera, division occurs at a well-defined cell mass and is strictly coordinated with cell division. In wild-type *E. coli*, the formation of cells lacking DNA is very rare and any physical, chemical or genetic interruption of DNA replication arrests cell division.

The molecular basis of this coupling between DNA replication and cell division remains elusive, although knowledge of other aspects is appreciable. Mechanisms of DNA synthesis have been discussed in Chapter 6, and here we are only concerned with how replication is coordinated with cell division. In a few bacteria studied in detail (*E. coli*, *Salmonella typhimurium*, *B. subtilis* and *Streptomyces coelicor*) there is one circular chromosome which, at least in *E. coli* and *B. subtilis*, replicates bidirectionally from a single origin. This single chromosome takes a relatively constant time to replicate at all except very slow growth rates: about 40 min in *E. coli* at 37°C. At high growth rates, replication is too slow to duplicate the entire chromosome in one generation time, hence new replication forks are initiated at the origin before previous ones are completed. This means that under conditions of

(a)

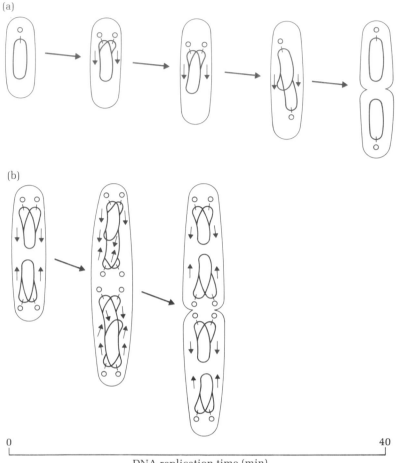

(b)

0   40

DNA replication time (min)

Fig. 8.4 Replication of bacterial (*Escherichia coli*) DNA. At low growth rates, there is a single chromosome per cell and no reinitiation at the origin before completion of a round of replication. At higher growth rates, there are multiple initiations of replication at the origin and more than one chromosome per cell. (a) Low growth rates (generation time greater than DNA replication time): single chromosome per cell, single replication loop, small cell size, O is origin of replication; (b) high growth rates (generation time less than DNA replication time): several chromosomes per cell, multifork replication, large cell size.

rapid growth there must be more than one chromosome per cell; this is best understood by reference to Fig. 8.4.

Chromosome replication must be synchronized in some way with cell division if each daughter cell is to receive at least one copy of the genome. One important finding in *E. coli* is that the time from the end of a round of DNA replication (termination) to the formation of a division septum is also constant at all except slow growth rates. How is this timing achieved? So far, the answer to this question has not been resolved, but Fig. 8.5 summarizes one model which takes into account much of the data from mutant and inhibitor studies as well as the constant times for DNA replication and for the interval from the end of replication to septum formation. In addition, it is based on the finding that the mass of a cell at the time of division (and its size) varies with growth rate, but that at times of initiation of DNA replication, the mass of a cell is constant regardless of growth rate.

Important features of this model are:

1 A new round of chromosome replication is initiated at a par-

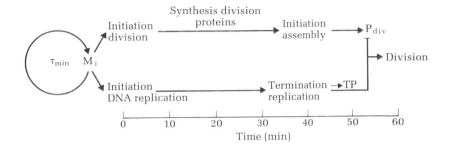

Fig. 8.5 Model for the coordination of DNA replication and cell division in *Escherichia coli*. M_i = mass at initiation; τ = mass doubling time; TP = termination protein; P_{div} = division protein. (Courtesy of Dr Donachie and the Society for General Microbiology.)

ticular cell mass, M_i, the 'initiation mass'. The initiation of replication depends on the synthesis of protein at this time. DNA replication then takes a constant time regardless of growth rate.

2 A second series of events concerned with cell division is initiated at the same time. A period of protein synthesis is followed by another which may involve the assembly of a septum precursor.

3 When replication of DNA is complete, a protein is synthesized and this interacts with the septum precursor leading to septum formation and cell division.

To explain these facts, alternative models have been proposed, based on the existence of an inhibitor of cell division which is broken down or decreased in activity when DNA replication is completed. With the advent of gene cloning, considerable work has been done on mutations which affect cell division. One of these, *sfiA*, has been found to identify an inhibitor of cell division. The *sfiA* gene is activated by the SOS repair system under the control of the *recA* and *lexA* genes (see p. 151) and its product inhibits cell division until DNA damage has been repaired. This inhibitor is subject to degradation by a protease in the cell, ensuring that division can resume when the *sfiA* protein is no longer being made. A related system accounts for part of the cell cycle control seen in eukaryotes. More details of this are known, and these are discussed below.

So far, relatively little is known about the mechanism which triggers DNA replication when a cell reaches a particular mass or size. Theories which have been proposed often include the concept of an inhibitor and/or initiator which is synthesized once per cell cycle and is diluted to a critical concentration by increase in cell volume.

Gene expression during the cell cycle

This has been studied mainly in terms of the synthesis of those RNA species which are most easily identified (rRNA) or of the synthesis of particular proteins, mainly enzymes. Usually there is a continuous synthesis of *total* protein and RNA during the bacterial cell cycle, but for a few individual proteins, the situation can be very different. If an enzyme were synthesized continuously throughout the cell cycle, in a synchronous culture its activity would increase linearly with time until the gene coding for the enzyme doubled; then, the rate should also double (provided the rate of enzyme synthesis is limited by the number of gene copies available for transcription). This is true for nearly all enzymes, and only a few appear to be synthesized discontinuously, since two-dimensional gel electrophoresis of proteins from cells labelled at different points during the cell cycle has confirmed that almost all proteins are synthesized continuously. One point, however, emerges very clearly; the composition of a microbial cell is in a considerable state of flux throughout its growth and division cycle, underlining the extensive heterogeneity of asynchronous populations.

EUKARYOTIC CELL CYCLE

In many respects, the patterns of control of cell division in eukaryotes resemble those found in bacteria, with additional complexity due to the presence of organelles, the nuclear arrangement of DNA and the differences in chromosome segregation. There are, however, more 'landmark' events which can be used to determine the stages reached in cell division and this has enabled a more detailed analysis of the mechanisms for cell cycle regulation.

Cell cycle events in yeasts

The eukaryotic cell cycle has been studied most extensively in the yeasts *S. cerevisiae* and *Schizosaccharomyces pombe*. The major events are concerned with *DNA replication, chromosome segregation, nuclear division* and *cell division*.

One main difference between prokaryotes and eukaryotes is that eukaryotic DNA replication occupies only a part of the cell cycle. This led early workers to split the cell cycle into phases: *S phase* for DNA synthesis and *M phase* for mitosis. Since there were gaps between these phases, they were termed *G1* and *G2*, as indicated in Fig. 8.6. The G phases were arbitrarily assigned without knowledge of events occurring during them, and the G1 phase at least can apparently be dispensed with (or be very short) under certain circumstances. The G1 phase appears to involve a period in which the cells grow to the correct size for another cell cycle to be initiated.

Once the cells have entered cell division, they undergo a series of landmark events determined by biochemical, genetic and ultrastructural analysis. For *S. cerevisiae*, which divides by budding, these events follow a defined order under normal growth conditions, as outlined in Fig. 8.6. These include the following.

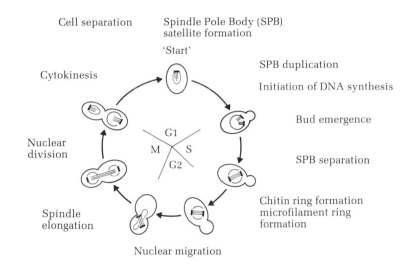

Cell separation

Spindle Pole Body (SPB)
satellite formation

'Start'

Cytokinesis

SPB duplication

Initiation of DNA synthesis

Nuclear
division

Bud emergence

SPB separation

Fig. 8.6 Schematic
representation of the
main events of the cell
division cycle in
*Saccharomyces
cerevisiae*. (Redrawn
from Dr Hartwell and
the American Society
for Microbiology.)

G1

M   S

G2

Chitin ring formation
microfilament ring
formation

Spindle
elongation

Nuclear migration

Initiation of DNA synthesis. As in bacteria, once initiated,
DNA synthesis occurs in a relatively constant time regardless of
nutritional conditions. There is evidence to indicate that most
origins of replication in yeast are triggered at about the same time,
but that telomeric regions are replicated later during S phase.
There is also a relatively constant time from the end of S phase to
the cell division process.

Bud emergence. Very soon after replication is initiated, a bud
begins to form on the mother cell surface. Associated with this
emerging bud is the formation of a ring of chitin at the neck
between the mother cell and the bud, and the appearance of a ring
of microfilaments in the cytoplasm in this region.

Spindle pole body changes. The spindle pole body (SPB) is a
plaque-like structure located in the nuclear membrane. It performs
in fungi the same function as the centriole in higher eukaryotes.
As one of the first recognizable events of the cell cycle, microtubules emanate from the SPB through the cytoplasm to the site
of bud formation on the cell surface. After bud emergence has
occurred, the SPB produces a small satellite structure which grows
to duplicate the whole structure, which then separates into two
distinct SPBs. A spindle develops between these as the nucleus
elongates.

Nuclear division. Unlike higher eukaryotes, the nuclear membrane does not break down during mitosis, nor do chromosomes
condense to give recognizable metaphase. As the spindle elongates,
the nucleus migrates and moves to a central position between the
parent and daughter. It undergoes considerable elongation across
the neck of the mother cell and bud, until it divides to leave one
nucleus in the mother and one in the daughter.

Cytokinesis and cell separation. Following nuclear division, the cytoplasm between the two cells is separated by the cell membrane (cytokinesis) and at a later time, after synthesis of wall material between the two cells, the cells separate.

S. pombe divides by binary fission and fewer of the events in this process have been characterized. The timing of the comparable cell cycle events differs slightly from that seen in *Saccharomyces*, with a shorter G1 phase and S phase occurring after cell plate formation (cytokinesis) but before cell division.

Regulation of the cell cycle

By isolating conditional mutants (*cdc*) which are blocked in cell division at the restrictive condition, and by using a few specific inhibitors (such as hydroxyurea, which blocks DNA replication), it has been possible to study some of the interrelationships between the various events in the cell cycle. These results are summarized for *S. cerevisiae* in Fig. 8.7, which illustrates where various *cdc* mutants are blocked and also how the cell division events can be

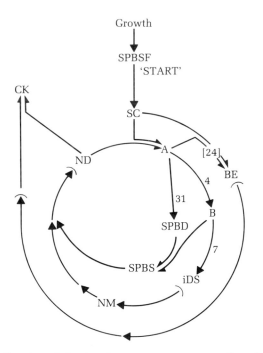

Fig. 8.7 Coordination of the *Saccharomyces cerevisiae* cell cycle events determined from studies of cell division cycle (*cdc*) mutants. The lines show how various landmark events depend on the occurrence of previous events in the cell cycle. Note that there are separate sequences which diverge and converge at later stages. Numbers refer to a few representative *cdc* mutants. BE = bud emergence; CK = cytokinesis; iDS = initiation of DNA synthesis; ND = nuclear division; NM = nuclear migration; SC = completion of start; SPBSF = spindle pole body satellite formation; SPBD = spindle pole body duplication; SPBS = spindle pole body separation. (Redrawn from Wheals (1987) *The Yeasts*, Vol 1, Rose & Harrison (eds.), p. 283–390. Diagram conceived by Dr Johnston.)

ordered into functional sequences in which some events can only occur if previous ones have taken place. Note the following points:

1 There are several 'cycles', e.g. one associated with DNA replication and nuclear division, another with morphological events such as bud emergence and nuclear migration. Either of these sequences can be blocked without affecting progression through the other.

2 The sequences are, however, coordinated since they merge at cytokinesis. Only the DNA replication/mitosis pathway need be completed for a second cycle to commence.

Coordination of growth with cell division: 'start'

The events described above are those directly concerned with cell division: while they are proceeding in an ordered way, the cells are growing by accumulating RNA, protein and other cellular components. How are these continuous growth processes coupled to the discontinuous ones associated with division?

In yeasts, this coupling occurs at the beginning of the cell cycle in the G1 phase during a process that is termed *start*. This has been defined by a group of mutations which all act at about the same point in G1, and by the fact that only during this phase is the cell cycle subject to nutritional conditions. Starved cells arrest at start. Moreover, it is only at this stage of the cell cycle that *S. cerevisiae* cells can be induced to undergo other developmental pathways such as mating (in haploids) or sporulation (in diploids).

It has also been shown that cells must grow to a critical size before they can traverse start, so that growth of cells is the rate-limiting step for cell proliferation rather than progress through the sequence of cell cycle events. The rate at which cells grow to the correct size and pass through start is the only factor determining the rate of division in this model. How cells monitor their size (volume) remains a mystery.

Some of the components of the start system have been identified, and all these point to protein modification by phosphorylations and dephosphorylations as being of importance to the cell. One of the crucial genes in *S. pombe* (*cdc2*) is highly homologous not only with the *S. cerevisiae* equivalent (*cdc28*), but also with regulated genes in higher eukaryotes. These encode a protein kinase whose activity is modulated by protein phosphorylation. Another set of genes in *S. cerevisiae* identifies a cascade of control leading to the activation of a cyclic AMP-dependent protein kinase (*cdc35* gene product). Mutations in this system lead to arrest of cells at start. This process is discussed in more detail in the next chapter.

Transition of cells from G2 to M phase

One of the best understood cell cycle controls at the molecular level comes from studies of the *cdc2* mutation in *S. pombe*. This

gene codes a protein kinase which functions at two points in the
cell division cycle—at start, and at the transition from G2 to M
phase. Figure 8.8 illustrates the known molecular events and genes
associated with this control and how they interact.

The *cdc2* protein kinase complexes with a protein (the *cdc13*
gene product, called cyclin). This complex triggers the cell into
mitosis. The *cdc2* protein kinase does not vary in concentration
throughout the cell cycle, but its activity does. At most other
times it is itself phosphorylated on a tyrosine residue within its
ATP-binding domain and this maintains the protein in an inactive
state. Just prior to mitosis, it is dephosphorylated by the action of
the *cdc25* gene (possibly encoding phosphatase) and this activates
its protein kinase activity. As a consequence of this, the *cdc13*
product (cyclin) begins to be degraded, probably as a result of
phosphorylation by the *cdc2* gene product. In higher eukaryotes,
the cell cycle is dependent on the accumulation of cyclin during
interphase and its destruction during mitosis. There has been a
high degree of conservation throughout eukaryotic evolution of
the *cdc2* gene product and cyclin, so that these fundamental
controls of cell division operate in all eukaryotes.

The activated *cdc2* protein kinase probably promotes mitotic
events by phosphorylation of proteins involved in spindle formation and chromosome condensation. Certain mutations in *cdc2*,
which prevent phosphorylation of its product, cause the cells to
progress into mitosis much earlier than usual. This creates a 'wee'
phenotype in which the cells divide at half their normal size, due
to an early mitosis. This entry into mitosis is regulated from the S

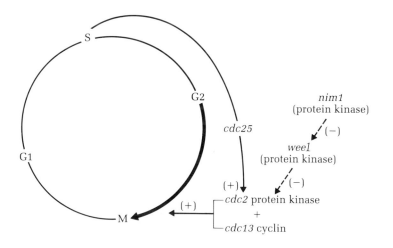

Fig. 8.8 Control of the G2 to mitosis transition in *Schizosaccharomyces pombe*. Genes involved in the
control are designated in italics. A (+) sign indicates that the gene product promotes the activity indicated
by the adjacent arrow, a (−) indicates inhibition. The *cdc2* protein kinase is activated by dephosphorylation
brought about by the activity of the *cdc25* gene product which may be a phosphoprotein phosphatase. This
activity is controlled by some event occurring in S phase. The precise role of the *nim1* and *wee1* pathway
is not known, but it presumably reflects another layer of control preventing mitosis.

phase via the *cdc25* gene product, which is in some way activated by the DNA replication process.

A similar process also occurs at start (G1 → S) since some mutations in *cdc2* (or *cdc28* in *S. cerevisiae*) arrest at start and there are homologues of cyclin which may be involved in this stage of the cell cycle as well.

In summary, the cell cycle is a series of dependent events which are entrained by fluctuating protein kinase activities. Many protein kinases in the cell are involved in this regulation—for example, two gene products that affect *cdc2* protein kinase activity (*nim1* and *wee1*) are themselves both protein kinases! Their function is yet to be determined.

Organelle duplication

Less is known about the mechanisms by which organelles, other than the nucleus, grow and divide during the cell cycle and how they are synchronized with nuclear or cell division.

Mitochondria and chloroplasts appear to divide by a fission process, seen most clearly in those small cukaryotes with a single representative organelle, e.g. the protozoan *Chromulina* and the alga *Chlorella*. In these, the fission of the organelle usually occurs at or about the time of cell division.

With organisms containing more than one mitochondrion, division is difficult to follow in detail, although there is no evidence for synchronous fission. In yeast, the mitochondria (from one to about ten per cell) are seen from serial sections to be sausage shaped. Usually one protrudes into the developing bud.

Replication of organelle DNA is not controlled in the same way as nuclear DNA, since in a number of microbial eukaryotes examined, including *Tetrahymena*, *Chlamydomonas* and *Saccharomyces*, the majority of the mitochondrial DNA is replicated at a different stage of the cell cycle from nuclear DNA. Some species of yeasts are ideally suited to studying the control of mitochondrial DNA replication since they can survive if grown on glucose in the absence of the mitochondrion. Petites (small colonies lacking mitochondria) are induced by a very wide range of physical and chemical treatments, including DNA intercalating dyes, mutagens and inhibitors of cytoplasmic and mitochondrial protein synthesis. This may indicate that the coordination between the nucleus (which codes for many mitochondrial proteins) and the mitochondrion is particularly sensitive to disruption.

9 Morphogenesis and differentiation

Morphogenesis is the *development of form*. The term was coined for the intriguing processes whereby structures in cells are produced and determined. Thus at a simple level, flagellar assembly is a morphogenetic process.

Differentiation is the process whereby a cell or group of cells changes from one shape and/or function to another; this involves a series of morphogenetic changes. In microbial life cycles, there are numerous examples of differentiation processes, including at the simplest level, the cyclic processes of cell division discussed in Chapter 8. At a slightly greater degree of complexity is the production of stalks by prosthecate bacteria, such as *Caulobacter*, which involves an asymmetric division to produce a sessile (stalked) cell and a motile cell (see Fig. 8.1). At the other end of the scale are examples of complicated multicellular growth and development seen in fruiting body formation in the myxobacteria and in members of the Basidiomycetes, or in the life cycle of *Volvox*.

Figure 9.1 illustrates a number of different life cycles found in microorganisms in which there are substantial changes in the form and function of the structures produced on passing from one stage of the life cycle to another. Rather than describing many of these life cycles in detail, we shall concentrate on the general principles to be learnt from several systems which have been studied in detail.

GENERAL CHARACTERISTICS OF DIFFERENTIATION SYSTEMS

Events occur as controlled sequences

Differentiation involves sequences of interrelated biochemical and morphological steps. Of these, the morphological changes are most easily studied by electron microscopy; the important biochemical events are often less easy to distinguish. Some, but by no means all of the steps require the expression of genes not used at any other phase of the organism's life cycle, since mutations can be obtained which affect only that one morphogenetic sequence. In microbial development systems, there is clearly no change in the *total* genetic information within the developing cell, since the final product (for example, a spore) often returns to the starting state (the vegetative cell), but there is control of the expression of this information. In the previous chapter, we have discussed the control of metabolic pathways; in this chapter, we are primarily concerned with how cells control the timing of sequential events and how they regulate the quantities of gene products formed.

Assembly

During morphogenesis and cellular development, new structures are formed on old foundations. This requires the assembly of subunit molecules into the correct spatial relationships relative to each other, and raises many interesting questions (some of which

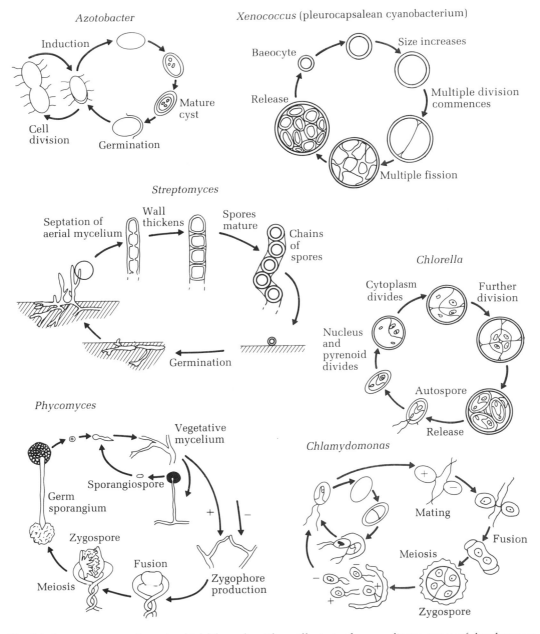

Fig. 9.1 Some representative microbial life cycles. These illustrate the very diverse types of development processes such as mating, sporulation and spore germination. *Azotobacter*, *Xenococcus* and *Streptomyces* are prokaryotes, the remaining genera are eukaryotic.

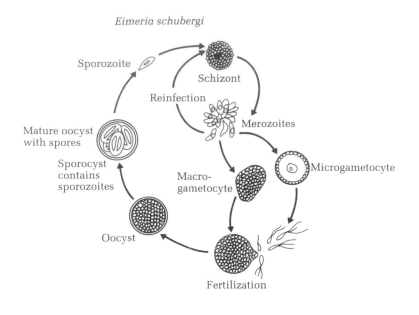

Eimeria schubergi

Sporozoite

Schizont

Reinfection

Merozoites

Mature oocyst
with spores

Microgametocyte

Sporocyst
contains
sporozoites

Macro-
gametocyte

Oocyst

Fertilization

Fig. 9.1 Cont.

have already been addressed). How are molecules transported from the site at which they are formed, to that at which they assemble into the structure (p. 173)? How do molecules aggregate correctly to form larger structures such as cell walls and flagella? Is this process of assembly spontaneous or is it controlled in some way? How are sequences introduced into assembly processes involving many components? What determines shape? (see p. 14 for cellular shape determination).

Cell–cell interactions

Some microbial differentiation systems involve only changes within a single cell (e.g. spore formation in bacteria, yeast sporulation, spore germination), but others, particularly those concerned with sexual fusion and/or fruiting body formation, depend on extensive cooperation between cells. These often involve initial communication and recognition stages, such as must occur in zygospore formation in *Mucor*, where aerial hyphae of different mating type grow inward towards each other along the most direct path. In some organisms, once aggregation has occurred, the individual cells do not fuse, but retain some integrity (as in cellular slime moulds), while in others, surface adsorption is followed by fusion of the cells. In eukaryotes, this fusion leads initially to heterokaryons (cells containing nuclei from different parents), and in some cases nuclear fusion also occurs to form heterozygotes. Here one can ask: how do fusing cells achieve synchrony with each other?

In such multicellular systems, there is also *pattern formation*. What determines the way cells (or hyphae) grow relative to each other to give rise to the delicate and intricate patterns that are characteristic to each particular species and structure?

Clearly, the study of morphogenesis needs an analysis of biochemical, cytological and genetic control processes, together with an understanding of how these interact with each other in function, time and space. When choosing an experimental system, there are several desirable features. Biochemical studies on microorganisms usually require large numbers of cells, hence synchrony of the morphogenetic process is essential. In order to study interactions in biology, it is common to interfere with the system in some way. This can be done using inhibitors, or more specifically, by mutation. The value of genetics in studying differentiation and how it is controlled is obvious if one considers the progress made in understanding metabolic control.

SEQUENTIAL EVENTS DURING MORPHOGENESIS

Morphological sequences

Bacterial endospore formation is the most extensively studied example of cellular development in a microbial system. It occurs in the genera *Bacillus*, *Clostridium*, *Sporosarcina*, *Thermoactinomyces*, *Sporolactobacillus* and *Desulfotomaculum* in vegetative cells facing starvation of either carbon or nitrogen substrates. The spore differs markedly from vegetative cells in shape and structure, as well as in being extremely resistant to heat, radiation, desiccation and most chemical disinfectants.

The changes seen by electron microscopy during sporulation in *Bacillus* species are outlined in Fig. 9.2. The process begins with the formation of an axial chromatin filament (*Stage I*), followed by an acentric membrane invagination (*Stage II*). Note that cell wall material is not formed between the now separate *prespore* and the mother cell. *Stage III* is characterized by engulfment of the prespore by the mother cell membrane, leading to inclusion of the prespore in the mother cell cytoplasm. This prespore is now surrounded by two membranes which have *opposite polarity*. Electron-transparent cortical material is next synthesized between these membranes (*Stage IV*), and if one considers the polarity of the membranes, it is apparent that the cortical membrane is laid down on the 'out' side of these (i.e. that facing into the medium before invagination took place). Not surprisingly, the *cortex* is composed of peptidoglycan which is modified. These modifications are important to the function of the cortex, which maintains the inside of the spore in a state of low water activity. The spore peptidoglycan is poorly crosslinked, and has fewer side-chains than the vegetative form. Some of the *N*-acetylmuramic acid residues are modified to form *N*-acetylmuramyl lactam, while others only carry an L-alanyl residue. Those side-chains that are present are negatively charged, and as the spore matures, the removal of Ca^{2+} from the cortex to

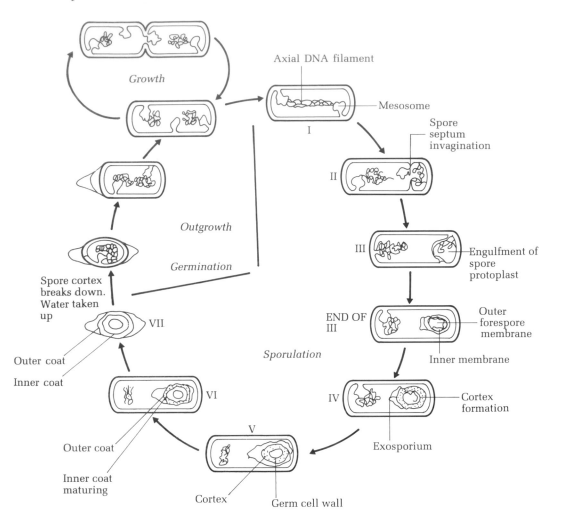

the spore protoplast leads to an expansion of this polymer and to maintenance of osmotic conditions which keep the spore protoplast effectively dry.

Once the cortex is almost complete, lysine- and cysteine-rich proteins condense in lamellae around the outside of the spore (*Stage V*) to form the coat which provides the mechanical strength against which the cortex tries to expand, and also provides protection against lytic enzymes. The spore subsequently matures to a very refractile, sometimes wrinkled structure (*Stage VI*; Fig. 9.3) and is released by lysis of the mother cell (*Stage VII*) to give a very heat- and solvent-resistant structure.

Fig. 9.2 Morphological stages during sporulation and germination in *Bacillus* species. (By courtesy of the Chemical Rubber Company (1972) *Critical Reviews in Microbiology* **1**, 479.)

Biochemical events also follow ordered sequences

Many biochemical changes have been detected during bacterial sporulation; some of these are summarized in Table 9.1. In many

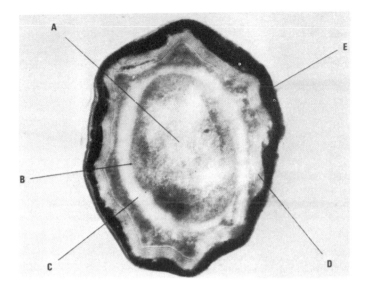

Fig. 9.3 Thin section of a mature *Bacillus subtilis* spore; × 3000. (A) DNA region; (B) protoplast membrane; (C) cortex; (D) inner spore coat; (E) outer spore coat.

Table 9.1 Some biochemical events occurring during sporulation in *Bacillus* species.

Synthesis of:	Morphological stage for onset
Proteases	0
Antibiotic(s)	0
Esterase	0
TCA cycle enzymes	0–I
Arginase	0–I
N-succinylglutamate	I
Alanine dehydrogenase	II
Alkaline phosphatase	III
Spore coat protein	III or IV
Glucose dehydrogenase	IV
Sulpholactic acid	IV
Ornithine transcarbamylase	IV
Cortex synthesizing enzymes	IV
Ca^{2+} incorporation into spore	IV
Cysteine incorporation (coats)	V
Lytic enzyme(s)	VI

cases, however, the relevance of these events to spore formation is not known. Any bacterial culture which is allowed to approach starvation will undergo numerous changes brought about by the relief of catabolite repression and the adaptive responses to starvation. These need not necessarily be associated with sporulation. There are, however, a few biochemical changes specific to spore formation, and these are useful 'marker' events in studying the process. Two compounds, *dipicolinic acid* (DPA) and the *muramic acid lactam*, have so far been found only in bacterial spores.

DPA chelates with calcium ions and forms about 10% of the spore dry weight; it may also be involved in heat resistance or maintaining dormancy. The muramyl lactam is a component of the cortical peptidoglycan, which also differs from the cell wall form in being less crosslinked. Another component of the spore, the *coat protein*, is antigenically distinct from proteins found in vegetative cells.

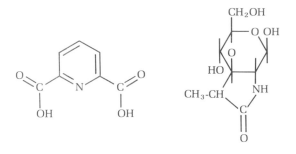

Dipicolinic acid   Muramyl lactam

The biochemical events that are always associated with sporulation occur in an ordered sequence which correlates with that for morphological changes, as indicated in Table 9.1.

How many functions are involved in sporulation?

This is a difficult question to answer, since some cellular processes are required for cells to grow vegetatively under certain conditions as well as for sporulation (e.g. CAC enzymes are essential for sporulation and for growth on minimal media). One way to try to answer this question is to isolate mutations which affect sporulation, to determine the number of functions that may be specific to the process. Many mutations affecting sporulation in *Bacillus subtilis* have been isolated; from mapping studies, at least 50 operons are known to be involved, and probably more remain to be identified. Sequencing of a number of these operons has shown that there are from one to five genes per operon, with two on average, so at least 100 and possibly 150 genes are involved in these sequential events. This constitutes about 5% of the *Bacillus* genome. In most cases, the precise biochemical function encoded by these genes has not been identified, and resolution of this problem is difficult in view of the complexity of the process. However, a number of gene products have been tentatively identified by sequencing of the cloned genes, and this has led to considerable advances in the study of control of the process.

Mutations causing asporogeny (inability to form normal heat-resistant endospores) usually lead to the cells undergoing normal development up to a particular stage of sporulation. Then there is an arrest, or sometimes an aberrant development from that stage (for example, one mutant overproduces the spore septum during invagination in Stage III). Such mutations are classified on the basis of the stage at which the block occurs, e.g. *spoII* mutants are blocked during the septation process, and the different mutations are known as *spoIIA*, *spoIIB*, etc.

Later events are dependent on successful completion of earlier ones

Studies with asporogenous mutants have shown that the morphological and biochemical sequences are tightly coupled to each other, since a mutation blocking sporulation at a particular morphological stage also prevents all biochemical changes normally occurring after that stage. For example, alkaline phosphatase in *B. subtilis* begins to appear towards the end of Stage II. No mutants blocked prior to Stage II produce the enzyme, but any which begin forespore invagination, do synthesize alkaline phosphatase.

These results also indicate that many events are dependent on the successful completion of all previous ones. There are some exceptions to this, since spore coat protein, which assembles on the developing spore at Stage V, can accumulate in cells blocked at Stage II. Moreover, once septation occurs, there are two chro-

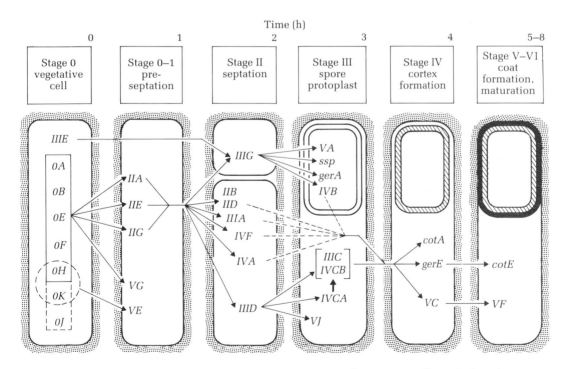

Fig. 9.4 Dependent sequences of operon expression during sporulation in *Bacillus subtilis*. The various stages of sporulation are designated 0, I, II, etc. Sporulation genes are indicated as 0A for *spo0A*, etc. Note that some genes are expressed only in the forespore, e.g. IIA, while others are only expressed in the mother cell, e.g. IIIG, as described in the text. Arrows indicate dependence of expression of later genes on successful expression of previous ones. (By courtesy of Dr Errington.)

mosomes each in the different protoplasts within the cell; both are active in protein synthesis and both are involved in separate sequences of events.

By cloning a large number of sporulation genes in *B. subtilis*, and fusing their promoter sequences to the *lacZ* gene of *Escherichia coli*, it has been possible to determine the timing, the order and the location (mother cell or forespore protoplast) of expression of each of these sporulation genes by monitoring the production of β-galactosidase. By studying this pattern in the various sporulation mutants blocked at different stages of development, a dependency pathway of gene expression has been constructed as shown in Fig. 9.4. These findings in bacterial sporulation have been confirmed in many other morphogenetic systems, including bacterial and yeast division cycles (p. 239) in which we have already seen that events are controlled as a pattern of branched interrelated sequences.

The cellular slime mould *Dictyostelium discoideum* provides an interesting insight into the strict correlation between morphology and biochemistry. The life cycle of this organism is shown in Fig. 9.5; amoeboid vegetative cells undergo aggregation

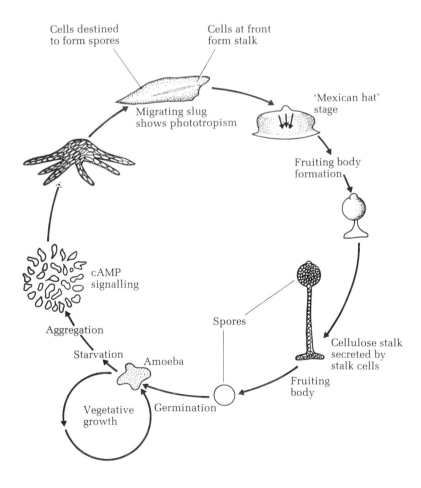

Fig. 9.5 Life cycle of the cellular slime mould *Dictyostelium discoideum*.

and subsequent multicellular stages following a period of starvation. During the programme leading to formation of the fruiting body with differentiated stalk cells and spore cells, a number of enzymes are synthesized following a given sequence. If, at the 'Mexican hat' stage, the multicellular mass is disaggregated, the amoebae re-aggregate and go through the usual sequence to produce twice the normal levels of these enzymes.

Control of sequences

Initiation

Sporulation in bacteria, and in yeast and other fungal systems, is usually induced by starvation of either carbon or nitrogen sources. It is not a general response to the cessation of growth, only to certain conditions. There are other examples in bacteria and fungi, in which sporulation is a specific response to CO_2 or light.

Spore germination, on the other hand, is usually triggered by the presence of one or more particular compounds; for example, some *Bacillus* spores are germinated in the presence of L-alanine, others by glucose–nitrate mixtures, and still others by K^+, fructose and glucose mixtures, or even Ca^{2+} dipicolinate.

Recently, much progress has been made in determining how yeast and slime mould cells respond to external conditions leading to morphogenesis. This work has received considerable stimulus since there are strong parallels between the way yeast cells control the initiation of cell development, and the way in which higher mammalian cells are controlled to prevent abnormal proliferation (i.e. tumour formation). For *Saccharomyces cerevisiae* cells to initiate sporulation, several sets of conditions have to be fulfilled:

1 The organism must be heterozygous for the mating-type alleles (*MATa/MATα*). *MATa* or *MATα* haploids do not sporulate.
2 The cells must reach a critical size of at least $23\,\mu m^3$.
3 The cells must be in the G1 phase of the cell division cycle.
4 The culture must be in conditions in which there is a poor carbon source which is non-fermentable (such as acetate) and low NH_4^+. Mitochondrial activity is a prerequisite.

A large number of mutations affect the ability of cells to initiate sporulation. Some of these bypass the intrinsic requirements for heterozygosity at the mating-type locus, while others affect the response to external nutritional conditions; there are clearly several control systems operating.

Mating-type control

Mating type in yeast is determined by a single gene *MAT* on chromosome III. There are two alleles, *MATa* and *MATα*, which are each transcribed divergently to give two transcripts; α1, α2 and **a**1 are the three which can encode proteins. Figure 9.6 illustrates

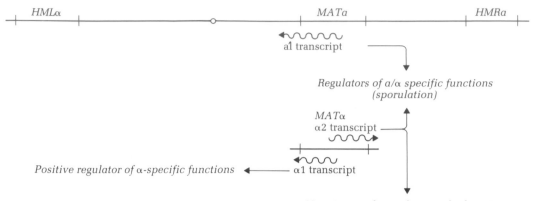

Fig. 9.6 Mating-type locus regulation of gene expression in yeast. Note that in the absence of any mating-type information, yeast cells behave as a type. The proteins formed from the *MATa1*, *MATa1* and *MATa2* transcripts are transcriptional regulators of other yeast genes associated with mating or sporulation.

how each of these transcripts controls the different mating-type and sporulation responses of the cell. In the absence of a functional mating-type gene, the cell behaves as an **a**. The α1 function activates α-mating behaviour, while the **a**1 and α2 transcripts turn on diploid **a**/α functions such as sporulation.

The products of the mating-type genes regulate a range of functions in the cell, concerned with mating in haploids as well as sporulation in diploids. One of the first, and main switches in sporulation is mediated via the *RME*1 gene, which is repressed in haploids and only turned on by both **a**1 and α2. Mutations in *RME*1 lead to sporulation being initiated independently of mating type.

Nutritional and cell division cycle control

From studies of mutants affected in the initiation of sporulation, it is clear that these controls, which make diploid cells respond to starvation and sporulate, are the same as those which control the decision made by a haploid cell in the G1 phase of the cell cycle whether to continue dividing, or arrest and adapt to starvation conditions.

One of the systems affecting this has been examined in some detail, and it is of considerable interest, since it parallels the controls found to prevent abnormal cell proliferation in higher eukaryotes. In fact, some of the yeast genes involved (*RAS*) were identified by cloning the yeast gene using the mammalian *ras* oncogene as a probe. The control centres on the activation of cAMP-dependent protein kinase by transduction of a signal (as yet undefined) activating adenyl cyclase. This pathway of activation involves the products of the *RAS*2 and *cdc*25 genes, as outlined in Fig. 9.7. Mutation of any of the genes encoding the components of this pathway leads either to derepressed sporulation or asporogeny. The *RAS* genes encode proteins with GTP-binding domains, and this might account for the finding that guanine deprivation can

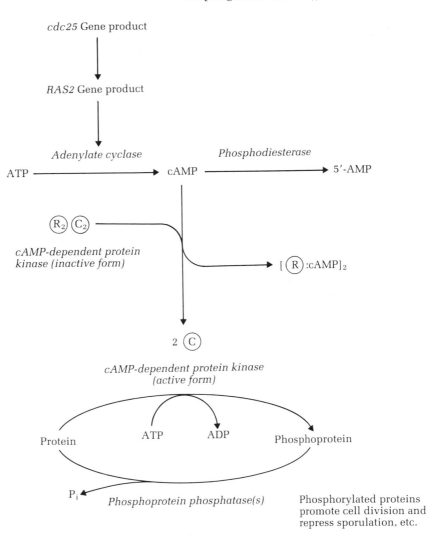

cdc25 Gene product

RAS2 Gene product

Adenylate cyclase   *Phosphodiesterase*

ATP $\longrightarrow$ cAMP $\longrightarrow$ 5′-AMP

R_2 C_2

*cAMP-dependent protein
kinase (inactive form)*

$[\, R :cAMP]_2$

2 C

*cAMP-dependent protein kinase
(active form)*

Protein   ATP   ADP   Phosphoprotein

P_i *Phosphoprotein phosphatase(s)*   Phosphorylated proteins
promote cell division and
repress sporulation, etc.

Fig. 9.7 The cAMP
pathway for activation
of protein kinases that
control cell division and
sporulation initiation in
the yeast
Saccharomyces. When
activated the kinases
maintain
phosphorylation of
proteins that allow the
cell to progress through
cell division and
prevent sporulation.
(Redrawn from
Matsumoto, Uno, &
Ishikawa (1985) *Yeast* **1**,
15–24.)

also lead to derepression of sporulation. As a result of the production of cAMP and the consequent activation of the protein kinase,
a number of enzymes and probably regulatory proteins are phosphorylated, and these allow the cell to progress into cell division
by mitosis. A good candidate for this phosphorylation is the *RAP*
gene protein which regulates many of the activities of the cell
associated with growth (p. 219). When the cell is starved, the
cAMP level falls and the protein kinase activity is reduced; in
some way, this promotes sporulation.

There are, however, other control systems which seem to operate,
since there are other mutations that derepress sporulation but
which do not fall into the above group. These may identify controls which respond to the nitrogen status of the cell rather than
the presence of appropriate carbon sources.

In the slime mould *Dictyostelium discoideum*, cells that are beginning to be starved also respond to cAMP, in this case as a signal molecule. This signalling is discussed on p. 267, from which it can be seen that there are strong parallels between the response of yeast to nutritional conditions and how slime moulds are affected by external stimuli at the onset of development.

In prokaryotic development, such as *Bacillus* sporulation, the mechanism of initiation is not fully understood. One hypothesis is based on the similarity between the conditions that alleviate catabolite repression, and those that initiate sporulation. It is usually assumed that there is a repressor or activator of early sporulation genes responding to some molecule in the cell which acts as a monitor of its ability to continue growth. This must also take into account the fact that sporulation can only be induced at a certain point during DNA replication.

A number of candidates for this type of molecule have been proposed. cAMP has been rejected and it seems clear from studies with inhibitors of guanine nucleotide biosynthesis that some molecule related to GTP may be involved. One group of compounds that has been mooted includes the highly phosphorylated nucleotides (ppGpp and pppGpp) produced by idling ribosomes during the stringent response. *Bacillus* cells do produce these nucleotides, but early in sporulation they begin to make the adenosine nucleotide pppAppp instead, in reactions catalysed by membrane-bound enzymes.

Regulation of sequences

Once initiated, a developmental process proceeds via the expression of genes unique to the process, so that the products of these genes are made in the right amount, at the right place, in the right order and at the right time.

Order and timing of sequences

There has been considerable recent progress in finding out how cellular systems control the timing of enzyme synthesis during development. There are also several examples of bacteriophage development which have been characterized very extensively, and from these a number of principles of development emerge.

Single-stranded RNA phages (R17, MS2, f2). These are very simple indeed, their RNA coding for only three proteins: a *replicase enzyme*, a *coat protein* and a *maturation protein*. These phages infect *E. coli* by attaching to sex pili and releasing their RNA through the pilus to the cytoplasm. Following infection, the three proteins do not appear in the same proportion, nor are they synthesized simultaneously. Moreover, during the late phases of infection, there is a marked reduction in the rate of replicase gene translation.

By *in vitro* protein synthesis studies, from the use of mutants affecting each phage gene, and by studying the interaction of the purified gene products with phage RNA, it has been found that:

1 The coat protein acts as a translational repressor of replicase synthesis, by binding to the start region of the replicase gene.

2 The replicase gene cannot be translated until part of the coat gene is translated. This may be due to the secondary structure of the phage RNA, which shows extensive intramolecular base pairing, hiding the initiation site from the replicase in the coat gene.

The important point here is that gene expression is controlled at the level of *translation*, regulating the amount of gene products synthesized (for R17, the ratio of coat protein:replicase:maturation protein is 20:5:1) rather than the timing of their synthesis. Translational repression can, however, account for some change in the rate of synthesis of a protein at a given time during development.

Bacteriophage lambda (λ). A much deeper insight into genetic regulation of phage development comes from studies of the double-stranded temperate DNA phage λ. Its DNA usually integrates into the chromosome of its host, *E. coli*, at a specific attachment site. The λ lysogens so formed are immune to further infection by other phages, including some unrelated to λ; they grow normally and the phage genome replicates along with the host genome. Control in this system is concerned with the maintenance of lysogeny and timing of the less frequent lytic development.

During lytic development in λ, the DNA is excised from the host chromosome and the previously unread genes coding for phage proteins are expressed. These phage-coded proteins are not all synthesized simultaneously. Some appear early after the induction of lytic development, while others are produced in significant amounts only at later stages.

What control systems coordinate protein synthesis in this way? In trying to answer this question, we should begin by considering the arrangement of genes on the genome, shown in Fig. 9.8. For our purposes, it is not necessary to know the function of every gene; what should be noticed is that genes coding for related functions (such as head synthesis, tail synthesis, recombination and DNA synthesis) are clustered into groups. Gene clustering, as we have already seen (p. 199), is one of the main characteristics of operon control, and in the following genetic 'control circuit' it should be possible to distinguish four interrelated operon-like systems. The following control activities have been identified:

1 *cI* gene: The product of this gene is the repressor protein which acts negatively at two operator sites (O_L and O_R) located on opposite strands of the phage genome, preventing reading of the remaining phage genes and thereby stopping lytic development.

2 O_L, O_R, P_L, P_R: When the activity of the repressor is decreased in some way (e.g. by UV treatment), transcription starts at two

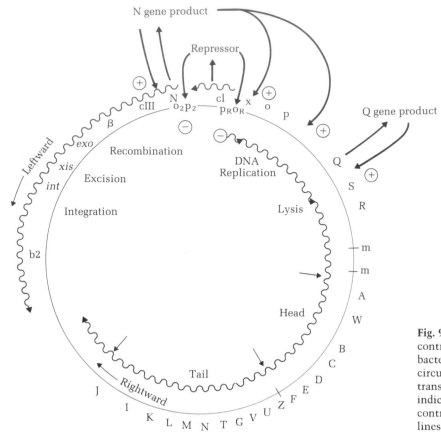

N gene product

Repressor

Q gene product

Recombination

DNA
Replication

Excision

Integration

Lysis

Leftward

Rightward

Tail

Head

Fig. 9.8 Genetics and control map of bacteriophage λ in circular form. RNA transcription is indicated by wavy lines; control circuits by solid lines.

promoters. From the leftward promoter, O_L, transcription proceeds leftward on the 'left' DNA strand, and in the early stages stops just after gene *N*. This termination appears to be brought about by the *E. coli* ρ factor (see Chapter 6). Similarly, rightward transcription from the O_R, P_R region occurs on the 'right' strand, and terminates between the *x* and *y* regions after reading about 1% of the genome.

3 *N* gene product: This most important control element acts at a number of sites to control the *timing* of the whole development. It is a positive control protein with 'antitermination' activity, permitting leftward transcription beyond *N* to continue indefinitely. This produces the proteins concerned with prophage excision and recombination. Similarly, it acts on rightward transcription allowing unhindered reading of genes *O* and *P*, and acts again later, beyond *P*, at a termination site just before gene *Q*.

4 *O*, *P* gene products: These proteins modify the host DNA polymerase so that λ DNA can be replicated, increasing the number of gene copies available for transcription, and amplifying the number of head and tail proteins made.

5 *Q* gene product: This protein in some way increases the transcription of late genes 'downstream' on the right strand, by a factor of about ten. Head and tail proteins are thus produced in large amounts as late events in lytic development. This protein may act as a phage-coded σ factor (see p. 157), which complements the *E. coli* RNA polymerase enabling it to recognize a promoter after *Q*.

We can now summarize the important concepts which arise from studies with λ:

1 Some proteins produced during phage development act as regulators controlling the timing of gene expression (e.g. *cI*, *N* and *Q*). These controls operate mainly at the level of transcription.

2 The arrangement of genes into sequences of operons is one way of coordinating the synthesis of proteins involved in a particular step or development.

3 Gene amplification can increase the production of proteins to levels needed for successful assembly.

4 Although control of the timing of protein synthesis is largely at transcription, there is probably some translational control similar to that found in R17. Thus the head and tail proteins, translated from the same messenger, are not produced in equimolar proportions.

Biochemical aspects of sequential control

So far, we have discussed genetic control circuits. How, in chemical terms, does the cell switch from using one set of information to another? One answer to this question was found not in λ, but in the lytic *E. coli* phage T4. The T-even phages have a complicated structure, shown in Fig. 9.9; many genes are involved

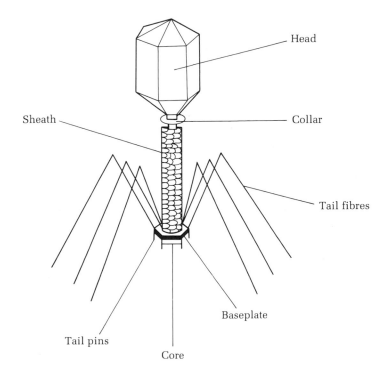

Fig. 9.9 Structure of bacteriophage T4.

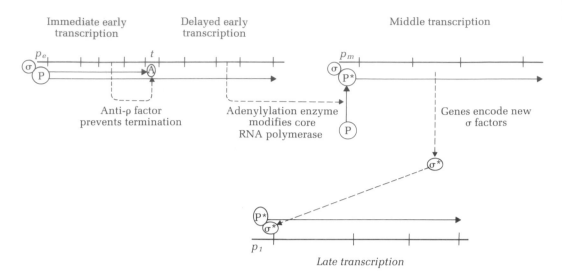

Fig. 9.10 Switching of gene transcription by phage-induced modification of *Escherichia coli* RNA polymerase and sigma factor. t = terminator; p_e = early promoter (*E. coli*); p_m = middle promoter (T4); p_l = late promoter (T4); Ⓟ = *E. coli* RNA polymerase; Ⓟ* = modified RNA polymerase; σ = *E. coli* factor; σ* = phage T4 coded σ factor; Ⓐ = antitermination protein.

in the assembly, and phage-coded proteins appear sequentially during the lytic development. Very soon after infection, the synthesis of bacterial proteins is shut off and only T4 genes are read. This switching is achieved quite simply; after infection, only a few phage genes (with bacterial-like promoters) are open to transcription by the *E. coli* RNA polymerase, most are not expressed. One of these 'early' genes encodes an antitermination factor which allows read through into 'delayed early' genes. One of the products of the delayed early genes is an enzyme which modifies the β subunit of the host RNA polymerase core enzyme by adding a diphosphoadenosyl group. This opens up new phage T4 promoters and 'middle' genes are read. At least two of these middle genes encode new σ factors which can recognize and promote transcription from late T4 promoters. A simplified outline of these interactions is shown in Fig. 9.10.

Timing control in cellular development

Modification of RNA polymerase is also important during bacterial sporulation. This was first indicated by the inability of lytic phage φe to develop in sporulating cells of *B. subtilis*, due to an alteration in the σ factor associated with RNA polymerase. Other evidence that RNA polymerase is somehow involved in sporulation control came from the finding that some mutations specifically affecting its β subunit (selected for resistance to the antibiotic rifamycin) also prevent sporulation in *B. subtilis* without affecting vegetative growth. This gave the clue to one of the mechanisms by which bacterial cells can switch from reading a set of genes needed in one phase of their life cycle to those required in another. Similar situations arise in *E. coli* cells subjected to heat shock (see p. 194).

It is now clear that there are a number of new σ factors that appear in sporulating cells of both *Bacillus* and *Streptomyces*. *Streptomyces* has a hyphal growth habit and when starved produces aerial hyphae that septate and develop into chains of spores. These new σ factors displace the vegetative forms from RNA polymerase and are responsible for selecting different sets of promoters. Vegetative *B. subtilis* cells have several σ factors, σ^{43} and σ^{37} and at low concentration, σ^{32} (the superscript indicates the molecular mass of the factor in kilodaltons). In vegetative cells, the main active form of the RNA polymerase is associated with σ^{43}, and as an early event in sporulation this is displaced in part by the less abundant σ^{37} form and new sporulation-associated genes are read. Once sporulation is under way, there are five new sporulation-specific σ factors produced: three of these, σ^H, σ^F and σ^E, are active early in sporulation, while σ^G and σ^K act later. Each of these sigma factors directs RNA polymerase core enzyme to different sets of promoters. Thus changes in sigma factors probably represent one of the major switching processes preventing transcription of unwanted vegetative genes and opening up sporulation genes.

Unlike the situation in phage λ, sporulation genes are scattered in at least 30 groups widely separated on the chromosome in random order in terms of the stage at which they act. Timing cannot therefore be explained in terms of *sequential transcription*. In addition to the changes in σ factors, one hypothesis suggests a process of *sequential induction* in which one product of a group of genes, switched on as an operon or set of operons, acts as an inducer for the next block of genes. Notice that this differs little from the hypothesis that new σ factors are formed for each block of genes since both inducers (or repressors) and σ factors are proteins acting at the operator–promoter region to regulate transcription. There is some evidence that at least one sporulation gene encodes a protein with the type of DNA-binding domain that would be expected of a repressor or activator protein. There are other possibilities, and some switching may occur at the level of translation, controlled by the relative affinities of mRNA binding sites for ribosome subunits.

Differential regulation in different compartments: communication between compartments

When *Bacillus* cells are sporulating, there are two different chromosomes, one in the mother cell and one in the forespore. After Stage II of sporulation these are in different compartments. Several types of experiment have shown that different genes are expressed in these two compartments and that this expression is coordinated so that the sequence of events in each is kept in 'synchrony'.

This switching and coordination is brought about in a very

interesting interaction which highlights the involvement of sigma factors in sporulation, and which also includes site-specific recombination, the action of a specific protease and transcriptional control.

The σ^K gene in *B. subtilis* controls transcription of genes only in the mother cell compartment. It is encoded by two genes, *spoIVCB* and *spoIIIC*, which are located 42 kb apart on the genome. During sporulation a site-specific recombination event occurs which leads to the fusion of these two regions to generate the complete σ^K gene. Recombination is brought about by the product of a recombinase gene (*spoIVCA*), which is located on the 42-kb segment that is excised. Since the mother cell chromosome does not survive at the end of sporulation this rearrangement is not inherited and represents a form of terminal differentiation.

The sigma factor σ^K is, however, synthesized in an inactive pro-protein form and has to be cleaved by a site-specific protease to become functional. This protease is encoded by the *spoIVF* gene, which is transcribed in the *forespore* compartment under the control of the forespore-specific σ^G factor.

This illustrates how the morphogenetic processes in the two compartments are coordinated. When the forespore begins to mature the σ^G factor directs synthesis of the protease, which is translocated to the outer forespore membrane. There it can cleave the pro-σ^K factor to activate it, ensuring that the late spore coat synthesis genes are not activated until the forespore is ready.

To add to this complexity, expression of the σ^K gene is under transcriptional control mediated by a protein produced by the *spoIIID* gene.

Site-specific recombination occurs in other terminally differentiating systems. The cyanobacterium *Anabaena* produces filaments composed of chains of cells. Under conditions of NH_4^+ limitation, some of the cells within the filament specialize to form N_2-fixing heterocysts. These heterocysts form at regular intervals along the filament of cells and lose the ability to divide. During heterocyst formation the genes for N_2 fixation are brought together by site-specific recombination in a similar way to the σ^K changes discussed above.

ASSEMBLY

Growth of cell surfaces involves the site-specific deposition of new wall material, and the control of assembly at this level is probably quite complicated. More is known, however, about the genesis of smaller and more regular structures such as pili, fimbriae and flagella. However, once again, viruses have been most extensively studied and can be used to illustrate fundamental concepts of assembly due to their simplicity of composition and regularity of shape.

Viral assembly

Viruses can be grouped in terms of their shape. Thus, animal and plant viruses can appear roughly spherical or filamentous in the electron microscope, while bacteriophages can be either spherical or have a more complicated head and tail arrangement exemplified by the T-even phages (Fig. 9.9).

Electron microscopic examination of simpler spherical viruses has shown that their coats, which surround and protect the nucleic acid, are composed of many apparently identical subunits. This illustrates an important principle of *morphopoiesis* (a term used for the process of assembly); large structures are constructed most efficiently by repetitive self-assembly of identical subunits. This efficiency is seen as a reduced need for genes to specify a large structure, and is clearly essential in the case of viruses with a very limited coding potential. The subunits, or *capsomeres*, are arranged in a particular type of cubic symmetry, icosahedral symmetry (an icosahedron has 20 faces, 12 vertices and 30 sides), which is the minimal energy arrangement of a closed shell built of regularly-bonded and identical subunits. That is, it approximates a sphere and produces a very strong structure. The subunit clusters in icosahedral viruses are arranged either as hexamers or pentamers, pentamers occurring only at vertices (there are only 12 in each spherical particle). If subunits can bond to each other by at least two different bonds, they can associate into a hexagonal array. Slight distortions of this bonding produces pentamers and forms a vertex rather than a flat sheet structure, as illustrated in Fig. 9.11. This introduces the principle of quasiequivalence, which implies that binding between subunits can be distorted non-randomly to give a more stable structure. When the phage coat (or *capsid*) of a spherical virus is composed of more than 60 subunits, then quasi-

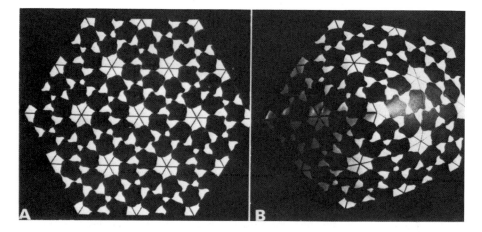

Fig. 9.11 Quasiequivalence and vertex formation in icosahedral assembly. (a) and (b) show vertex formation by introducing slight distortion in a flat icosahedral array of subunits leading to a pentamer.

equivalent bonding is necessary to provide both pentamers for vertices and hexamers between the vertices.

Filamentous viruses are formed by helical arrangements of identical subunits; helices are the natural consequence of joining subunits by a single type of bond arrangement. This is found not only in viruses such as tobacco mosaic virus and in the tails of more complicated bacteriophages, but also in cellular structures including microtubules and actin microfilaments of eukaryotic cells and in bacterial flagella and pili.

Cellular assembly during development

This is a very difficult area of research, since many of the techniques for studying cells lead to a disruption of the principal architectural features of the cell, and, unlike viruses, cells develop by modifying a pre-existing vegetative structure. Considerable progress has been made in determining how proteins made in the cytoplasm of the cell are targeted to particular locations (see p. 173) and this must play an essential role in developmental assembly processes.

One system that has been amenable to study is that of assembly of the spore coats in *B. subtilis*. The spore coat has a lamellar structure and is made up of two layers distinguishable in the electron microscope. There are four major proteins, and at least eight others, that appear in the spore coats. From radioactive labelling studies, it has been shown that some of these are synthesized as early as Stage II of sporulation, although they assemble on the spore surface during Stage V; others begin to be synthesized at Stage IV or even later. The assembly of these onto the spore surface has been studied by surface labelling with ^{125}I, using a lactoperoxidase-catalysed reaction. Since lactoperoxidase cannot penetrate beyond the surface of the spore, this technique labels only those proteins which are exposed. This has shown that there is order in the assembly of the various polypeptides onto the surface: some of them are labelled in early spores, then as sporulation progresses these are buried and other proteins become labelled.

Control of assembly

Is subunit assembly controlled? The simplest possibility is that, once formed, subunits undergo automatic self-assembly into the final structure. This is true for simpler cellular structures such as flagella and viruses, and *in vitro* assembly of capsid structures has been achieved using dissociated capsomeres. For more complicated phages built from several different structures, the picture is more complex, since sequences are introduced into the assembly line.

Morphopoiesis of T4 has been extensively studied. A large number of phage genes are involved in the assembly, but by no means all of them code for polypeptides appearing in the completed particle. Some, presumably, exert control over and above that of direct self-assembly. For example, eight genes are known to be involved in the assembly of the T4 head, although the final head is composed largely of a single protein species arranged into an elongated version of an icosahedron. Other genes ensure correct assembly, and mutations in these lead to aberrant development, including the production of elongated heads, short heads or heads unable to package DNA. Initially, a procapsid is formed by assembly of the gene 23 product on a core protein, involving the participation of shape-specifying proteins. Subsequently, a phage-coded protease specifically cleaves the gene 23 polypeptide, inducing a conformational change in the major subunit. At the same time, other proteins complex with the procapsid and phage DNA is taken up. Here again, we see how the modification of proteins by specific cleavage can be important in controlling morphogenesis. In this case, the limited proteolysis may give rise to irreversibility of the process, or effect a conformational change in the structural protein needed at a particular stage in the structural assembly.

INTERCELLULAR INTERACTION

Cooperation between cells during morphogenesis is seen most clearly in eukaryotic microorganisms; there are fewer examples in bacteria and blue–green algae. However, in one group of bacteria, the myxobacteria, there is extensive interaction between cells during the development of multicellular fruiting bodies. The process in *Myxococcus xanthus* is typical and is illustrated in Fig. 9.12. In the presence of an adequate supply of nutrients, these bacteria multiply and glide over the surface of the substrate. Even at this vegetative stage, individual cells are attracted to the colony from which they are derived. Cells at the edge of the colony can move away, but return eventually or stop until the colony catches up, so that the whole colony moves as a loose, dynamic conglomerate. When nutrients are exhausted, the organisms aggregate into a mound and eventually form up into a more or less complex fruiting structure, characteristic for each species. In *M. xanthus*, this structure is relatively less differentiated, forming a single spherical structure. In *Stigmatella*, the fruiting body comprises a stalk from the top of which radiate *macrocysts*; within these, the vegetative cells develop into *microcysts* (also called myxospores).

This illustrates some of the important elements of intercellular interaction: communication between cells to maintain contact; recognition associated with this communication and the later stages of aggregation into the fruiting body; and pattern formation. In the following discussion, in moving from description to consider the physiology of interactions between cells, we will concentrate on those systems most extensively studied. These are mainly

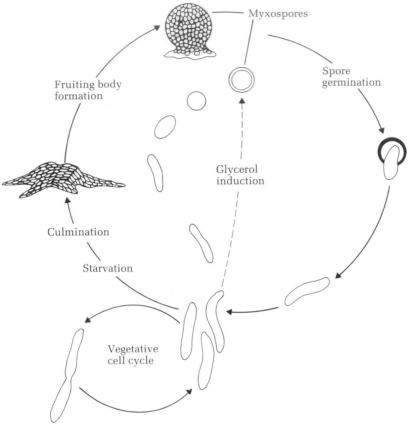

Fig. 9.12 Life cycle of
Myxococcus xanthus.

eukaryotic, but again we find bacteriophages provide useful models.

Communication and recognition

Recognition at cell surfaces

In liquid suspension, interacting cells can make contact, even if non-motile, by a process of random diffusion and collision. This occurs in algal and yeast mating (in which the two cells of opposite mating type recognize each other and fuse), mating during bacterial conjugation (recognition between the sex pilus and recipient cell surface) and during bacteriophage adsorption to its host. In each system, recognition occurs at the cell surface.

Bacteriophage adsorption to the host illustrates clearly how this recognition occurs. Most phages show a very restricted host range, often infecting only a few strains of one species. Moreover, different phages adsorb to different surface structures of the host: sex pili, flagella or bacterial surface polymers. In the case of phages attaching to the host surface lipopolysaccharide (including T4 and *Salmonella* phage P22), recognition involves a protein of the phage tail fibre binding to a specific sequence of sugar residues in the lipopolysaccharide. This is probably very similar to enzyme–substrate interactions, such as that between lysozyme and its peptidoglycan substrate in which six aminosugar residues lie within a long groove of the lysozyme molecule, or antigen–antibody recognition. The specificity is illustrated by the host range of *Salmonella typhimurium* phages against various bacterial mutants blocked at different stages of completion of lipopolysaccharide. For example, P22 recognizes the O-specific side-chains only, while phage 6SR adsorbs to the outer core region exposed in mutants lacking the O-antigen (Fig. 9.13).

This principle of surface interaction between complementary molecules, one of which is often carbohydrate in nature, the other a lectin-like carbohydrate-binding protein, occurs often in other, higher systems. During mating in yeast, recognition between opposite mating types involves agglutinins which are *mannan–protein* complexes—this is most pronounced in *Hansenula wingei*, which agglutinates very strongly. In the alga *Chlamydomonas*, recognition between (+) and (−) gametes involves a sugar sequence

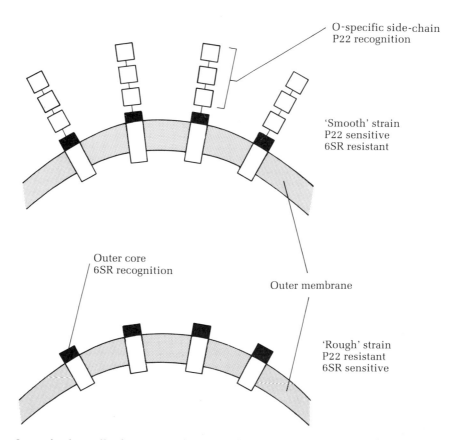

Fig. 9.13 Host specificity of *Salmonella* phage P22 and 6SR and the nature of the lipopolysaccharide in the host outer membrane.

of a glycoprotein present on the tip of flagella of (+) strains and probably a protein conformation on the (−) gamete flagella. This phenomenon is not restricted to mating systems, since a mutation altering the function of a carbohydrate-binding protein blocks cell–cell cohesion in developing cells of the slime mould, *D. discoideum*.

Communications at a distance

When cells interact at an interface, or in the atmosphere above a substrate, there is a need for communication and/or recognition over a distance. This is seen clearly in two systems: in *D. discoideum* during aggregation of amoebae prior to the multicellular phase of fruiting body formation, and in the formation of zygospores in *Mucor* and related genera.

In the cellular slime moulds, amoebae multiply singly but begin to aggregate when they reach starvation. This occurs at surfaces, and is a chemotactic response to a low-molecular weight compound (acrasin) identified for *Dictyostelium* as cyclic AMP. The cAMP acts as a messenger molecule across the whole spectrum of biological complexity (see discussion on catabolite repression, p. 215). In the vegetative phase of growth, slime moulds are attracted by folates, but at the onset of starvation they respond to pulses of cAMP produced at about 5-minute intervals and this causes aggregation. Slime mould aggregation has been extensively studied as a model for intracellular communication and the findings can be summarized:

1 Soon after the onset of starvation, 'pacemaker' cells secrete cAMP in pulses.

2 All amoebae have a receptor protein for cAMP located in the surface membrane and, in addition, a potent phosphodiesterase that hydrolyses cAMP.

3 Cells stimulated by a pulse of cAMP move briefly towards the source of the pulse and then secrete a pulse of cAMP themselves. This leads to waves of inward movement (Fig. 9.14), which are gradually changed into radial 'streams' of cells moving towards aggregation centres.

4 Each pulse of cAMP elicits profound changes in the shape and cohesive properties of the amoebae, leading to strong end-to-end contact.

Clearly, this communication system (and probably that in the myxobacteria, which also display wave-like propagation of signals) depends on the synthesis by cells of a diffusible molecule which can be detected, relayed and broken down by the receiving cells.

Signal reception

There has been considerable progress in determining how slime mould cells receive and respond to cAMP, and in many ways this

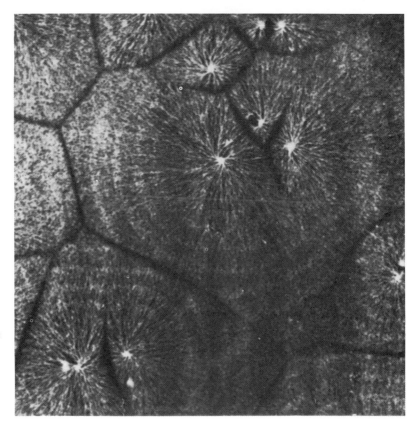

Fig. 9.14 Outward wave propagation from pacemaker cells in aggregating *Dictyostelium* amoebae. (Courtesy of Dr Monk.)

conforms to the pattern used by higher cells to respond to hormones. In *D. discoideum* amoebae, there are two pathways involved in reception of the signal and its transduction to functions altering cell behaviour. These are outlined in Fig. 9.15. One pathway is analogous to that seen in the regulation of yeast's response to nutrients. In this, a cAMP pulse is received at a receptor which may become phosphorylated. The signal is passed on via a G (GTP/GDP binding) protein to activate adenylate cyclase. This leads to activation of transcription, in the nucleus, of a set of genes expressed during development and to the relay of the cAMP pulse, probably via the activation of cAMP-dependent protein kinase.

The second pathway also involves a membrane receptor and a G protein, which activates phospholipase C. This enzyme catalyses the cleavage of phosphatidyl inositol 4,5-bisphosphate in the membrane to the soluble inositol-1,4,5-triphosphate (IP$_3$) and 1,2-diacylglycerol. Both of these may be signal molecules, although it is probably the IP$_3$ which transmits a signal causing Ca^{2+} release from storage. This in turn leads to polymerization of actin, which causes the formation of pseudopodia. It also, possibly via the production of cyclic GMP, leads to cell elongation as the cells move forward in response to the cAMP signal.

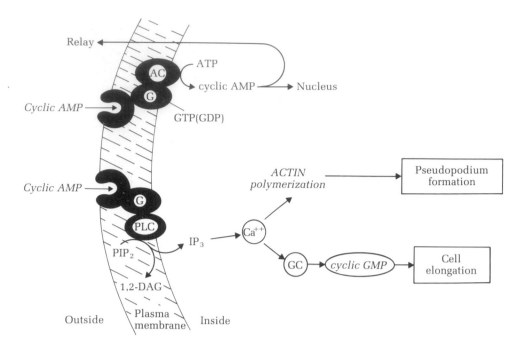

Note that for these steps there is an amplification of the incoming signal. For example, the reception of a single molecule of cAMP leads to the activation of adenylate cyclase and, therefore, the production of many molecules of cAMP. These, in turn, may activate protein kinases which can convert even more molecules of protein to the phosphorylated form.

Aerial communication

Zygospore formation in *Mucor* occurs above the surface of the growth medium; (+) and (−) hyphae in proximity are induced to produce specialized hyphae, *zygophores*, which grow towards each other with a high degree of recognition of both direction and mating type, illustrated in Fig. 9.16. This zygotrophism is presumed to be mediated by the synthesis of distinctive molecules by each type of zygophore; these must diffuse in the vapour phase, and be detected by the zygophore of opposite mating type to elicit the correct growth response.

The presence of a single chemical, *trisporic acid*, controls the induction of zygophores in unmated cultures of either (+) or (−) strains. This 'hormone' acts at very low concentration ($<10^{-8}$ M). How can the production of a single compound elicit the specific response of both (+) and (−) strains, when neither alone can synthesize it, but both together can? One suggestion is that each mating type produces intermediates in trisporic acid synthesis up to a particular step. To complete formation of the hormone, two reactions are needed, and these can occur in any order. When close

Fig. 9.15 Model of the signal transduction pathways for the transmission of the cAMP signal in *Dictyostelium discoideum*. The pathways involve regeneration of the signal and the induction of pseudopodium formation and cell elongation associated with chemotaxis. G = GTP/GDP-binding protein; PLC = phospholipase C; PIP$_2$ = phosphatidyl inositol 4,5-bisphosphate; IP$_3$ = inositol 1,4,5-triphosphate; 1,2-DAG = 1,2-diacylglycerol; GC = guanyl cyclase. (From Newall, Europe-Finner & Small (1987) *Microbiological Sciences* **4**, 5–11.)

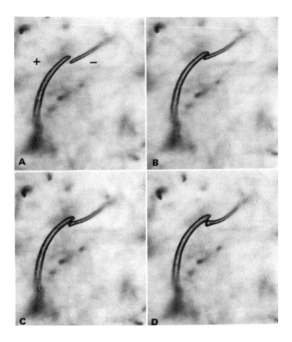

Fig. 9.16 Zygophore formation in *Mucor mucedo*. (a) The two zygophores attracted by zygotrophism; (b) 4 min later; (c) contact 1 min later; (d) swelling at point of contact, 10 min later. (Courtesy of Professor Gooday.)

to each other, both mating types can complement each other in the complete synthesis of trisporic acid.

Trisporic acid may be involved in zygotropism as well as zygophore induction. If not, volatile hormones which are complementary and specific to both transmitters and receivers must be involved together with a mechanism for chemoreception and for transducing the reception to a directed growth response. Many intriguing problems remain to be solved.

Phasing of cells

Another form of communication found during mating is exemplified by the mating hormones in *S. cerevisiae*. Haploid cells of opposite mating type (**a** and α) fuse to form heterokaryons briefly, followed by heterozygosis. If two cells were not at the same stage of the cell cycle, then fusion would present problems. However, **a** cells excrete a diffusible polypeptide (− factors) into the medium, which arrests α cells at the beginning of the cell cycle, and similarly α cells produce α factor which has comparable effects on **a** cells. The factor also induces temporary shape changes in **a** cells, causing an elongation of one 'end' of the ellipsoidal cells, which may be essential for the mating process.

Fusion of cells

Cell fusion occurs during mating in eukaryotic microorganisms following the recognition and surface adsorption processes. In fungi and algae with rigid cell walls, there is a need for specific breakdown and in some cases resynthesis at the site of contact. Once wall breakdown has been accomplished, membrane fusion appears to occur spontaneously, since it can be induced in some organisms by mixing protoplasts.

Pattern formation

Less is known about the intricate way in which cells are organized into complicated patterns. At a simple level, the cyanobacteria, such as *Anabaena*, are of interest. These dinitrogen-fixing photo-synthetic bacteria form a number of differentiated structures, including akinetes and heterocysts. Heterocysts are interesting since they occur at regularly spaced intervals along the chain of cells, and are the sites at which the essentially anaerobic process of N_2 fixation occurs in an O_2-producing organism. Heterocysts are non-reproducing cells which differentiate from vegetative cells when the concentration of NH_4^+ in the medium is low. The spacing between heterocysts in the chain is less as the NH_4^+ available to the cells diminishes. It is thought that this simple example of pattern formation is caused by gradients of NH_4^+ diffusing from the heterocysts along the chain of vegetative cells. As the vegetative cells divide to increase the length of the chain, the cells distal from the heterocyst will eventually become limited for fixed nitrogen, and this triggers formation of a new heterocyst. Thus diffusible factors passing from one cell to another can also give rise to pattern formation by causing cells to enter alternative developmental pathways.

Similar effects probably occur in slime moulds as the front cells in the migrating slug stage develop into stalk cells, while the anterior slug cells develop into spores. Morphogens (i.e. mol-ecules acting as signals from one cell to another to alter its course of development) other than cAMP have been identified in *D. discoideum*. These lead to changes in gene expression within the target cells with a new programme of developmental gene ex-pression. One such molecule identified in slime moulds is DIF (differentiation factor), with the chemical structure:

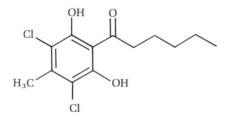

There are many aspects of morphogenesis which we have not touched on—for example, the cooperation of cells in fruiting structures so that some form spores, others form stalks (as in *Dictyostelium* and some myxobacteria)—in which cell position and even 'history' may play important roles. At its highest level in microorganisms is the behaviour of organisms such as *Volvox*, in which groups of cells are beginning to behave almost as tissues, having specific functions within the organism as a whole. In general, less is known about these phenomena and space does not permit extensive discussion; there are, however, some interesting reviews listed under 'Further reading'.

The points which we have discussed are general to developmental biology and are not confined to microbiology. Ultimately, one wants to be able to find answers to such questions as: 'how does a fertilized egg give rise to all the various cell types found in the mammalian body?' This is obviously extremely complicated and microorganisms provide a way of analysing development in simpler systems to formulate principles testable in higher organisms.

This is, however, not the sole justification for this type of research. Microbial development is intrinsically a fascinating subject and worthy of study for its own sake. For those seeking economic reasons, bacterial spore formation and germination are of considerable importance in food processing and other sterilization industries due to the extreme resistance of spores to desiccation, heat, radiation and disinfectants. Moreover, for many fungal pathogens of both plants and animals, morphogenetic processes seem to play a role in pathogenicity, exemplified by the yeast to pseudomycelial transition in *Candida* species.

Further reading

General sources of review articles covering most aspects of microbial physiology are given in the Introduction.

CHAPTER 1

ALBERTS, B., BRAY, D., LEWIS, J., RAFF, M., ROBERTS, K. & WATSON, J.D. (1989) *Molecular Biology of the Cell*, 2nd edn. Garland Publishing, New York & London.

MANDELSTAM, J., MCQUILLEN, K. & DAWES, I.W. (1983) *Biochemistry of Bacterial Growth*, 3rd edn. Blackwell Scientific Publications, Oxford. (The major bacterial cell structures are covered in some detail in Chapter 1.)

WOLFE, S.L. (1981) *Biology of the Cell*. Wadswarth, California.

CHAPTER 2

ACTOR, P., DANEO-MOORE, L., HIGGINS, M.L., SALTON, M.R.J. & SHOCKMAN, G.D. (1988) *Antibiotic Inhibition of Bacterial Cell Surface Assembly and Function*. American Society for Microbiology, Washington.

GALE, E.F., CUNDLIFFE, E., REYNOLDS, P.E., RICHMOND, M.H. & WARING, M.J. (1981) *The Molecular Basis of Antibiotic Action*, 2nd edn. John Wiley & Sons, London and New York.

CHAPTER 3

INOUYE, M. (1987) *Bacterial Outer Membranes as Model Systems*. Academic Press, Orlando.

SAIER, M.H. (1985) *Mechanisms and Regulation of Carbohydrate Transport in Bacteria*. Academic Press, Orlando and San Diego. (An excellent discussion of carbohydrate uptake and metabolism in prokaryotes.)

CHAPTER 4

MOAT, A.G. & FOSTER, J.W. (1988) *Microbial Physiology*. John Wiley, New York.

NEIDHART, F.C., INGRAHAM, J.L. & SCHAECHTER, M. (1990) *Physiology of the Bacterial Cell*. Sinauer, Sunderland, Massachusetts.

CHAPTER 5

MANDELSTAM, J., MCQUILLEN, K. & DAWES, I.W. (1983) *Biochemistry of Bacterial Growth*, 3rd edn. Blackwell Scientific Publications, Oxford. (Chapters 3, 4 and 8 give a detailed picture not only of the biosynthetic pathways in bacteria but also of the way in which they are regulated.)

CHAPTER 6

CASKEY, C.T. (1980) Peptide chain termination. *Trends in Biochemical Sciences* **5**, 234–7.

CLARK, B. (1980) The elongation step of protein synthesis. *Trends in Biochemical Sciences* **5**, 207–10.

FIRSHEIN, W. (1989) Role of the DNA/membrane complex in prokaryotic DNA replication. *Annual Reviews of Microbiology* **43**, 89–120.

HELMAN, J.D. & CHAMBERLIN, M.J. (1988) Structure and function of bacterial sigma factors. *Annual Reviews of Biochemistry* **57**, 839–72.

HUNT, T. (1980) The initiation of protein synthesis. *Trends in Biochemical Sciences* **5**, 178–81.

LEWIN, B. (1990) *Genes IV*. Oxford University Press, Oxford.

MICHAELIS, S. & BECKWITH, J. (1982) Mechanism of incorporation of cell envelope proteins in *Escherichia coli*. *Annual Reviews of Microbiology* **36**, 435–65.

NANNINGA, N. (1985) *Molecular Cytology of Escherichia coli*. Academic Press, Orlando.

SANCAR, A. & SANCAR, G.B. (1988) DNA repair enzymes. *Annual Reviews of Biochemistry* **57**, 29–67.

SAWADOGO, M. & SENTENAC, A. (1990) RNA polymerase B (II) and general transcription factors. *Annual Reviews of Biochemistry* **59**, 711–54.

SHOCKMAN, G.D. & BARRETT, J.F. (1983) Structure, assembly and function of cell walls of Gram positive bacteria. *Annual Reviews of Microbiology* **37**, 501–28.

CHAPTER 7

ALBRIGHT, L.M., HUALA, E. & AUSUBEL, F.M. (1989) Prokaryotic signal transduction mediated by sensor and regulator protein pairs. *Annual Reviews of Genetics* **23**, 311–36.

BUSBY, S. & BUC, H. (1987) Positive regulation of gene expression by cAMP and its receptor protein in *Escherichia coli*. *Microbial Sciences* **4**, 371–5.

COZZONE, A.J. (1988) Protein phosphorylation in prokaryotes. *Annual Reviews of Microbiology* **42**, 97–125.

GOTTESMAN, S. (1984) Bacterial regulation: global regulatory networks. *Annual Reviews of Genetics* **18**, 415–41.

HIRST, T.R. & WELCH, R.A. (1988) Mechanisms for secretion of extracellular proteases by Gram negative bacteria. *Trends in Biochemical Sciences* **13**, 265–9.

INOUYE, M. (1987) *Bacterial Outer Membranes as Model Systems*. John Wiley, New York.

MEYER, D.I. (1988) Preproteins conformation: the year's major theme in translocation studies. *Trends in Biochemical Sciences* **13**, 471–4.

STRUHL, K. (1989) Molecular mechanisms of transcriptional regulation in yeast. *Annual Reviews of Biochemistry* **58**, 1051–77.

WANDERSMAN, C. (1989) Secretion, processing and activation of bac-

terial extracellular proteases. *Molecular Microbiology* **3**, 1825–31.
YANOFSKY, C. (1987) Attenuation in the control of expression of bacterial operons. *Nature* **289**, 751–8.

CHAPTER 8

DONACHIE, W.D. & ROBINSON, A.C. (1987) Cell division: parameter values and the process in *Escherichia coli* and *Salmonella typhimurium*. In: Neidhart, F.C. (ed.) *Cellular and Molecular Biology*, pp. 1578–93. American Society for Microbiology, Washington, DC.
LUTKENHAUS, J. (1988) Genetic analysis of bacterial cell division. *Microbiological Sciences* **5**, 88–91.
NURSE, P. (1985) Cell cycle control genes in yeast. *Trends in Genetics* **1**, 51–5.
WHEALS, A.E. (1987) Biology of the cell cycle in yeasts. In: Rose, A.H. & Harrison, J.S. (eds.) *The Yeasts*, Vol. I, pp. 283–390. Academic Press, London.

CHAPTER 9

MANDELSTAM, J. & ERRINGTON, J. (1987) Dependent sequence of gene expression controlling spore formation in *Bacillus subtilis*. *Microbiological Sciences* **4**, 238–44.
NEWELL, P.C., EUROPE-FINNER, G.N. & SMALL, N.V. (1987) Signal transduction during amoebal chemotaxis of *Dictyostelium discoideum*. *Microbiological Sciences* **4**, 5–11.
NEWTON, A. (1987) Temporal and spatial regulation of differentiation in *Caulobacter crescentens*. *Microbiological Sciences* **4**, 338–41.

Glossary

alleles Different forms of the same gene; e.g. different mutations within the one coding sequence are different alleles.

allosteric protein A protein, usually an enzyme, which undergoes an alteration in conformation on binding low-molecular weight molecules (ligands). The binding alters the (catalytic) activity of the protein (see p. 220).

autotroph An organism which does not require any organic carbon for its energy source or for its growth.

auxotroph An organism requiring a particular organic molecule for growth. Often used to refer to mutants with a specific growth requirement, such as an amino acid.

cap A structure at the 5' end of eukaryotic messenger RNA involved in selection of the message by the ribosome.

cistron The functional unit of heredity, which in physical terms is a region of DNA coding for a single polypeptide chain or ribosomal or transfer RNA species.

conjugation The process of mating between two compatible cells. In bacteria part of the chromosome is transferred, while in eukaryotes the process involves complete fusion of (usually) haploid cells to form a diploid.

consensus sequence The ideal DNA base sequence for a particular function derived by comparison of as large a number of different sequences performing that function as possible.

domain A functional region of a protein; e.g. the part involved in the binding of a substrate.

exons Sequences in a split gene that are retained after splicing to provide the mature messenger RNA that is translated by the ribosome.

fruiting body A structure produced by most fungi, and a few bacteria, which bears the spores or other reproductive structures.

gel electrophoresis The process of separating charged species by subjecting them to a voltage gradient. The gel (usually of agarose or polyacrylamide) provides mechanical support and prevents mixing of the molecules being separated.

gene probe A labelled sequence of single-stranded nucleic acid (DNA or RNA) which can be used to detect the complementary nucleic acid sequence by a hybridization reaction.

genotype The genetic constitution of an organism.

heat shock response A coordinated response of the cell involving the increased expression of a number of genes in response to injury by heat, osmotic change and certain other forms of stress.

heterokaryosis The process whereby cells fuse to form a multinucleate cell containing nuclei from different parents. Nuclear fusion *does not* take place.

heterologous gene A gene from one organism which has been introduced into a different organism by suitable recombinant DNA techniques.

heterotroph   An organism requiring organic nutrients.

heterozygosis   The process whereby cells and their nuclei fuse to form a cell containing a single nucleus with chromosomes from each parent.

homothallism   A process occurring in some yeasts and other fungal strains whereby haploid spores formed during meiosis undergo self-diploidization due to the switching of mating type by some of the progeny of the spore.

intercalating dye   A dye which can insert between the bases of nucleic acids; e.g. ethidium bromide and acridine dyes, which can be used to stain DNA or cause mutation.

intron   A sequence of a gene which is transcribed but which is excised by a splicing reaction before the mature messenger is translated.

ligation   The formation of a phosphodiester bond to link together two strands of nucleic acid.

lysogen   A bacterium containing a bacteriophage chromosome integrated into and replicating with its own chromosome.

meiosis   The process of nuclear division associated with the formation of gametes or of haploid cells from a diploid.

mitosis   The normal process of nuclear division in a eukaryote, whereby nuclear division occurs on a spindle structure without reduction in the chromosome number in the daughter nuclei.

mixotrophic growth   (of hydrogen bacteria)   The process whereby organic nutrients are assimilated for anabolism to cell material while energy required for synthetic processes is derived from oxidation of hydrogen.

murein   A synonym for peptidoglycan (q.v.).

mutagen   A compound which causes damage to nucleic acid leading to the induction of mutations.

Park nucleotides   Bacterial peptidoglycan precursors, including UDP-*N*-acetylmuramic acid and its aminoacyl derivatives, which are found to accumulate in the presence of certain inhibitors of cell wall synthesis.

palindromic sequence   This term is frequently but incorrectly applied to DNA sequences that show rotational symmetry; i.e. the sequence 5′ to 3′ on one strand is the same as the (antiparallel) 5′ to 3′ sequence on the other strand. Also described as an inverted repeat or a sequence showing dyad symmetry.

peptidoglycan   The structural component of most prokaryotic cell walls, except archaebacteria.

peroxisomes   Structures in eukaryotic organisms which contain various oxidative and other enzymes.

phenotype   The observable characteristics displayed by an organism due to the presence of the particular forms of its genes (e.g. its wild-type or mutant alleles).

plasmid   A piece of extrachromosomal DNA capable of replication independent of the host chromosome.

poly(A) A polymer of adenylic acid residues found attached terminally to messenger RNA fractions.

polycistronic message A messenger RNA species which has been transcribed from a DNA sequence which encodes more than one gene (cistron).

primer A sequence of nucleotides needed to initiate polymerization of complementary DNA from a single-stranded template.

promoter A region of DNA necessary for the correct binding of RNA polymerase to initiate transcription of a gene.

pseudomurein A polymer with some similarities to peptidoglycan, found in the walls of some species of archaebacteria.

signal sequence A specific sequence of amino acids which is involved in the targeting of a protein to the membrane or an extracellular location.

spindle plaque A structure in some lower eukaryotes replacing the centriole. The spindle plaque lies on the nuclear membrane and from it radiates the spindle fibres on which chromosomes segregate during meiosis or mitosis.

splicing The process whereby introns are removed from primary RNA transcripts leading to the joining of adjacent exons or coding sequences.

TATA box A conserved sequence found within about 30 bp of the start of transcription of a eukaryotic gene transcribed by RNA polymerase II. It is involved as the site for binding some of the proteins needed to initiate transcription.

temperate bacteriophage A bacteriophage that, after infection, may either integrate its DNA into the host chromosome or undergo lytic development.

transformation In microorganisms, the transfer of naked DNA into a host organism leading to the transfer of genetic markers into the host.

transposon A DNA sequence containing at least one phenotypically functional gene flanked by either an IS element or an inverted repeat sequence; it can change its position by the process of integration.

Index